Essential Quick Review

ORAL MEDICINE AND RADIOLOGY

Essential Quick Review

ORAL MEDICINE AND RADIOLOGY

Editior-in-Chief

Priya Verma Gupta MDS FPFA
Professor
Department of Pedodontics and Preventive Dentistry
Divya Jyoti College of Dental Sciences and Research
Ghaziabad, Uttar Pradesh, India

Co-Author

Jyoti Gupta BDS MDS
Professor
Department of Orthodontics
Career Post Graduate Institution of Dental Science and Hospital
Lucknow, Uttar Pradesh, India

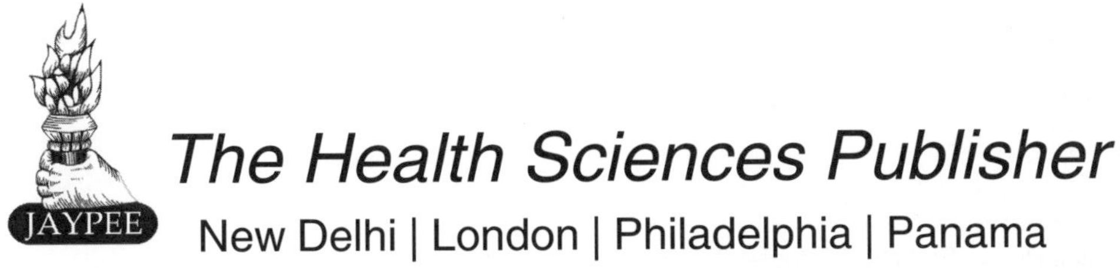

The Health Sciences Publisher
New Delhi | London | Philadelphia | Panama

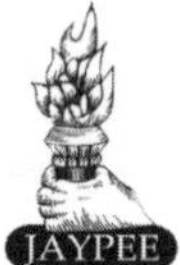

Jaypee Brothers Medical Publishers (P) Ltd

Headquarters

Jaypee Brothers Medical Publishers (P) Ltd
4838/24, Ansari Road, Daryaganj
New Delhi 110 002, India
Phone: +91-11-43574357
Fax: +91-11-43574314
Email: jaypee@jaypeebrothers.com

Overseas Offices

J.P. Medical Ltd
83 Victoria Street, London
SW1H 0HW (UK)
Phone: +44 20 3170 8910
Fax: +44 (0)20 3008 6180
Email: info@jpmedpub.com

Jaypee-Highlights Medical Publishers Inc.
City of Knowledge, Bld. 235, 2nd Floor, Clayton
Panama City, Panama
Phone: +1 507-301-0496
Fax: +1 507-301-0499
Email: cservice@jphmedical.com

Jaypee Medical Inc.
325 Chestnut Street
Suite 412, Philadelphia, PA 19106, USA
Phone: +1 267-519-9789
Email: support@jpmedus.com

Jaypee Brothers Medical Publishers (P) Ltd
17/1-B Babar Road, Block-B, Shaymali
Mohammadpur, Dhaka-1207
Bangladesh
Mobile: +08801912003485
Email: jaypeedhaka@gmail.com

Jaypee Brothers Medical Publishers (P) Ltd
Bhotahity, Kathmandu, Nepal
Phone: +977-9741283608
Email: kathmandu@jaypeebrothers.com

Website: www.jaypeebrothers.com
Website: www.jaypeedigital.com

Inquiries for bulk sales may be solicited at: jaypee@jaypeebrothers.com

Essential Quick Review: Oral Medicine and Radiology

First Edition: **2016**

ISBN: 978-93-86056-20-7

Printed at Rajkamal Electric Press, Plot No. 2, Phase-IV, Kundli, Haryana.

Editorial Board

Preface

I am very pleased to introduce you to the first edition of Essential Quick Review; A series for final year undergraduate students.

The series will be available in eight subjects, i.e., Periodontics, Operative Dentistry and Endodontics, Pedodontics, Prosthodontics, Oral Surgery, Oral Medicine and Radiology, Orthodontics and Public Health Dentistry covering essential parts of each subject. This book will not only help the student to attain the knowledge, but will also give an idea how to attempt a question during the examination, covering entire syllabus in a limited period of time.

The book gives a complete outline for writing an essay type, a short answer type or a viva-voce type of question. The language used is very simple enabling a better understanding with well-illustrated diagrams wherever possible. Each book also carries a section that contains recently asked questions covering majority of the universities in India.

What makes it different from other books is, that it is supported with a supplementary booklet for each subject that contains three sections, i.e., definitions, classifications and viva-voce covering the entire syllabus enabling the student to undergo a quick revision.

The study material provided in this book is an attempt to provide an additional help to students for easy retention and reproduction of subject in the examination. This book is in no way a replacement to standard text books.

I thank all my subject matter experts for their valued suggestions and contributions. A very special word of thanks to my family for being the source of constant encouragement. I profusely thank Shri Jitendar P Vij (CEO), Mr Ankit Vij (Group President), and production team of M/S Jaypee Brothers Medical Publishers (P) Ltd, New Delhi for their enthusiasm and constant efforts in bringing out this book.

Dr Priya Verma Gupta

Contents

Section 1 Oral Medicine

1. Ulcerative, Vesicular and Bullous Lesions 3-7
2. Red and White Lesions 8-14
3. Keratotic and Non-keratotic White Lesions 15-20
4. Oral Pigmentation 21-25
5. Oral Cancer 26-31
6. Diseases of Tongue and Lips 32-36
7. Salivary Gland Diseases 37-41
8. Disorder of TMJ and MPDS 42-49
9. Ionising Radiation and Regressive Alterations of the Oral Cavity 50-52
10. Odontogenic and Non-odontogenic Tumours 53-57
11. Orofacial Pain 58-65
12. Aids, Bacterial and Viral Infections 66-71
13. Metabolic Disorders 72-78
14. Haematological Disorders 79-86
15. Diagnostic Laboratory Procedure 87-89

Section 2 Radiology

16. Radiation Physics 93-96
17. Radiation Biology 97-106
18. X-Ray Films 107-109
19. Processing of X-Ray Films 110-113
20. Intraoral Radiographic Techniques 114-119
21. Extraoral Radiography 120-129
22. Specialized Radiographic Techniques 130-136
23. Image Principles and Characteristics 137-140
24. Radiolucencies of Jaws 141-155

Section 3 Recently Asked Questions

25. Recently Asked Questions 159-193

SECTION 1

ORAL MEDICINE

CHAPTER 1 Ulcerative, Vesicular and Bullous Lesions

LONG ESSAYS

Question 1

Give the classification of vesiculobullous lesions. Discuss in detail the aetiology, clinical features and management of erythema multiforme?

Answer

Classification by Fitz and Patrick is as follows

- According to anatomical plane
  - Intra epidermal blister granular layer
    - Pemphigus foliaceous
    - Frictional blisters
    - Staphylococcus scalded syndrome.
  - Spinous layer
    - Eczematous dermatitis
    - Secondary to heat and cold
    - Herpes virus infection
    - Familial benign pemphigus.
  - Suprabasal
    - Pemphigus vulgaris
    - Pemphigus vegetans
    - Darier's disease.
  - Basal layer.
    - Erythema multiforme
    - Toxic epidermolysis necrolysis
    - Lupus erythematosis
    - Lichen planus
    - Epidermolysis bullosa simplex.
- Derma-epidermal junction zone.
  - Lamina lucida
    - Bullous pemphigoid
    - Cicatricial pemphigoid
    - Epidermolysis bullosa junctional.
  - Below basal layer.
    - Erythema multiforme
    - Epidermolysis bullosa dystrophica.

Erythema Multiforme

It is an inflammatory, acute and self limiting dermatological disorder, involving skin, mucous membrane and occasionally internal organs.

Aetiology

- Infectious agents: Herpes simplex, Mycoplasma pneumoniae
- Drug hypersensitivity: Anticonvulsants like carbamazepine, phenobarbital, sulpha drugs, salicylates, oxicam-non-steroidal anti-inflammatory drugs (NSAIDS) and penicillin
- Hyperimmunereaction: It is an immune-mediated disease. It is caused due to deposition of immune complexes in the superficial microvasculatures of skin and mucosa or cell-mediated immunity.

Types

- Erythema multiforme minor: are localised eruptions of skin with mild or no mucosal involvement
- Erythema multiforme major: is also referred to as Stevens-Johnson syndrome (SJS). It is a more severe form of skin and mucosal disease can be life-threatening disorder.

Clinical Manifestations

General Features

- Seen mainly in children and young adults—age range of 15–40 years
- Males are more commonly affected than females
- It is generally characterised by the occurrence of asymptomatic vividly erythematous discrete macule, papules and rarely vesicles and bullae which are symmetrically distributed over arms and hands, legs, feet, face and neck

- Classical lesions which commonly appear on extremities are concentric ring which results from varying shades of erythema giving rise to terms 'iris', 'target' or 'bull's eye' lesions
- It is a self-limiting form of disease
- Over the mucosal surface, the vesicles develop rapidly and are short lived
- These vesicles become eroded or ulcerated and bleed profusely
- Recurrence is common and patient may also have tracheobronchial ulceration and pneumonia
- Stevens–Johnson syndrome is a variant of erythema multiforme which is a life-threatening and debilitating hypersensitivity
- Skin lesions involve the necrosis of scrotal skin, penile skin or vulvar and labial surfaces
- Patient ulcers described as having 'ocular-genital lesions'
- There is epithelial necrosis of the cornea and conjunctiva, which develop prominent ulceration and necrosis
- It generally leads to blindness directly or to visual loss caused by secondary infection.

Intra-oral Features

- Oral lesions occur in only 50% of cases with skin lesions and are observed concurrently
- Oral lesions are large, painful, haemorrhagic, crusting ulcers, especially lips and labial mucosa
- Oral lesions can cause secondary drooling leading to excess fluid and electrolytes loss and would lead to secondary infection, causing cervical lymphadenitis
- Oral lesions suggestive of erythema multiforme without concomitant skin lesions probably do not represent true erythema multiforme, they often represent a lichenoid drug eruption or an immune-based disease.

Histopathology

- There is an intercellular or intracellular oedema along with necrosis of epithelium
- Prickle cell necrosis is a significant finding
- Vesicles may be seen either within the epithelium or at epithelial connective tissue junction
- There is oedema and perivascular infiltration of macrophages and lymphocytes in the subepithelial connective tissue.

Diagnosis

- Both the types of erythema multiforme are clinically diagnosed
- Skin or a mucosal biopsy is recommended to rule out immune-based and viral diseases.

Differential Diagnosis

- Toxic epidermal necrolysis
- Pemphigus
- Cutaneous pemphigoid.

Management

- Aetiology should be identified and removed
- Erythema multiforme is self-limiting, and usually not requires any treatment
- It would improve after 5–8 days, and will completely resolve within 2–4 weeks
- Few cases require antibiotics to treat secondary skin or oral infections appropriately
- Symptomatic treatment is advocated for all forms of erythema multiforme
- Treatment includes oral anti-histamines, analgesics, local skin care and soothing mouthwashes
- Skinwhichisnecrosedistreatedwithtopicalantimicrobial creams (1% silver sulphadiazine, silvadene, Aventis), and the eyes are irrigated and patched
- Erythema multiforme major requires systemic corticosteroids
- Antibiotics along with topical steroids can be considered, on the other hand systemic steroid therapy is controversial
- Corticosteroids can be stopped, once the intensity of the disease decreases and there is no development of new skin lesions.

Question 2

Discuss in detail the classification, aetiology, clinical features, histopathological features, differential diagnosis and management of aphthous stomatitis?

Answer

Aphthous Stomatitis

It is a painful condition which has recurrent, solitary or multiple lesions restricted to the mouth with no other signs of any other disease.

Classification

- Minor aphthae: It is also known as canker sores. Ulcers are less than 1 cm in diameter and they heal without scar
- Major aphthae: It is also known as Sutton's disease, or periadenitis mucosa necrotica recurrens. Ulcers are 1 cm in diameter and heal with scarring
- Herpetiform ulcers: Recurrent, many small ulcers are seen throughout the oral mucosa
- Recurrent ulcers associated with Behcet's syndrome.

Aetiology

- Bacterial infection: Alpha-haemolytic Streptococcus and Streptococcus sanguis are suggestive of causing this disease
- Iron deficiency or folic acid deficiency
- Immunologic abnormalities
- Haematological deficiency, serum iron or vitamin B12 deficiency, secondary malabsorption syndrome, such as celiac disease
- Hereditary: Increased susceptibility to RAS is seen among the children of RAS-positive parents.

Precipitating Factors

- Trauma: trauma such as self-inflicted bites, oral surgical procedures, tooth brushing, needle injections and dental trauma
- Endocrine conditions: A relationship between pregnancy and aphthous ulcer has been seen. Aphthous ulcer is also associated with menstruation and menopause
- Cessation of smoking increases the frequency and severity and RAS
- Psychic factors: Aphthous ulcers are precipitated by acute psychological problems and under stress and anxiety
- Allergy: Aphthous ulcers can also be seen in patients with history of asthma, hay fever and food or any drug allergy.

Clinical Features

- It is seen mainly between second and third decades of life
- More commonly seen in women than men
- It occurs generally on buccal and labial mucosa, tongue, soft palate, buccal and lingual sulci, pharynx and gingiva
- Prodromal symptoms: It starts with prodromal burning for 24–48 hours, before the ulcer appears
- It starts as a single or multiple superficial erosions which are covered by a grey membrane
- Lesions appear as round, symmetric and shallow in shape
- No tissue tags are present from the ruptured vesicles
- Aphthous ulcers are seen as localised areas of erythema and within hours small white papules are formed, that ulcerate and enlarge over next 48–72 hours
- Lesions are very painful; therefore, it interferes with eating
- Multiple lesions at a time can also occur but number and size varies
- Lesions remain for about 7–14 days.

Minor Aphthae

- They are 0.3–1 cm in size
- Within 10–14 days, heal without scarring.

Major Aphthae

- Their size is larger than 1 cm and may increase to 5 cm in diameter
- They interfere with speech and mastication
- Lesions may be covered with deep painful ulcers
- Lesions heal slowly and leave scars, which result in decreased mobility of uvula and tongue and destruction of some areas of oral mucosa.

Histopathological Features

- Ulcerated areas are covered with fibrinopurulent membrane
- This membrane can consist of superficial colonies of microorganisms
- Within the connective tissue, intense inflammatory cell infiltrate is present
- Neutrophils are predominantly present
- Anitschkow cells consist of cells with elongated nuclei
- It consists of a linear bar of chromatin with radiating processes of chromatin that intends towards the nuclear membrane.

Differential Diagnosis

- Pemphigus
- Cyclic neutropenia
- Bednar's aphthae
- Erythema multiforme
- Lupus erythematosus
- Necrotising sialometaplasia
- Psoriasis
- Erosive lichen planus
- Atrophic candidiasis
- Primary syphilitic lesions
- Herpetic stomatitis
- Herpangina
- Herpetiform gingiva stomatitis
- Hand, foot and mouth disease.

Management

Based on the severity of lesion, management is divided into two parts:

1. Mild
2. Severe cases.

Mild Cases

- Topical protective emollient base (Orabase)
- Tetracycline mouthwash (250 mg/mL)—it should be used four times daily for 5–7 days
- Topical corticosteroid, i.e., triamcinolone acetonide can be given three to four times daily

- Replacement therapy can also be given using vitamin B12, ferritin, folate and iron
- Tetracycline can be applied topically, followed by cortisone ointment
- Chlorhexidine mouthwash should be used.

Severe Cases

- Clobetasol cream or beclomethasone spray or fluocinolone gel can be used
- Corticosteroid injections can be given directly into the lesion along with systemic cortisone
- In few cases, dapsone or thalidomide can also be used
- Chlortetracycline can be used as a mouth rinse
- Nicotine tablets, colchicine and interferon-alpha can also be used
- Biostimulation using soft-tissue lasers can also be done
- In extremely severe cases, excision with primary closure or cryosurgery can be done.

Question 3

What are vesicles? Discuss the pathogenesis, clinical features, differential diagnosis, investigations and management of primary herpetic infection?

Answer

Vesicles

They are elevated blisters which contain clear fluid that are beyond 1 cm in diameter.

Primary Herpetic Infection

Pathogenesis

- Primary herpetic gingivostomatitis is caused due to herpes simplex virus type I infection
- Herpes simplex virus enters into the patient's body through:
  - Direct or airborne
  - Water droplet transmission via an infected person.

Clinical Features

- Incubation period is 5–7 days
- First prodromal symptom will appear for 2 days before appearance of oral lesions
- It is seen commonly in children and young adults
- Vesicular lesions that are painful develop on all mucosal surfaces
- Since these lesions are very thin, they can rupture easily, producing foul-smelling ulcers
- It can appear as generalised acute marginal gingivitis
- Patient has an acute illness, which lasts about 10 days and resolves with scar formation
- The patient is generally febrile, drool and has significant maliase, feels miserable and will have tender cervical lymphadenopathy.

Differential Diagnosis

- Necrotising ulcerative periodontitis
- Pemphigus vulgaris
- Erythema multiforme
- Aphthous ulcers
- Herpes zoster.

Management

- Acyclovir is very effective against HSV
- It is self-limiting condition and can be managed by supportive care like hydration, nutrition, antipyretics and possibly antibiotics if secondary bacterial infections arise
- Topical 5% acyclovir is used for immunocompromised patient
- These patients may also require intravenous therapy
- Foscarnet (Foscavir) is used in acyclovir-resistant strains as a substitute to acyclovir or as an addition to it at dose of 40–60 mg/kg IV thrice a day.

SHORT NOTES

Question 1

Describe clinical features of ANUG along with its treatment plan?

Answer

Acute Necrotising Ulcerative Gingivitis

- It is a destructive and an inflammatory oral condition in which there is necrosis of gingival tissue
- It is commonly known as trench mouth or Vincent's infection.

Clinical Features

- It presents as an acute disease and symptoms are sudden in onset
- In some cases, it can resolve on its own, and shows milder symptoms which lead to subacute stage
- Some common predisposing factor could be debilitating disease or acute respiratory tract infection, psychological

stress, nutritional deficiencies use of tobacco, smoking and continuous work without rest.

Characteristics Clinical Signs are as follows

- This infection shows punched out, crater like depressions at the crest of the interdental papillae and it might involve the marginal gingiva
- Attached gingiva and oral mucosa are rarely involved
- A slough which is grey in colour and pseudomembranous in nature, cover the gingival craters
- It can be demarcated from the healthy gingiva by a pronounced linear erythema
- In some cases lesions may be denuded of the pseudomembrane, exposing red, shiny and haemorrhagic gingival surface
- Lesion bleeds even on slightest provocation
- Fetid odour
- Increased salivation
- Pasty saliva
- Metallic foul taset
- Generally patient complains off a constant radiating, gnawing pain that is aggravated upon taking hot and spicy food and upon chewing
- Extraoral and systemic sign and symptoms are local lymphadenopathy and mild fever
- In very severe cases following signs can be seen: High fever, increased pulse rates, leukocytosis, loss of appetite, and general lassitude
- These signs and symptoms are more severe in children.

Treatment

- Local debridement and irrigation along with antibiotics
- Oral cavity should be cleaned superficially and should be irrigated with a 3% solution of hydrogen peroxide mixed with 1:1 saline or chlorhexidine or warm salt water scaling should be done so as to remove superficial plaque and calculus under local or topical anaesthesia
- Plaque control instructions should be given for home care
- Antibiotics are effective, with penicillin being the drug of choice, i.e., 500 mg four times daily for 7–10 days
- In penicillin-allergic patient, erythromycin can be given, i.e., 400 mg twice a day for 7–10 days, or doxycycline 100 mg once daily for 7–10 days
- Vitamin B and C should be given additionally.

CHAPTER 2 Red and White Lesions

LONG ESSAYS

Question 1

Discuss the aetiology, clinical features, differential diagnosis and treatment of oral lichen planus (OLP)?

Answer

Lichen Planus

Lichen planus is a chronic disease of skin and mucous membrane, with different etiologies with a common clinical and histological appearance.

Oral lichenoid reactions include the following disorders:

- Lichen planus
- Lichenoid contact reactions
- Lichenoid drug eruptions
- Lichenoid reactions of graft versus host disease (GVHD).

Aetiology

- It is mainly an immunologic disorder, which can occur due to variety of reasons
- Emotional stress is one of the major causes for exacerbation or remission of the condition
- Such cases are common following psychological stress.

Clinical Features

- It is seen in middle aged and elderly patients
- More commonly seen in females
- It most commonly involves buccal mucosa, tongue, lips, vestibule, gingiva, floor of mouth and palate
- There may be burning sensation of oral mucosa
- Generally, the oral lesion is characterised by radiating white and grey velvety thread-like papules in linear, angular or retiform arrangement
- At the intersection of these white lines, tiny white elevated dots are usually present which are known as wickham striae
- Patterns or types of lichen planus are as follows:
  - Linear pattern
  - Papular pattern
  - Reticular pattern
  - Annular or circular pattern
  - Vesicular or bullous pattern
  - Erosive or atrophic pattern
  - Hypertrophic pattern.

Histopathology

- Hyperorthokeratosis or parakeratosis is seen over the overlying surface
- Granular cell layer becomes thickened
- There is acanthosis of spinous cell layer and saw-tooth appearance of rete pegs
- Band-like subepithelial mononuclear infiltrate is present which consists of T-cells and histiocytes
- There is presence of necrosis or liquefaction degeneration of basal cell layer of epithelium
- In juxtraepithelial region, chronic inflammatory cell infiltrate is present
- Degenerating basal keratinocytes form rounded or ovoid, amorphous eosinophilic bodies known as Civatte, hyaline, cytoid bodies
- Degeneration of basal keratinocytes and disruption of anchoring elements of epithelial basement membrane weakens the epithelial-connective tissue interface resulting in histological cleft known as Max-Joseph space.

Differential Diagnosis

- Leukoplakia
- Lichenoid Reaction
- Mucous patches of secondary syphilis
- Candidiasis (thrush)

- Pemphigus
- Recurrent aphthae (ulcer)
- Erythema multiforme
- Lupus erythematosus.

Treatment

- Most predictable and successful medications for OLP are corticosteroids
- Topical or systemic corticosteroids can be given to patients
- Topical corticosteroids help in reducing pain and inflammation
- Topical medications are:
  - 0.05% fluocinonide (Lidex), triamcinolone acetonide 0.1% in orabase and 0.05% clobetasol (Temovate)
  - High-potency steroid mouthwash can also be used effectively like betamethasone valerate 0.1%, fluocinolone acetonide 0.1% and clobetasol propionate 0.05%.
- Occlusive splints as carriers can be used for topical steroids
- Topical or systemic antifungal therapy can be given in cases of candida overgrowth
- Bacterial growth can be avoided by using an antibacterial rinse, such as chlorhexidine before steroid application
- Systemic administration of prednisone tablets may be given of varying dosages, i.e., between 10 mg and 80 mg daily for less than 10 days without tapering
- When underlying medical problems are present, then it is advisable to consult with patient's physician
- Retinoids can be given along with topical corticosteroids as an adjunctive therapy for OLP
- Topical application of a retinoid cream or gel can eliminate reticular and plaque-like lesions
- Systemic and topically-administered beta all-trans retinoic acid, vitamin A acid, systemic etretinate and systemic and topical isotretinoin are all very effective
- Other medications which can be used topically and systemically are dapsone, doxycycline and antimalarials
- Cyclosprorine can also be applied topically for managing recalcitrant extensive and otherwise intractable oral lesions of OLP
- In cases where concomitant dysplasia has been identified, in those case surgical excision is indicated.

Question 2

Classify white lesions of the oral cavity? Discuss the aetiology, clinical features and management of leukoplakia?

Answer

Classification of White Lesions

According to Ghom, classification of white lesions is as follows:

- Normal variation
  - Leukoedema
  - Fordyce's granules
  - Linea alba.
- Non-keratotic white lesion
  - Habitual cheek biting
  - Uremic stomatitis
  - Koplik's spot
  - Burns
  - Radiation mucositis.
- Candidiasis
  - Thrush
  - Acute atrophic candidiasis
  - Id reaction
  - Extraoral candidiasis
  - Chronic mucocutaneous candidiasis (CMC)
  - Systemic candidiasis.
- Keratotic white lesions
  - Traumatic keratosis
  - Stomatitis nicotina
  - Intraoral skin graft
  - Focal epithelial hyperplasia
  - Keratosis associated with dental restoration
  - Psoriasis.
- Oral genodermatoses.
  - White sponge nevus
  - Pachyonychia congenita
  - Hereditary benign intraepithelial dyskeratosis
  - Porokeratosis
  - Keratosis follicularis
  - Hereditary mucoepithelial dysplasia
  - Warty dyskeratoma
  - Pseudoxanthoma elasticum
  - Hyalinosis cutis et mucosa oris.

Leukoplakia

- It can be of two types.
  - Which shows history of atypia (dysplasia)
  - Which shows different degrees of atypia.
- A leukoplakia lesion can show severe atypia with malignant change throughout the depth of epithelial layer, but its basement membrane may still be intact, such lesion is referred to as carcinoma in situ or intraepithelial carcinoma

- Leukoplakia can also be categorised into two types depending on its spontaneous disappearance, following removal of chronic irritant as follows:
  - Reversible leukoplakia: Lesions of leukoplakia become infeasible after removing the chronic irritants
  - Irreversible leukoplakia: Even after removal of the irritants, lesion is persistent.

Clinical Features

- It is asymptomatic and generally found during routine oral examination
- Most commonly seen in older age group of greater than 35 years (40–70 years)
- Most commonly seen in males
- Frequently seen sites are lips, vermilion border, buccal mucosa, tongue, hard palate, floor of the mouth, gingiva of maxilla
- Floor of mouth and lateral border of tongue are high-risk sites for malignant transformation
- Lesions vary in size, shape, and distribution
- Borders can be distinct or indistinct smoothly contoured or ragged
- Typical homogeneous leukoplakia is characterised as white, well-demarcated plaque with an identical reaction pattern throughout the lesion
- The surface texture can vary from smaller thin surface to leathery appearance with surface fissures referred to as 'cracked mud'
- Erythroleukoplakia or speckled leukoplakia is a non-homogeneous type of oral leukoplakia, having white patches or plaque intermixed with red tissue elements
- In verrucous or verruciform leukoplakia, lesion, white component is dominated by papillary projections similar to oral papilomas
- This variety of leukoplakia which has more aggressive proliferation pattern and recurrent rate and is referred to as proliferative verrucous leukoplakia (PVL)
- It is more common in older women and most common prediction site is mandibular gingiva
- Lesions which are located in the high-risk areas like central surface of tongue, floor of mouth, margins of the tongue and retromolar areas have high risk for malignant transformation.

Differential Diagnosis

- Lichen planus
- Leukoedema
- Smokeless tobacco lesion
- Cheek biting lesion
- Lupus erythematosus
- Hyperplastic or hypertrophic candidiasis
- Verrucous or squamous cell carcinoma
- Verruca vulgaris
- White sponge nevus.

Management

Removal of Aetiological or Causative Factors

- No appropriate treatment has been established for sanguinaria-induced leukoplakia
- Therefore, complete discontinuation of sanguinaria-containing products is important and declining of any other harmful habits like alcohol or smoking is mandatory.

Conservative Approach

- Vitamin therapy with vitamin A and vitamin E, B complex, 13-cis-retinoic acid, antioxidant therapy has proved to be effective
- Nystatin is given in candidal leukoplakia.

Surgical Therapy

- Cold-knife surgical excision
- Cryosurgery (liquid nitrogen or CO_2 now is used)
- Laser surgery
- Fulguration (electrocautery or electrosurgery)
- Laser (light amplification by specially CO_2 lasers stimulated fusion of radiation)
- Re-examination should be done every 3 months for first year irrespective of surgical excision
- Follow-up should be done every 6 months
- Self examination is reasonable approach if there is no relapse for 5 years
- An initial biopsy is necessary
- Careful clinical follow-ups should be given to all patients with a biopsy of any recurrent or worsening lesions.

Question 3

What are the precancerous lesions and conditions? Discuss definition, aetiopathogenesis, clinical features, differential diagnosis and management of oral submucous fibrosis?

Answer

The premalignant lesions are defined as morphologically altered tissue in which cancer is more likely to occur than in the apparently normal counterpart. For example,

- Leukoplakia
- Erythroplakia
- Nicotiana palati
- Stomatitis
- Dyskeratosis congenitis.

Premalignant condition is defined as generalised state of body, which is associated with significantly increased risk of cancer. For example,

- Oral submucous fibrosis
- Syphilis
- White sponge nevus
- Lichen planus.

Oral Submucous Fibrosis

It is a chronic and a high-risk precancerous condition.

Definition

It is an insidious, chronic disease affecting any part of the oral cavity and sometimes pharynx, although occasionally preceded by and/or associated with vesicle formation.

It is always associated with juxtraepithelial inflammatory reaction followed by fibroelastic changes of lamina propria with epithelial atrophy leading to stiffness of oral mucosa thereby trismus and inability to eat.

Aetiopathogenesis

Chronic Irritation

- Chillies: Chillies have been thought to be an important aetiological factor for OSMF. It consists of capsaicin, which is the vanillylamide of 8-methyl-6-nonenic acid, which is the active irritant of the chillies
- Lime: It acts as a local irritant. It is used along with betel nut for chewing. It causes local irritation and damage to the mucosa along with ulcer and vesicle formation in susceptible individuals
- Betel nut: Areca nut is the unhusked whole fruit of the areca nut tree and betel nut is the inner kernel or seed which is obtained after removing husk. Betel nut has areca alkaloids, mainly arecolines which have a psychotropic and antihelmintic property. These alkaloids have a powerful parasympathetic property which causes euphoria and counteract fatigue. Areca nut contains different types of alkaloids, such as arecoline, arecadine, arecalidine, guvacoline, guvacine and isoguvacine. Betel nut consists of tannic acid, which causes OSMF. Mixed calcium powder and the conditional action of arecoline content in betel nut, affects the vascular supply of oral mucosa and causes neutrotropic disorder. Metabolism of areca nut-specific nitrosamine will cause formation of cyanoethyl, which adducts with o'methyl guanine in DNA. Prolonged exposure to this irritant will cause malignant transformation
- Tobacco: It is responsible for causing oral malignancy. It may act as a local irritant.

Nutritional Deficiency

- Repeated vesiculations and ulcerations of oral cavity are seen
- Subclinical vitamin B complex deficiency is seen
- Deficient nutrient intake can precipitate the condition because of impaired food intake in advanced cases and can be an effect, rather than the cause of the disease.

Defective Iron Metabolism

Microcytic hypochronic anaemia along with high serum iron have been reported in OSMF, but there is no definite proof available to support this cause.

Collagen Disorders

- Oral submucous fibrosis is believed to be a localised collagen disease of oral cavity
- Scleroderma, Duputreyen's contracture, intestinal fibrosis and rheumatoid arthritis have been linked to OSMF.

Bacterial Infections

- Streptococcal bacteria is considered a factor in aetiology of OSMF, as seen in some collagen disorder like rheumatic disease
- Klebsiella rhinoscleromatis can be a aetiological factor in cause of OSMF.

Immunological Disorders

- Increased ESR and globulin levels are indicative of immunodeficiency disorder
- In OSMF, there is an increase in levels of serum immunoglobulin like IgA, IgG and IgM
- These raised levels are suggestive of an antigenic stimulus in the absence of any infection.

Altered Salivary Composition

There is an increase in pH of saliva, increase in salivary amylase, low levels of calcium, increase in alkaline phosphatase and potassium and normal levels of salivary immunoglobulin.

Genetic Susceptibility

The familial occurrence of OSMF has been reported.

Clinical Features

- Age and sex distribution
  - Both sexes are affected
  - Most commonly affects 20–40 years of age.

- Site distribution
  - Most commonly affected site is buccal mucosa and the retromolar area
  - Other sites involved are soft palate, faucial pillars, uvula, tongue and lateral mucosa
  - It may also involve the floor of mouth and gingiva.
- Symptoms.
  - Onset of condition is insidious and duration is of 2–5 years
  - Initial symptoms are burning sensation of oral mucosa, which is generally aggravated by spicy food, is followed by hypersalivation or dryness of mouth
  - Early symptoms also include vesiculation, pigmentation, ulceration, recurrent stomatitis and defective gustatory sensation
  - After the initial symptoms have occurred, gradual stiffening of oral mucosa is seen
  - It causes difficulty in opening the mouth and protruding the tongue
  - Patient experiences difficulty in swallowing the food due to extension of fibroids to pharynx and oesophagus
  - Occlusion of eustachian tube can occur thereby causing referred pain in ears and deafness
  - Typical nasal voice has also been reported.

Signs

- Blanching of mucosa is the earliest and most common sign
- It occurs due to decrease in vascular supply
- Blanched mucosa appears opaque and white
- On progression of disease, there is stiffness of mucosa and vertical bands may also appear
- Loss of pigmentation or hypopigmentation may be seen occasionally
- Vesicle formation is seen in the areas of erythema in the soft palate, anterior faucial pillar, buccal mucosa or the mucosal surface of lip, especially the lower one
- Vesicles are painful and rupture soon leaving a superficial ulceration behind
- During the course of disease ulceration is commonly seen, especially in advanced cases
- Epithelium becomes atrophic
- Small, raised, reddish-blue spots known as petechiae are seen in OSMF.

Clinical Stages of OSMF

There are three stages:

1. Stage of stomatitis and vesiculation
   - It is the earliest stage
   - It is characterised by recurrent stomatitis and vesiculation
   - Patient is unable to eat spicy food and complains of burning sensation
   - Vesicle formation is seen especially on palate
   - They can rupture and superficial ulceration may be seen, which can cause difficulty in mastication
   - Fibrosis is seen in this stage and whitish streaks are seen on the mucosa.
2. Stage of fibrosis
   - There is stiffness and inability to open the mouth completely
   - Difficulty in blowing out the cheeks
   - Tongue movements are difficult too
   - Pain in ear may occur occasionally
   - Due to restriction of jaw movement speech may become indistinct
   - There is fibrosis of submucosal tissue
   - It appears whitish and blanched
   - Vestibule of mouth is gradually reduced and obliterated and also the lip and cheek become stiff
   - This leads to difficulty in placing the fingers between lips, cheeks and teeth in advanced cases
   - Blanching is seen over the palate also
   - Atrophy of papillae is seen on the dorsum of this tongue.
3. Stage of sequelae and complications.
   - Patient complaints are similar to stage 2
   - There is presence of white leucoplakic changes and rarely an ulcerating malignant lesion may be seen.

Histopathologic Features

- Epithelium is atrophic in nature
- Epithelium exhibits intercellular oedema, epithelial atypia and signet cells
- Liquefaction degeneration of the basal cells can also be seen
- Hyperorthokeratosis and pyknotic changes can be seen occasionally
- There is complete loss of retipegs
- Due to subepithelial accumulation of fluid, there is formation of vesicles
- Inflammatory cells are mainly mononuclear, eosinophils and plasma cells can be seen occasionally
- In early stages, collagen becomes moderately hyalinised and amorphous, changes start from the juxtraepithelial basement membrane
- In advanced stages, collagen gets completely hyalinised and is seen as a smooth sheath with separate bundles.

Management

Restriction of Habit or Behavioural Therapy

- Habit should be stopped
- Patient should be made aware about the disease and its malignant potential
- Patients who discontinue the habit, there is a gradual increase in inter-incisal opening.

Medical Therapy

Supportive treatment:
- Vitamin-rich diet along with iron preparation is given
- Iodine-B complex (injection Ranodine) is a combination of iodine preparation with synthetic vitamin B complex
- Dose IM injection starting with small doses and continuing with larger doses (2 mL ampule daily)
- It is a five-injection course which is repeated after 7 days
- Arsina typhoid and iodine injection can also be given since arsenal typhoid is a fibrin dissolving agent.

Steroids

Local

Hydrocortisone injection along with procaine hydro chloride injection can be applied locally in the area of fibrosis.

Systemic

- Cortisone
- 25 mg hydrocortisone tablet in a dose of 100 mg/day is beneficial in relieving burning sensation
- Triamcinolone or 90 mg of dexamethasone can be given
- It is given in conjugation with injection of 25 mg hydrocortisone daily.

Placental Extract

- Placentrex is an important biogenic stimulator
- It is believed that it stimulates pituitary adrenal cortex and regulates metabolism of tissue.

Hyaluronidase

It reduces the burning sensation and trismus.

Vitamin E

Vitamin E in combination with dexamethasone and hyaluronidase injections produces better results.

Other Therapies

- Injection of vitamin A, collagenese and gold
- Vasodilator injections.

Surgical Treatment

Conventional:
- It is the treatment of choice, in case of marked limitation of opening of mouth
- Fibrous bands are excised followed by use of tongue flap as a graft gives good results because tongue flap is highly vascular and resists further fibrosis
- Excision of fibrotic bands is followed by reconstruction using bilateral full-thickness nasolabial flap.

Laser

- Laser has proved to be very useful for treating OSMF
- CO_2 laser surgery is useful in alleviating the functional restriction, when compared to traditional surgical technique, followed by grafting.

Cryosurgery

- It causes local destruction of tissue by freezing it in situ
- Open liquid sprays are used for this purpose.

Oral Physiotherapy

- Prescribed in early and moderately advanced cases
- In this, mouth opening exercises are done alongwith forceful opening of mouth and ballooning
- The therapy places pressure on fibrous bands.

Diathermy

- It is useful in early or moderately advanced stages
- In this, a low-level current of 20 watts × 2,450 cycles is used
- It acts by physiofibriolysis of bands.

SHORT ESSAYS

Question 1

Discuss systemic and discoid lupus erythematosus with histological features?

Answer

Systemic Lupus Erythematosus (SLE)

- It is an immunologically mediated inflammatory condition which causes multiorgan damage
- Oral lesions of systemic lupus are almost similar to discoid lupus
- They are most commonly seen on buccal mucosa followed by gingival tissue, vermilion border of lip and the palate
- Lesions are symptomatic, mainly when the patients ingests hot or spicy foods
- It represents erythema, keratotic plaques, surface ulce ation and white striae or papules
- These lesions appear lichenoid, they may be nonspecific and resemble leukoplakia, vesiculobullous disease or even a granulomatous lesion
- They respond well to topical or systemic steroids.

Discoid Lupus Erythematosus

- It is relatively common
- It occurs more commonly in females in the 3rd or 4th decade of life
- It can occur as a localised or disseminated forms and is also known as chronic cutaneous lupus erythematosus (CCL)
- It is restricted to oral mucous membrane and skin, and has a better prognosis than SLE
- Lesions appear as red and scaly patches which favour sun-exposed areas like face, back, chest and extremities
- Lesions appear as disc-shaped
- Oral lesions can be seen in the absence of skin lesions
- As there is expansion of lesion in the periphery, there is central atrophy, scar formation, and occasional loss of surface pigmentations are seen
- Oral mucosal lesions of DLE resemble reticular or erosive lichen planus
- Common locations of these lesions are buccal mucosa, palate, tongue and vermilion border of lips
- Lesions can be atrophic, erythematous or ulcerated and are often painful.

Histopathologic Features

- There is hyperorthokeratosis with keratotic plugs, atrophy of the rete ridges and liquefactive degeneration of the basal cell layer
- In the lamina propria, superficial oedema is seen
- Direct immunofluorescence testing of lesion shows deposition of various immunoglobulins and C3 in a granular band involving the zone of basement membrane
- Direct immunofluorescence testing of uninvolved skin in SLE has a same kind of deposition of immunoglobulins
- This is known as positive lupus band test
- Discoid lesions will not show this result.

SHORT NOTES

Question 1

Short note on Stevens–Johnson syndrome?

Answer

Stevens–Johnson Syndrome

It is a bullous form of erythema multiforme involving the skin, oral cavity, genitalia and eyes.

Clinical Features

- Fever
- Malaise
- Photophobia
- Purulent conjunctivitis (eye)
- Erythematous eruptions of oral mucosa, genitalia and skin
- Constitutional disturbance
- Painful lesions
- Difficulty in mastication
- Haemorrhagic lesions which are often vesicular or bullous.

CHAPTER 3

Keratotic and Non-keratotic White Lesions

LONG ESSAYS

Question 1

Give the classification of white lesions. Explain in detail about oral candidiasis?

Answer

Classification of White Lesions

According to Ghom, classification of white lesions is as follows:

I. Normal variation
  - Leukoedema
  - Fordyce's granules
  - Linea alba.

II. Non-keratotic white lesion
  - Habitual cheek biting
  - Uremic stomatitis
  - Koplik's spot
  - Burns
  - Radiation mucositis.

III. Candidiasis
  - Thrush
  - Acute atrophic candidiasis
  - Id reaction
  - Extraoral candidiasis
  - Chronic mucocutaneous candidiasis (CMC)
  - Systemic candidiasis.

IV. Keratotic white lesions
  - Traumatic keratosis
  - Stomatitis nicotina
  - Intraoral skin graft
  - Focal epithelial hyperplasia
  - Keratosis associated with dental restoration
  - Psoriasis.

V. Oral genodermatoses
  - White sponge nevus
  - Pachyonychia congenita
  - Hereditary benign intraepithelial dyskeratosis
  - Porokeratosis
  - Keratosis follicularis
  - Hereditary mucoepithelial dysplasia
  - Warty dyskeratoma
  - Pseudoxanthoma elasticum
  - Hyalinosis cutis et mucosa oris.

Candidiasis

Candidiasis is the disease caused by yeast-like fungus Candida albicans.

Oral Candidiasis

It is one of the most common manifestations of human candidal infection.

Classification (According to Ghom)

I. Oral Candidiasis

Acute

- Acute pseudomembranous candidiasis (thrush)
- Acute atrophic candidiasis (antibiotics sore mouth).

Chronic

- Chronic atrophic candidiasis
  - Denture stomatitis
  - Median rhomboid glossitis
  - Angular cheilitis.
- Id reaction
- Chronic hyperplastic candidiasis.

II. Chronic Mucocutaneous Candidiasis

- Familial CMC
- Localised CMC

- Diffuse CMC
- Candidiasis endocrinopathy syndrome.

III. Extraoral Candidiasis

- Oral candidiasis associated with intraoral lesions orofacial and intertriginous sites (candidal vulvovaginitis, intertriginous candidiasis)
- Gastrointestinal candidiasis
- Candida hypersensitivity syndrome.

IV. Systemic Candidiasis

Eye, skin and kidneys are affected.

Causative Organisms

Candida albicans, Candida stellatoidea, Candida tropicalis, Candida parapsilosis, Candida farnata, Candida krusei, etc.

Predisposing Factors

- Changes in oral microbial flora: Antibiotics (broad spectrum), xerostomia secondary to anticholinergic agents or salivary gland disease or excessive use of antibacterial mouth rinse—all these factors can cause change in the oral microbial flora, which could predispose to candidiasis
- Local irritant: Chronic local irritational factors, such as orthodontic appliance, denture and heavy smoke
- Drug therapy: Administration of drugs, such as corticosteroids, cytotoxic drugs, immunosuppressive agents and radiation to head and neck
- Malnutrition: Decreased levels of serum vitamin A, pyridoxine and iron levels can predispose to candidiasis
- Acute and chronic disease: Acute and chronic disease, like leukaemia, lymphoma, diabetes and tuberculosis can predispose to candidiasis
- Age: Commonly seen in infants, old age and pregnancy
- Immunodeficiency state: Primary and acquired immunodeficiency states like hypogammaglobulinemia
- Endocrinopathy: For example, hypoparathyroidism, hypothyroidism and Addison's disease
- Others: Tightly fitted clothes can promote the growth of Candida
- Areas around the indwelling catheter, hospitalization and oral epithelial dysplasia.

Thrush

- It is an oral infection which occurs due to yeast-like fungus
- It causes formation of patchy white plaque or flicks on mucosal surface
- It is a superficial infection seen on the upper layer of oral mucous membrane.

Clinical Features

- In infants
  - Age: 6th and 10th day after birth, in neonates
  - Aetiology: can be caused from the internal vaginal canal, as Candida albicans flourishes during pregnancy
  - Appearance: It appears as soft white or bluish white adherent patches which can be seen on oral mucosa that can reach up to the circumoral tissue
  - Symptoms: They are usually painless, they can be easily removed.
- In adults.
  - Sites: Roof of the mouth, retromolar area and mucobuccal fold
  - Sex: More common in females than in males
  - Prodormal symptoms: Bad taste, discomfort by spicy food
  - Symptoms: Burning sensation in mouth
  - Also, there can be history of dryness of the mouth.

Signs

- Erythema, inflammation and painful eroded areas can be seen
- Loosely adherent patches which can be multiple and curdy in appearance
- There is presence of red and moderately-swollen mucosa adjacent to the patch
- Sometimes there is appearance of pearly-white or bluish-white plaque
- White patches can be easily removed with a wet gauze which causes a normal or a erythematous area can also be seen
- Ulcerative lesions can also be seen
- White or erythematous area can be seen below the partial or complete denture
- It can be associated with dysplastic or carcinomatous change.

Histopathological Features

- Yeast cells can be seen. Hyphae or mycelia are also seen in the superficial and deeper layer of the epithelium
- Submucosa may contain a chronic inflammatory cell infiltrate.

Differential Diagnosis

- Leukoplakia
- Plaque form of lichen planus
- Gangrenous stomatitis

- Genodermatoses
- Chemical burns.

Acute Atrophic Candidiasis

It is also known as antibiotics sore mouth. When white plaque of psuedomembranous candidiasis is removed, generally red atrophic and painful mucosa remains.

Clinical Features

- It appears as a red or erythematous rather than white, therefore resembles the pseudomembranous type
- It can be seen normally on the tongue and tissues beneath on appliance
- Patient complains of vague pain or a burning sensation
- Pain can be elicited by mild abrasive pressure with cotton gauze
- Few white thickened foci can be seen which can be rubbed off leaving a painful surface
- It resembles erosive lichen planus and erythroplakia.

Histopathological Features

- Atrophic epithelium can be seen which has a few hyphae in the superficial layer
- There is a mild acute inflammatory infiltrate in the lamina propria and increased vascularity
- Microabscesses can be seen in superficial areas.

Differential Diagnosis

- Drug reaction
- Chemical burn
- Necrotic ulcer and gangrenous stomatitis
- Traumatic ulcer
- Syphilitic mucous patches.

Chronic Hyperplastic Candidiasis

It is also known as candidal leukoplakia as it appears as firm and adherent white patches in the oral mucosa.

Clinical Features

- It is most commonly seen in males of middle age or more
- Patients are generally heavy smokers
- It occurs most commonly on cheek, lips and tongue
- It appears as white leathery plaques
- Lesion may remain asymptomatic for many years
- In women suffering from oral candidiasis, vaginal itching and discharge suggestive of vaginal candidiasis
- It does not rub off easily upon applying pressure
- Lesions are slightly white to dense white with cracks and fissures present occasionally
- Borders are not well defined, and mimic the appearance of epithelial dysplasia
- It can also occur as a part of chronic mucocutaneous candidiasis.

Histopathological Features

- Epithelial dysplasia is seen
- Mycelial invasion of the deeper layers of mucosa and skin is seen
- Epithelium is generally parakeratinised
- Acanthosis is seen in the spinous layer and bulbous elongated rete pegs
- There is pseudoepitheliomatous hyperplasia and microabscesses formation
- There is presence of inflammatory exudates and chronic inflammatory cell infiltration of polymorphonuclear neutrophils in the corneum layer.

Differential Diagnosis

- Hairy leukoplakia
- Lichen planus
- Superficial bacterial infection.

Candida-associated Lesion (Denture Stomatitis)

It is also known as chronic atrophic candidiasis.

Clinical Features

- It is mainly found under the denture either complete or partial
- More common in females than in males
- It appears as patchy, often associated with speckled curd-like white lesion
- Patient complains of dryness and soreness of mouth
- Palatal tissue is erythematous and granular and therefore appears as bright red in colour
- Reddened mucosa is restricted to the tissue actually which is in contact with the denture
- In the maxilla, there are pinpoint foci of hyperemia.

Histopathological Features

- Superficially oriented mycelia are present
- Epithelium is atrophic
- Inflammatory infiltrate is present.

Differential Diagnosis

- Allergic reaction due to denture base
- Erosive lichen planus
- Dermatitis herpetiformis.

Treatment

Troches that contain clotrimazole and nystatin four to five times after meal and bed time.

Lab Diagnosis

Smear

- Smear from infected area is taken by scraping and smeared directly onto the slide
- It is a simple and a quick method
- It has a low sensitivity.

Imprint Culture

- Sterile plastic foam pads dipped into Sabouraud broth are placed over the lesion for 60 seconds
- Pad is pressed over Sabouraud agar plate, and incubated, and a colony counter is then used to count the microorganisms
- It is a sensitive and a reliable method
- It can differentiate between infected and carrier states.

Impression Culture

- Maxillary and mandibular impressions are made with alginate
- Casting is done in an agar fortified with Sabouraud broth
- It is then incubated
- Thismethodhelpsindeterminingtherelativedistribution of yeasts on mucosal surfaces
- It is generally used as a research tool.

Salivary Culture

- 2 mL of saliva is taken from the patient and converted into a sterile container
- It is vibrated and cultured on Sabouraud agar by a spiral plating and counting
- It is a sensitive and reliable method
- It requires more chair side time
- It is not very helpful in xerostomic patients.

Swabs

Swabs can also be used.

Oral Rinse

- Patient is given phosphate-buffered saline (PBS) for rinsing for 60 seconds at a pH of 7.2, 0.1 M
- Patient returns it to the original container which is then concentrated by centrifugation
- Culturing is done and then the microorganisms are counted in a colony counter
- It is a simple method
- It shows better results if CFU is greater than 50/cm2
- This method is generally performed for surveillance cultures in the abscence of focal lesions
- Site of infection cannot be identified.

Management

- Both topical and systemic medications are given for the treatment of oropharyngeal candidiasis
- Drugs should be given for at least 1 week after signs and symptoms have disappeared.

Before the administration of any drug, the underlying cause should be eliminated.

- The dentures should be replaced or relined or mycostatin suspension should be applied beneath the denture during insertion in the mouth in cases of angular cheilitis and denture sore mouth
- Thorough cleaning of the dentures should be done regularly
- Dentures should be kept outside the mouth at night in a hypochlorite solution.

Topical Management

It is given in cases which are mild and superficial, where patients have a good resistance against microorganisms and have a good immune system.

Drugs Given are as follows

Nystatin:

- Most frequently given drug
- It works by destroying the cell membrane by binding to ergosterol in them
- It cannot be absorbed through gastrointestinal tract (GIT)
- It is available as oral ointment, suspension/cream, vaginal troche, powder, tablets
- Pastilles: It is the most frequently used form—200,000 units/each pastilles, 1–2 pastilles dissolved in mouth four to five times per day.

Clotrimazole:

- It is derivative of imidazole which can be used topically
- It is an azole which acts by changing the membrane permeability of Candida by blocking the production of ergosterol
- It is available as 10 mg oral troche (Mycelex), dissolves slowly in mouth, five times per day
- This should be continued for 2–4 weeks or at least week after manifestations have disappeared.

Gentian Violet:

- It is a deep-violet alcohol solution, which can be directly painted on the lesions
- It is cheap and can be easily made by the clinician.

Chlorhexidine:

- It is used as a mouth rinse 0.1–0.2%
- It is active against Candida and some bacteria
- It is responsible for increasing the cell membrane permeability
- It acts by interfering with candidal adhesion to oral mucosa.

Yogurt:

- Yogurt can also be consumed two to three times per week
- Oral hygiene should be maintained.

Systemic Therapy

It involves mainly use of these three drugs:

1. Ketoconazole
2. Fluconazole
3. Amphotericin B.

Systemic drugs are given in deep-seated cases and superfical cases that are refractory to topical agents.

Ketoconazole:

- Most commonly used
- It acts by affecting the cell membrane permeability of the fungal cell
- Ketoconazole (Nizoral) is available as 200 mg tablets and as an intravenous preparation
- One to two tablets per day for at least 2 weeks and at least for a week after the symptoms have subsided
- Intravenous administration is given in refractory cases. For example, AIDS patients
- Liver profile test should be done before chronic administration
- It can cause liver toxicity.

Fluconazole:

- It is more effective than ketoconazole
- Its frequent usage can lead to drug resistance
- It is available as Diflucan—50 mg tablets
- Dosage—50 mg/day a single dose
- In difficult cases, 400 mg/day can be given
- It is very effective in AIDS patients for prophylaxis and treatment
- It can be used intravenously in the treatment of resistant lesions.

Amphotericin B:

- It is majorly given as intravenous drug in serious cases of systemic distribution
- It can cause severe toxicity to many organs, especially kidneys.

SHORT ESSAYS

Question 1

Discuss psoriasis?

Answer

Definition

It is a common dermatological disease characterised by white, scaly papules and plaque on an erythematous base that mainly affects the scalp and the extremities. .

Aetiology

- Hereditary: It has a possible familial pattern, transmitted as a dominant trait
- Infection: Alpha-haemolytic streptococcal infection is most commonly associated infection
- Drugs: Such as beta-blocker, antimalarials may precipitate psoriasis and the rash may rebound after stopping systemic corticosteroids
- Emotion: Anxiety may precipitate the condition
- Neurogenic factor: Stress and mental anxiety can increase the disease severity
- Trauma: Surgical wounds or scratches can worsen psoriasis
- Others: Metabolic disturbances and endocrine disturbances can precede psoriasis.

Clinical Features

- It is commonly seen in 2nd and 3rd decades of life
- Most frequently occurs on extremities and scalp
- It is generally chronic with acute generalised exacerbations
- It is more severe in winter
- It appears as small sharply defined, dry papules each covered by delicate silvery scale which resembles a thin layer of mica
- When the deep scales are removed, one or more bleeding points are created
- They are referred to as Auspitz 'sign

- At the periphery, the papules are enlarged and can form large plaques that are roughly symmetrical
- The skin appears red and dusky upon the removal of the scale.

Clinical Types

- Stable plaque psoriasis
  - It is the most common type
  - It appears as red with dry, silvery white scaling, which can be appreciated after scraping the surface.
- Guttate psoriasis
  - It is commonly seen in children and adolescents
  - It may follow a streptococcal sore throat
  - Lesions individually appear as droplet-shaped, small and scaly.
- Erythrodermic psoriasis
  - In this, the skin becomes red all over and scaly.
- Pustular psoriasis.
  - It is a severe form
  - There is eruption of small pustule with shedding of nails.

Oral Manifestations

- It is most commonly seen on lips, buccal mucosa, palate, gingiva and floor of the mouth
- It appears as plaques which are silvery, scaly having an erythematous base
- They are multiple papular eruptions that can be ulcerated or can be as papillary elevated lesions with scaly surface
- Generally, there are four kinds of oral manifestations which can be seen in a patient having psoriasis:
  - Small, well-defined grey to yellowish white lesion which can be oval or round
  - White, lacy, elevated, circinate lesion can be seen on the oral mucosa involving the tongue also
  - There can also be a fiery-red erythematous surface of the oral mucosa
  - Geographic tongue—frequently seen in patients with psoriasis.

Histopathological Features

- Munro's abscess: They are intraepithelial microabcess which can be formed over the skin surface
- It is characterised by uniform parakeratosis, absence of stratum granulosum and elongation and clubbing of rate pegs
- Capillaries are dilated and tortuous, extending high in the papillae
- Epithelium over the connective tissue is thin and it is from this point bleeding occurs when the scales are removed.

Management

- Topical agents:
  - Emollient: They help in reducing the scale
  - Dithranol: It inhibits proliferation and normalised differentiation
  - Tar: It has a proinflammatory effect
  - Calcipotriol: It is a vitamin D agonist and it reduces the thickness of plaque
  - Corticosteroid: It is also effective.
- Ultraviolet light: It uses three to seven times in a week
- PUVA therapy: It includes clearance to greater degree than any other therapy
- Systemic treatment: Methotrexates, oral retinoid and cyclosporine are commonly used.

CHAPTER 4 Oral Pigmentation

LONG ESSAYS

Question 1

Describe the aetiology, clinical features, oral manifestations and treatment of Kaposi's sarcoma?

Answer

- It was first described by Moritz Kaposi in 1872
- It is a tumour of putative origin and was rarely encountered in oral cavity prior to 1983.

Aetiology

- It is a proliferation of endothelial cell
- Dermal/submucosal dendrocytes, macrophages, lymphocytes and mast cell play an important role
- Other factors are:
  - Infections
  - Enviornmental influences
  - Reduced immunosurveillance
  - Human herpesvirus 8 (HHV8).

Clinical Features

Three clinical patterns have been emerged and they are as follows:

- Classic type
- Endemic type
- Immunodeficiency type.

Classic Type

- Most common in Mediterranean Basin
- Prevalence is rare
- Usually occur in old age
- Multiple bluish-purple macule and plaque
- Skin lesions occur in lower extremities
- Other organs occasionally involved
- Oral lesions are rare, mainly in palate.

Endemic Type

Benign Nodular Type

- Aggressive type: Progressive development of locally invasive lesions that involve the underlying soft tissue and bone
- Florid form: Rapidly progressive and widely disseminated aggressive lesions with frequent visceral involvement
- Lymphadenopathic type: Occurs mainly in young black children and exhibits generalised rapidly growing tumours of lymph nodes, occasional visceral organ lesion and sparse skin involvement.

Immunodeficiency Type

- Most common in metropolitan areas
- Prevalence is relatively common
- Mostly occur in adults
- Any site of skin may get involved
- Other organs are frequently involved.

Oral Manifestations

- Palate, gingiva and tongue are common sites
- Lesion may be flat, ominous or nodular exophytic type
- Lesion may be single or multifocal
- Colour is usually red or blue
- Other features can be present:
  - Candidiasis
  - Hairy leucoplakia
  - Advanced periodontal condition
  - Xerostomia.

Treatment

- Electrocautery
- Intralesional injection of 1% sodium tetradecyl sulphate
- Intralesional 1% vinblastinesulphate, biweeklyinjections.

Question 2

Discuss the diseases causing oral pigmentation?

Answer

- Pigmentation is a discolouration of the oral mucosa or gingiva due to the wide variety of lesions and conditions
- Oral pigmentation has been associated with a variety of endogenous, exogenous biochemical substances and metabolic products. For example,
  - Melanin
  - Melanoid
  - Oxyhaemoglobin and reduced haemoglobin
  - Carotene
  - Haemosiderin
  - Bilirubin
  - Porphyrins.

Melanin

- Most common endogenous pigment
- Present in basal layer of epithelium
- Derivative of tyrosine and synthesised in melanocytes.

Melanoid

- Granules are scattered in stratum lucidum and stratum corneum of skin
- Imparts a clear yellow shade to the skin.

Oxyhaemoglobin and Reduced Haemoglobin

- They results from haemosiderin deposits
- Skin colour is affected by the capillary and venom plexuses shining through the skin.

Carotene

- Distributed in the lipids of the stratum corneum and stratum lucidum
- Deep yellow colour to the skin.

Haemosiderin

- Gives brown colour
- Deposited as a consequence of blood extravasations
- May occur as a consequence of trauma or a defect in haemostatic mechanism.

Classification of Oral Pigmentation

- Endogenous pigmentations **(Table 4.1)**
- Exogenous pigmentations **(Table 4.2)**
- Clinical classification **(Table 4.3)**.

Table 4.1: Endogenous pigmentation in oral mucosal disease

Pigment	Colour	Disease
Haemoglobin	Blue/red/purple	Varix, haemangioma, Kaposi's sarcoma, angiosarcoma
Melanin	Brown/black/grey	Melanotic macule, nevus, melanoma, basilar melanosis with incontinence
Haemosiderin	Brown	Ecchymosis, petechiae, thrombosed varix, haemorrhagic, mucocele, haemochromatosis

Table 4.2: Exogenous pigmentation of oral mucosa

Source	Colour	Disease
Silver amalgam	Grey/black	Tattoo, iatrogenic trauma
Lead, mercury, bismuth	Grey	Ingestion of paint and medicines
Graphite	Grey/black	Tattoo, trauma

Table 4.3: Clinical classification of oral pigmentation

Colour	Focal lesion	Diffuse lesion	Multifocal lesion
Blue/purple	Varix, haemangioma	Haemangioma	Kaposi's sarcoma, hereditary haemorrhagic telangiectasia
Brown	Melanotic macule, nevus, melanoma	Ecchymosis, melanoma, hairy tongue, drug induced	Physiologic pigment, neurofibromatosis, haemochromatosis, Addison's disease, drug induced, Peutz–Jeghers syndrome, petechiae
Grey/black	Amalgam, nevus, graphite, melanoma	Amalgam, melanoma, hairy tongue	Heavy metal ingestion

SHORT ESSAYS

Question 1

Describe the aetiology, clinical features, oral manifestations, investigations, radiographic features and treatment of haemangioma.

Answer

- It is a common tumour characterised by proliferation of blood vessels
- Usually congenital in nature.

Aetiology

- Abnormality of endothelial cell proliferation
- Results from increased number of capillaries.

Clinical Features

- Usually occur at birth or at early age
- Female: Male = 3 : 1
- Head and neck region most common (60%)
- In very few cases, total body surface is involved
- More in white people
- Lesion may be single or multiple
- Lesion may be bright red and lobular surface
- Lesion is firm in consistency
- Blood cannot be evacuated on pressure.

Oral Manifestations

- Flat or raised lesion of oral mucosa
- Deep red or bluish red in colour
- Well circumscribed
- Lips, tongue, buccal mucosa are common sites.

Investigations

- Diascopy
- Radiographs
- Biopsy
- Angiogram
- Doppler and conventional ultrasonography
- Radionuclide-labelled red blood cell scintigraphic scanning.

Radiographic Features

- Honeycomb appearance may be present
- Resorption of roots may be seen.

Treatment

- Congenital: Undergoes spontaneous regression at an early age
- Radiation therapy
- Surgery: Lasers or cryosurgery
- Sclerosing: 1% sodium tetradecyl sulphate
- Intralesional steroids in children.

Question 2

Write briefly about Sturge–Weber syndrome?

Answer

- It is also known as encephalofacial or encephalo-trigeminal angiomatosis
- It is a rare, non-hereditary developmental condition that is characterised by a hamartomatous vascular proliferation involving the tissues of brain and face
- It is believed to be caused by the persistence of a vascular plexus around the cephalic portion of the neural tube
- This plexus develops during the 6th week of intrauterine development but normally undergoes regression during the 9th week.

Clinical Features

- Dermal capillary vascular malformation of the face known as port-wine stain or nevus flammeus, because of its deep purple colour
- Unilateral distribution along with one or more segments of trigeminal nerve
- Patient may also have leptomeningeal angiomas
- Convulsive disorders may be present
- Mental retardation or contralateral hemiplegia may also be present.

Oral Manifestations

- Gingiva may show vascular hyperplasia or more massive haemangiomatous proliferation
- Unilateral involvement of oral mucosa
- Asymmetric jaw growth
- Alter tooth eruption sequence.

Radiographic Features

Radiograph of the skull shows gyriform 'tramline' calcifications on the affected side.

Question 3

Describe the aetiology, clinical features, oral manifestations and management of hereditary haemorrhagic telangiectasia/ Osler-Weber-Rendu disease?

Answer

It is a form of haemangioma, congenital hereditary disease characterised by numerous telangiectatic or angiomatous areas which are widely distributed on the skin and mucosa of the oral cavity and which tend to undergo repeated haemorrhage.

Aetiology

- Hereditary haemorrhagic telangiectasia type 1 (HHT1) is caused by mutation of the endoglin gene on chromosome 9, whereas activin receptor-like kinase 1 (ALK1) mutation produces HHT2
- Transmitted by both sexes as a simple autosomal dominant.

Clinical Features

- Male : Female = 1:1
- Spider-like telangiectasia is present at or shortly after birth
- Skin lesions are most common on face/neck and chest
- Most important sign—epistaxis as well as bleeding from oral cavity.

Oral Manifestations

- Characterised by multiple round or oval purple papules measuring less than 0.5 mm in diameter
- Common sites are:
  - Vermilion border of lip
  - Gingiva
  - Buccal mucosa
  - Palate
  - Floor of mouth
  - Tongue.

Management

- Pressure packs
- Electrocauterisation
- Radiation therapy
- Surgical excision
- Septal dermoplasty
- Iron supplement therapy.

Question 4

Write briefly about heavy-metal pigmentation?

Answer

- Ingestion or exposure to any one of several heavy metals can cause significant systemic and oral abnormalities
- Exposure to heavy metals may be massive, resulting in acute reactions or it may be minimal over a longer period producing chronic changes
- Oral alterations can be produced by ingestion of following metals:
  - Lead
  - Mercury
  - Silver
  - Bismuth
  - Arsenic
  - Gold.

Mercury

- Mercury poisoning may be acute or chronic
- Increased flow of saliva
- Metallic taste
- Swelling of gingiva may be seen
- Grey to black colour of mucosa may be seen
- Loosening of teeth.

Acrodynia (Pink Disease, Swift's Disease)

- Chronic mercury exposure to infants and children
- Profuse salivation
- Gingiva becomes sensitive and painful
- Premature shedding of teeth.

Silver (Argyria)

- Subepithelial deposits in skin
- Diffuse greyish-black discolouration is seen
- Sclerae and nails may be affected
- In oral mucosa, slate-blue lines are seen along the gingival margin.

Bismuth

- Mostly used for treating dermatologic disorders
- Usually occurs in buccal mucosa and gingiva
- Characteristic 'bismuth line' is seen, thin blue-black along with marginal gingiva
- May be seen on lips, ventral surface of tongue.

SHORT NOTES

Question 1

Write briefly about café au-lait pigmentation?

Answer

- Bronze and tan diffuse multifocal macular pigmented lesions are present
- Macule may be several centimetres wide
- They are present over face, neck
- Occasionally present in oral mucosa
- Associated disease are:
  - Neurofibromatosis
  - McCune Albright syndrome
  - Fibrous dysplasia.

Question 2

Describe the aetiology and oral manifestations of amalgam tattoo?

Answer

It is a clinically evident pigmented lesion.

Aetiology

- Dentist's bur loaded with small amalgam particles
- Traumatically introduces metal flecks
- At the time of multiple tooth extraction
- Metal particles may fall unnoticed in the extraction socket.

Oral Manifestations

- Solitary or focal pigmentation of oral mucosa
- Lesion may appear as macule
- Bluish grey or black in colour
- Most commonly on buccal mucosa, gingiva and palate.

Question 3

Write briefly about drug-induced melanosis?

Answer

- Lesion may be large but localised
- Usually to hard palate
- It may be multifocal throughout the mucosa
- Lesions are flat
- Various drugs:
  - Antimalarials
  - Quinidine
  - Zidovudine
  - Minocycline
  - Tetracycline
  - Oral contraceptives
  - Ketoconazole.

Chapter 5 Oral Cancer

LONG ESSAYS

Question 1

Describe the aetiology, clinical features, staging and treatment of oral submucous fibrosis?

Answer

- Oral submucous fibrosis is a disease of the oral cavity which is characterised by inflammation and fibrosis of the submucosal tissues
- The fibrosis involves lamina propria and deeper connective tissues
- Oral submucous fibrosis leads to rigidity and eventual inability to open the mouth
- Most common site of involvement is buccal mucosa but any part of oral cavity can be affected.

Aetiology

- Areca nut chewing
- Nutritional deficiencies
- Ingestion of chillies
- Genetic and immunologic processes.

Clinical Features

- There is a progressive inability to open the mouth (trismus) due to fibrosis and scarring or oral mucosa
- Burning sensation and pain upon eating of spicy foodstuffs
- Change of gustatory sensation
- Mouth movements are impaired like eating, whistling, blowing, sucking
- Increased salivation
- Dryness of the mouth is commonly seen
- Dysphagia to solid food when oesophagus is involved.

Staging of Oral Submucous Fibrosis

Oral submucous fibrosis is divided into three stages:

1. First Stage: Stomatitis which includes erythematous mucosa, mucosal petechiae, vesicles, mucosal ulcers and melanotic pigmentation in mucosa
2. Second Stage: Fibrosis is seen in ruptured vesicles and ulcers when they heal
   - Blanching of the oral mucosa is seen in early lesions
   - Older lesions exhibit vertical and circular palpable fibrous bands in the buccal mucosa leading to mottled, marble-like appearance of the mucosa.
     - Reduction of the mouth opening (trismus) is seen
     - Tongue is stiff and small
     - Floor of the mouth appears blanched and leathery
     - Fibrotic and depigmented gingiva is seen.
3. Third Stage: In this, the oral submucous fibrosis has evolved into:
   - Leucoplakia
   - Speech and hearing defects due to involvement of the tongue and the eustachian tubes.

Treatment

The treatment depends on the degree of clinical involvement:

- If detected at a very early stage, cessation of the habit generally is sufficient
- In moderate-to-severe conditions, oral submucous fibrosis is irreversible
- Medical treatment is symptomatic and is mainly aimed at improving mouth movements.

Steroids: Submucosal intralesional injections or topical application of steroids weekly help in preventing further damage.

Placental Extracts: Submucosal administration of aqueous extract of healthy human placental extract (Placentrex) along with the cessation of the habit of chewing areca nut has shown marked improvement of the condition.

Hyaluronidase: Hyaluronidase in conjunction with steroids show marked improvement in the condition.

Interferon-gamma: It helps in the condition due to immunoregulatory effect.

Lycopene: Oral nutritional supplement at 16 mg daily.

Pentoxifylline: 400 mg three times daily.

Surgical Management

- Simple excision of the fibrous bands
- Split-thicknessskingraftingfollowingbilateraltemporalis myotomy or coronoidectomy in cases of trismus
- Nasolabial flaps andlingualpedicle flaps: Surgery to create flaps is performed in cases where tongue is not involved
- Use of a KTP-532 laser release procedure helps in increasing mouth opening.

Question 2

Describe in detail squamous cell carcinoma?

Answer

- Squamous cell carcinoma, the most common oral malignancy, may be defined as a malignant tumour originating from surface epithelium
- It is characterised initially by invasion of malignant epithelial cells into the underlying connective tissue with subsequent spread into deeper soft tissues, adjacent bone, local-regional lymph nodes and ultimately to distant sites, such as the lung, liver and skeleton.

Squamous Cell Carcinoma Originating in Soft Tissues

Clinical Features

- Appears initially as white or red (sometimes mixed) irregular patchy lesions of the affected epithelium
- With time, these lesions exhibit central ulceration; a rolled or indurated border, which represents peripheral invasion of malignant cells
- Palpable infiltration into adjacent muscle or bone
- Pain may be variable
- Regional lymphadenopathy, characterised by rubberyhard lymph nodes that may be fixed to underlying structures, may be present.

Radiographic Features

Location

- Commonly involves the lateral border of the tongue
- Therefore, a common site to observe bone invasion is the posterior mandible
- Lesions of the lip and floor of the mouth may invade the anterior mandible
- Lesions involving attached gingiva and underlying alveolar bone may mimic inflammatory disease, such as periodontal disease.

Periphery and Shape

- It may erode into underlying bone from any direction, producing a radiolucency that is polymorphous and irregular in outline
- Invasion occurs in one half of cases and is characterised most commonly by an ill-defined, non-corticated border
- If bone involvement is extensive, the periphery appears to have finger-like extensions preceding a zone of impressive osseous destruction
- If pathological fracture occurs, the borders show sharpened thinned bone ends with displacement of segments and adjacent soft tissue mass.

Effects on Surrounding Structures

- Evidence of invasion of bone around teeth may first appear as widening of the periodontal ligament space with loss of adjacent lamina dura
- Teeth may appear to float in a mass of radiolucent soft tissue without any bony support.

Differential Diagnosis

Osteomyelitis.

Management

- It is usually managed using a combination of surgery and radiation therapy
- The choice of which modality to use depends on the protocol of the treating centre and the location and severity of the tumour.

Squamous Cell Carcinoma Originating in Bone

Clinical Features

- These neoplasms are rare and may remain silent until they have reached a fairly large size
- Pain, pathologic fracture and sensory nerve abnormalities, such as lip paraesthesia and lymphadenopathy may occur with this tumour
- It is more common in men and in patients in their 4th to 8th decade of life
- The surface epithelium is invariably normal in appearance.

Radiographic Features

Location

- The mandible is far more commonly involved than the maxilla, with most cases being present in the molar region
- Because the lesion is by definition associated with remnants of the dental lamina, it originates only in tooth-bearing parts of the oral cavity.

Periphery and Shape

- The periphery of the majority of lesions is ill-defined, although some have been described as well-defined
- They are most often rounded or irregular in shape and have a border that demonstrates osseous destruction and varying degrees of extension at the periphery
- The degree of raggedness of the border may reflect the aggressiveness of the lesion
- If sufficient in size, pathologic fracture occurs, with its associated step defects, thinned cortical borders and subsequent soft tissue mass.

Effects on Surrounding Structures

- Capable of causing destruction of the antral or nasal floors, loss of the cortical outline of the mandibular neurovascular canal, and effacement of the lamina dura
- Root resorption is unusual
- Teeth that lose both lamina dura and supporting bone appear to be floating in space.

Management

- Generally these tumours are excised with their surrounding osseous structure in an en bloc resection
- Radiation and chemotherapy may be used as adjunctive therapies.

Squamous Cell Carcinoma Originating in a Cyst

Synonyms

- Epidermoid cell carcinoma
- Carcinoma ex odontogenic cyst.

Definition

- It arises in a pre-existing dental cyst, is uncommon and excludes invasion from surface epithelial carcinomas, metastatic tumours and primary intraosseous carcinoma
- This condition may arise from inflammatory periapical, residual, dentigerous and odontogenic keratocysts
- Histologically the lining squamous epithelium of the cyst gives rise to the malignant neoplasm.

Clinical Features

- The most common presenting sign or symptom associated with this condition is pain
- The pain may be characterised as dull and of several months duration
- Swelling is occasionally reported
- Pathologic fracture
- Fistula formation
- Regional lymphadenopathy.

Radiographic Features

Location

- This tumour may occur anywhere an odontogenic cyst is found, namely the tooth-bearing portions of the jaws
- Most cases occur in the mandible.

Periphery and Shape

- Because the lesion arises from a cyst, the shape is often round or ovoid
- If it is a small lesion in a cyst wall, the periphery may be mostly well-defined and even corticated
- In this case, the radiographic differentiation from a normal cyst is impossible
- As the malignant tissue progressively replaces cyst lining, the smooth border is lost or becomes ill-defined.

Internal Structure

- This lesion lacks any ability to produce bone
- It is wholly radiolucent, perhaps more so than invasive surface carcinoma, owing to prior osteolysis from the cyst.

Effects on Surrounding Structures

- Carcinoma arising in dental cysts is capable of thinning and destroying the lamina dura of adjacent teeth or adjacent cortical boundaries, such as the inferior border of the jaw
- It can produce complete destruction of the alveolar process.

Differential Diagnosis

Infected dental cyst.

Management

The treatment of squamous cell carcinoma originating in a cyst is identical to that described with primary intraosseous carcinoma.

Question 3

Define osteosarcoma. Discuss the clinical features, radiographic features, differential diagnosis and management of the same?

Answer

Definition

- It is a malignant neoplasm of bone in which osteoid is produced directly by malignant stroma as opposed to adjacent reactive bone formation
- The three major histologic types are:
  1. Chondroblastic
  2. Osteoblastic
  3. Fibroblastic.

Clinical Features

- Osteosarcoma of the jaws is quite rare and accounts for approximately 7% of all other sarcomas
- The lesion occurs in all racial groups worldwide
- In males twice as frequently as females
- A peak in the 4th decade of life
- The most commonly reported symptom or sign is swelling, which may be present as long as 6 months before diagnosis; the swelling is usually rapid.

Radiographic Features

Location

- The mandible is more affected than maxilla
- Although the lesion can occur in any part of either jaw, the posterior mandible, including the tooth-bearing region, angle and vertical ramus, is most commonly affected
- The posterior areas are also more commonly affected in the maxilla, with the most frequent sites being the alveolar ridge, antrum and palate
- The lesion may cross the midline.

Periphery and Shape

- Osteosarcoma has an ill-defined border in most instances
- When viewed against normal bone, the lesion is usually radiolucent with no peripheral sclerosis or encapsulation
- If the lesion involves the periosteum directly or by extension, one may see the typical sunray spicules or 'hair- on-end' trabeculae
- This occurs when the periosteum is displaced, partially destroyed and disorganised
- If the periosteum is elevated and maintains its osteogenic potential but is breached in the centre, a Codman's triangle at the edges is formed.

Internal Structure

- Osteosarcoma may be entirely radiolucent, mixed radiolucent-radiopaque, or quite radiopaque
- The internal osseous structure may take the appearance of granular- or sclerotic-appearing bone, cotton balls, wisps, or honeycombed.

Effects on Surrounding Structures

- Widening of the periodontal membrane is present
- The antral or nasal wall cortices may be lost in maxillary lesions
- Mandibular lesions may destroy the cortex of the neurovascular canal and adjacent lamina dura.

Differential Diagnosis

- Chondrosarcoma
- Ewing's sarcoma
- Fibrosarcoma.

Management

- Resection with a large border of adjacent normal bone
- Generally radiation therapy and chemotherapy are used only for controlling metastatic spread or for palliation.

Question 4

Describe the aetiology, clinical features, oral manifestations and treatment of Kaposi's sarcoma?

Answer

- It was first described by Moritz Kaposi in 1872
- It is a tumour of putative origin and was rarely encountered in oral cavity prior to 1983.

Aetiology

- It is a proliferation of endothelial cell
- Dermal/submucosal dendrocytes, macrophages, lymphyocytes and mast cell play an important role
- Other factors are:
  - Infections
  - Enviornmental influences
  - Reduced immunosurveillance
  - Human herpesvirus 8 (HHV8).

Clinical Features

Three clinical patterns have been emerged and they are as follows:

1. Classic type
2. Endemic type
3. Immunodeficiency type.

Classic Type

- Most common in Mediterranean Basin
- Prevalence is rare
- Usually occur in old age
- Multiple bluish-purple macule and plaque
- Skin lesions occur in lower extremities
- Other organs occasionally involved
- Oral lesions are rare, mainly in palate.

Endemic Type

Benign nodular type:

- Aggressive type:
  - Progressive development of locally invasive lesions that involve the underlying soft tissue and bone.
- Florid form:
  - Rapidly progressive and widely disseminated aggressive lesions with frequent visceral involvement.
- Lymphadenopathic type:
  - Occurs mainly in young black children and exhibits generalised rapidly growing tumours of lymph nodes, occasional visceral organ lesion and sparse skin involvement.

Immunodeficiency Type

- Most common in metropolitan areas
- Prevalence is relatively common
- Mostly occur in adults
- Any site of skin may get involved
- Other organs are frequently involved.

Oral Manifestations

- Palate, gingiva and tongue are common sites
- Lesion may be flat, ominous or nodular exophytic type
- Lesion may be single or multifocal
- Colour is usually red or blue
- Other features can be present:
  - Candidiasis
  - Hairy leucoplakia
  - Advanced periodontal condition
  - Xerostomia.

Treatment

- Electrocautery
- Intralesional injection of 1% sodium tetradecyl sulphate
- Intralesional 1% vinblastine sulphate, biweekly injections.

SHORT ESSAYS

Question 1

Write about TNM staging?

Answer

TNM classification/staging of malignant tumours is a notation system that gives codes in order to identify the stage, malignancy and spread of the tumour.

T describes the size of the original (primary) tumour and whether it has invaded nearby tissue.

N describes nearby (regional) lymph nodes that are involved.

M describes distant metastasis (spread of cancer from one part of the body to another).

- T: Size or direct extent of the primary tumour
  - Tx: Tumour cannot be evaluated
  - Tis: Carcinoma in situ
  - T0: No signs of tumour
  - T1, T2, T3, T4: Size and/or extension of the primary tumour.
- N: Degree of spread to regional lymph nodes
  - Nx: Lymph nodes cannot be evaluated
  - N0: Tumour cells absent from regional lymph nodes
  - N1: Regional lymph node metastasis present (at some sites: Tumour spread to closest or small number of regional lymph nodes)
  - N2: Tumour spread to an extent between N1 and N3 (N2 is not used at all sites)
  - N3: Tumour spread to more distant or numerous regional lymph nodes (N3 is not used at all sites).
- M: Presence of distant metastasis.
  - M0: No distant metastasis
  - M1: Metastasis to distant organs (beyond regional lymph nodes).

Question 2

Discuss the aetiology, predisposing factors, clinical features and management of basal cell carcinoma/rodent ulcer?

Answer

- It is a non-melanoma type of skin cancer
- Most common of all skin cancers (>80%).

Aetiology

- Exposure to UV rays
- Damage to skin by burns, scars or ulcers.

Predisposing Factors

- People with freckles or with pale skin and blonde or red hair
- Those who have had a lot of exposure to the sun, such as people with outdoor hobbies or who work out of doors, and people who have lived in sunny climates
- People who use sunbeds
- People who have previously had a basal cell carcinoma.

Clinical Features

- Most basal cell carcinomas are painless
- Scab that bleeds occasionally and does not heal completely
- Some lesions are superficial with flat scaly red appearance while some are pearl like with crater in the centre
- If left unattended, the latter one, develops into an ulcer by eroding the underlying skin, thus termed as 'rodent' ulcer.

Management

- Surgical excision
- Radiotherapy
- Chemotherapy.

Question 3

Describe the malignant melanoma?

Answer

It is a malignant neoplasm of melanocytic origin that arises from a benign melanocytic lesion from melanocytes within otherwise normal skin or mucosa.

Clinical Features

Four histopathologic types of melanoma have been described:

1. Superficial spreading
2. Nodular
3. Lentigo
4. Acral lentiginous.

Oral Melanoma

- Early lesion may be flat
- Macular lesion with irregular borders
- Brown to black in colour
- Focal/diffuse in nature
- Anterior labial gingiva, hard palate.

Management

- Surgical excision
- Chemotherapy, e.g., interferon-gamma, vinblastine, dacarbazine, etc.

SHORT NOTES

Question 1

What are precancerous lesions and precancerous conditions?

Answer

Definition

- A precancerous lesion is a morphologically altered tissue in which oral cancer is more likely to occur than in its apparently normal counterpart
- A precancerous condition is a generalised state associated with a significantly increased risk of cancer.

Classification

Classification according to WHO is as follows **(Table 5.1)**:

Table 5.1: Endogenous pigmentation in oral mucosal disease

Precancerous lesions	Precancerous conditions
Leucoplakia	Submucous fibrosis
Erythroplakia	Actinic keratosis
Palatal lesions in reverse smokers	Lichen planus, Discoid lupus erythematosus

CHAPTER 6

Diseases of Tongue and Lips

LONG ESSAYS

Question 1

Classify disorders of lips. Discuss about cleft lip and palate?

Answer

Disorders of lips are classified below:

- Developmental
  - Cleft lip and palate
  - Congenital lip pits
  - Double lip
  - Commissural lip pits.
- Cheilitis
  - Granulomatous cheilitis
  - Glandular cheilitis
  - Angular cheilitis
  - Eczematous cheilitis
  - Contact cheilitis
  - Exfoliative cheilitis
  - Actinic cheilitis
  - Plasma cell cheilitis
  - Cheilitis due to drugs.
- Carcinoma of lips
- Miscellaneous.
  - Actinic Elastosis
  - Chapping of lips
  - Lip ulcers due to caliber persistent artery.

Cleft Lip and Palate

Definition

- It is a congenital defect which results in an unilateral or bilateral opening of the upper lip between the mouth and the nose
- It is also known as hare lip
- Occurs due to developmental defect
- The defect occurs along many planes.

Development

- Cleft lip in the mandible occurs due to the failure of copula that give rise to mandibular arch or persistence of the central groove of mandibular process
- Cleft lip in the maxilla occurs due to failure of mesodermal mass, which actually constitutes the facial process
- Deficiency or absence of these mesodermal masses or their failure to penetrate the ectodermal grooves leads to breakdown of the ectoderm, causing cleft formation.

Classification

First Classification

- Unilateral incomplete
- Unilateral complete
- Bilateral incomplete
- Bilateral complete.

Veau's Classification

- Cleft lip
  - Class I: A unilateral notching of vermilion not extending into the lip
  - Class II: A unilateral notching of vermilion with cleft extending into lip but not including the floor of the nose
  - Class III: A unilateral cleft of vermilion extending into the floor of the nose
  - Class IV: Any bilateral cleft of the lip, whether this is complete or incomplete.
- Cleft palate.
  - Class I:Involving only soft palate
  - Class II:Involving soft and hard palate but not alveolus
  - Class III:Involving soft and hard palate and alveolus of one side
  - Class IV:Involving both the soft and hard palate and alveolus on both sides of the pre-maxilla.

Etiology

- Hereditary is the most common and important factor
- Nutritional disturbances, such as, riboflavin deficient diet can lead to cleft formation
- Ischaemia may occur due to defective vascular supply to the related area, which in turn causes cleft formation
- Physiological, emotional and traumatic stress during the developmental stages can cause cleft lip
- Mechanical disturbances, like size of tongue might prevent union of parts
- Lack of inherent developmental force and infection can lead to cleft lip
- Steroid therapy during pregnancy, or alcohol and toxins in circulation are some of the causes which can also cause cleft formation.

Formation of Cleft

- Patients with clefts have a deficiency of tissue and it is just not merely a displacement of normal tissue
- When an epithelial bridge fails, due to lack of mesoderm delivery proliferation from the maxilla and nasal processes, a cleft lip may occur
- Cleft lip occurs earlier and inhibits tongue migration, which can prevent horizontal alignment and fusion of the palatal shelves
- In case of a unilateral cleft lip, the floor of the nose communicates.

Clinical Features

General

- More commonly seen in boys than in girls
- Seen more commonly on the left side than on the right side
- It appears as a large defect with a direct opening in the nasal cavity
- Teeth can be deformed, missing, displaced or divided, producing supernumerary teeth.

Specific Features of Cleft Lip

- A unilateral cleft involves only one side and bilateral involves both sides
- Incomplete cleft lip: It extends for varying distances forward to the nostril, but not up to the nostril
- Complete cleft lip: It extends into nostril and palate is involved commonly
- Cleft is commonly associated with fattening and widening of the nostril of the affected side
- Patient has difficulty in sucking
- There is defective speech, especially with labial letters, like B, F, M, P and V
- Mandibular cleft lips are rare
- There is presence of soft tissue mass between the ends of the bone, uniting the tongue to the lip, so that tongue is bound down.

Radiographic Features

- Presence and absence of unerupted teeth would be determined
- Maxillary lateral incisiors are the most commonly missing teeth
- Supernumerary teeth are also present
- Teeth are poorly positioned and are malformed.

Management

- Its management requires a complete rehabilitation
- Cheiloplasty: It refers to surgical closure of lip
- Orthodontic treatment is done to treat malocclusion
- Cleft rhinoplasty is done to improve nasal function and correct the distortion
- Speech therapy is given to improve pronunciation of the words
- Psychologic therapy is also important
- Freely with the oral cavity, maxilla on the cleft side is hypoplastic, columella is displaced to the normal side and the nasal ala on the cleft side is displaced laterally, posteriorly and inferiorly
- The lower lateral cartilage of the nose is lower on the cleft side, its lateral cruz is longer and the angle between the medial and lateral cruz is more obtuse.

Question 2

Classify tongue diseases and discuss about ankyloglossia?

Answer

Classification (According to Ghom's)

- Congenital and developmental disorders
    - Aglossia and microglossia
    - Macroglossia
    - Ankyloglossia
    - Cleft tongue
    - Ankyloglossia superior syndrome
    - Lingual varices
    - Lingual thyroid module
    - Variations in tongue movement
    - Patent thyroglossal duct cyst
    - Tongue thrusting
    - Lingual polyp

- Reactive lymphoid aggregate
- Lingual cyst.

- Local tongue disorders
  - Median rhomboidal glossitis
  - Fissured tongue
  - Benign migratory glossitis
  - Hairy tongue
  - Crenated tongue
  - Foliate papillitis
  - Leukokeratosis nicotina glossi.
- Depapillation of tongue
  - Local disease
    - Eosinophilic granuloma
    - Traumatic injuries
    - Lesions due to automutilation
    - Allergic stomatitis
    - Facial hemiatrophy
    - Cranial arteritis
    - Chronic candidiasis.
  - Systemic disease.
    - Iron deficiency anaemia
    - Plummer–Vinson syndrome
    - Pernicious anaemia
    - Niacin deficiency
    - Folic acid deficiency
    - Peripheral vascular diseases
    - Dermatomyositis
    - Diabetes
    - Syphilis
    - Zoster infection
    - Tuberculosis.
- Neurological disease
  - Glossodynia
  - Paralysis
  - Dyskinesia
  - Oropharyngeal dysphagia.
- Cyst
  - Bronchogenic cyst
  - Anterior median lingual cyst
  - Gastric mucosal cyst
  - Epidermoid and dermoid cyst
  - Thyroglossal cyst
  - Parasitic cyst.
- Benign tumours
  - Fibroma
  - Granular cell tumour
  - Glomus tumour
  - Leiomyoma
  - Plasmacytoma
  - Rhabdomyoma.
- Premalignant lesions and condition
  - Leukoplakia
  - Lichen planus
  - Oral submucous fibrosis.
- Malignant tumour
  - Squamous cell carcinoma
  - Malignant lymphoma
  - Malignant melanoma
  - Metastatic tumour
  - Sarcoma.
- Miscellaneous.
  - Phlebectasia
  - Pigmentation of tongue.

Ankyloglossia

- It is also referred to as tongue tie
- In this condition, the lingual frenulum is either too short or placed anteriorly which limits the tongue mobility.

Types

- Complete: There is complete fusion of tongue and the floor of mouth
- Partial: Short lingual frenum.

Clinical Features

Symptoms

- Tongue movement is limited
- Nursing and feeding problems may occur in extreme cases
- Inability to chew, poor suckig and recurrent tongue biting can be observed
- It can lead to speech abnormalities.

Signs

- There can be a V-shaped notch at the tip, when there is an attempt to stick the tongue out
- On physical examination, there is short or anteriorly placed lingual frenulum
- There is a mandibular midline diastema and inability to clean teeth.

Associated syndromes are

- Ankyloglossum superius syndrome
- Rainbow syndrome
- Orofacial digital syndrome.

Management

- Parentel education
- Physician education
- Reassurance to the patient.

Surgery

Frenectomy can be done. Indications for frenectomy are as follows:

- In case of complete fusion of tongue
- In cases when nursing and feeding becomes a problem
- Patients who have poor speech
- In cases where tongue tie has recurred after snipping.

Complications of Surgery

- Injudicious cutting of the frenum can cause haemorrhage and the tongue may become very mobile and may be swallowed, which causes asphyxia
- There can be subsequent infection at the base of the tongue, with formation of large ulcer and spreading stomatitis.

Question 3

Explain benign migratory glossitis/geographic tongue.

Answer

- It is a psoriasiform mucositis of the dorsum of the tongue that has a constantly changing pattern of serpiginous white lines surrounding areas of smooth and depapillated mucosa
- Also known as wandering rash, glossitis areata exfoliativa and erythema migrans.

Etiology

Allergic reaction, immunological reaction, hereditary factors, emotional stress, nutritional deficiencies and infections.

Classification

- Type I: Lesion is confined to tongue. It has both active and remission phases
- Type II: Similar to type I, with similar lesions elsewhere in the mouth
- Type III: Lesions on the tongue that are not typical and may be accompanied by lesions elsewhere in the mouth. It has two forms:
  1. Fixed form: Few areas of the tongue are affected, but no movement is observed
  2. Abortive form: Intially, occurs as yellow-white patches, but disappear before acquiring the typical appearance of geographic tongue.
- Type IV: No tongue lesions are present, but geographic areas present elsewhere in the mouth.

Clinical Features

Symptoms

- It is most commonly seen in young and middle-aged adults, with an age range of 5–84 years with female predilection
- Most commonly seen on the dorsal surface and lateral borders of the tongue, but can be seen on the ventral surfaces as well
- Varies in size and diameter and may be single or multiple
- Generally asymptomatic, but patient may complain of burning sensation that is worsened by spicy or citrus food
- Appears as small, non-indurated, erythematous, atrophic lesion in the initial stages that is bordered by an elvated distinct rim which varies from grey to white to light yellow
- Appears as pink to red in colour with smooth shiny surface due to loss of filiform papillae.

Signs

- Multiple areas of desquamation of filiform papillae are seen
- Borders of the lesion are outlined by thin yellowish white line or band and central portion occasionally appears inflamed
- Fungi form papillae persist in the desquamated areas as small elevated red rods.

Histopathological Features

- There is loss of filiform papillae at the margins of the lesions
- Hyper parakeratosis along with same acanthosis is seen
- There is marked migration of polymorphonuclear leukocytes (PMNs) and lymphocytes into the epithelium
- There is desquamation of parakeratin
- There is degeneration of epithelial cells and microabscess formation
- This is known as Monroe's abscess
- There is an inflammatory cell infiltration of neutrophils, lymphocytes and plasma cells in the underlying connective tissue.

Differential Diagnosis

- Reiter's syndrome
- Psoriasis
- Lichen planus
- Pityriasis rosea
- Anaemic condition.

Management

- Topical local anaesthetic agents, like lidocaine can be applied to control burning
- Diet should be kept bland, irritants should be removed and psychological reassurance should be given
- Topical corticosteroids and topical application of salicylic acid and tretinoin should be done.

SHORT NOTES

Question 1

Define cleft tongue?

Answer

- It is also known as bifid tongue
- There is a cleavage of the tongue, due to lack of fusion of the lateral halves
- It is caused because of incomplete blending and failure of groove obliteration by underlying mesenchymal proliferation
- Completely cleft tongue or bifid tongue is rare
- It happens due to lack of merging of lateral swellings of the organs
- Deep grooves can be seen in the midline of dorsal surface
- Food debris and microorganisms may collect in the base of cleft and causes irritation
- It can be seen with oral-facial-digital syndrome, with thick fibrous bands in lower anterior mucobuccal fold, which eliminates sulcus and is related with clefting of hypoplastic mandibular alveolar process.

CHAPTER 7

Salivary Gland Diseases

LONG ESSAYS

Question 1

What are salivary gland tumours? Give its classification? Discuss pleomorphic adenoma in detail?

Answer

- Tumours originating from salivary glands are described as salivary gland tumours
- Salivary gland tumours (SGTs) arise from:
  - Parotid
  - Submandibular
  - Sublingual
  - Minor salivary glands
  - Ectopic salivary gland tissue.

Incidence

1–6.5 cases/100,000 people.

Common Site

- Parotid gland: 64–80% of all cases
- Rate: 2/3–3/4
- Benign: 2/3–3/4.

Submandibular Gland

- Rate: 8–11% of all cases
- Rate of malignancy: 2 times of parotid (37–45%).

Sublingual Gland

- Rate: 1%
- Rate of malignancy: 70–90%.

Minor Salivary Glands

- Second most common site
- Rate: 9–23%
- Palate most common site (42–54%)
- Most tumours occur on posterior lateral hard or soft palate
- Other sites: lips > buccal mucosa.

Rate of Malignancy

- Palate: 42–50%
- Buccal mucosa: 42–50%
- Upper lip: 14–25%
- Lower lip: 50–86%
- Retromolar area: 91%.

Hence, common sites in decreasing order are: parotid, minor salivary glands, submandibular and sublingual.

Etiology

- Viruse
  - Epstein–Barr virus (EBV)
  - Polyomavirus
  - Cytomegalovirus
  - Human papillomavirus (HPV): Types 16 and 18.
- Radiation
  - Ionising radiation
  - Tumorigenic dose: Controversial
  - 483 rad: Risk of tumour development.
- Occupation
  - Certain occupations: Increase risk
  - Example:
    - Asbestos mining
    - Plumbing
    - Wood working
    - Manufacturing rubber products.
- Lifestyle
  - Severe malnutrition
  - Enlarged salivary gland
  - No tumorogenic effect observed.
- Hormones.

Classification

Classification of salivary gland neoplasms is as follows:

Benign

- Mixed tumour
- Papillary cystadenoma lymphomatosum
- Oxyphil adenoma
- Sebaceous cell adenoma
- Benign lymphoepithelial lesion
- Unclassified.

Malignant

- Malignant mixed tumour
- Mucoepidermoid tumour: Low grade and High grade
- Squamous cell carcinoma
- Adenocarcinoma
  - Adenoid cystic
  - Trabecular or solid
  - Anaplastic
  - Mucous cell
  - Pseudoadamantine
  - Acinic cell.
- Unclassified.

Revised Classification WHO 1991

- Adenomas
  - Pleomorphic adenoma
  - Myoepithelioma (myoepithelial adenoma)
  - Warthin's tumour (adenolymphoma)
  - Oncocytoma (oncocytic adenoma)
  - Basal cell adenoma
  - Canalicular adenoma
  - Sebaceous adenoma
  - Ductal papilloma:
    - Inverted ductal papilloma
    - Intraductal papilloma
    - Sialadenoma papilliferum.
  - Cystadenoma:
    - Papillary cyst adenoma
    - Mucinous cyst adenoma.
- Carcinomas
  - Acinic cell carcinoma
  - Mucoepidermoid carcinoma
  - Adenoid cystic carcinoma
  - Epithelial: Myoepithelial carcinoma
  - Polymorphous low-grade adenocarcinoma (terminal duct adenocarcinoma)
  - Basal cell adenocarcinoma
  - Mucinous adenocarcinoma
  - Papillary cyst adenocarcinoma
  - Oncocytic carcinoma
  - Salivary duct carcinoma
  - Adenocarcinoma
  - Malignant myoepithelioma (myoepithelial carcinoma)
  - Carcinoma in pleomorphic adenoma (malignant mixed tumour)
  - Squamous cell carcinoma
  - Small cell carcinoma
  - Undifferentiated carcinoma
  - Other carcinomas.
- Non-epithelial tumours
- Malignant lymphomas
- Secondary tumours
- Unclassified tumours
- Tumour-like lesions.
  - Sialadenosis
  - Oncocytosi
  - Necrotising sialometaplasia (salivary gland infarction)
  - Benign lymphoepithelial lesion
  - Salivary gland cysts
  - Chronic sclerosing sialadenitis of submandibular gland (Küttner's tumour)
  - Cystic lymphoid hyperplasia in acquired immune deficiency syndrome (AIDS).

Pleomorphic Adenoma/Mixed Tumour

Synonyms

- Branchioma
- Enclavoma
- Endothelioma
- Enchondroma.

Most common Salivary gland tumours are:

- Mixed tumour named by Minssen (1874)
- Pleomorphic adenoma named by Willis.

Cells differentiate into:

- Epithelial
- Mesenchymal cells.

Mixed tumour shows combined features of epithelioid and connective tissue, like growth.

- Not derived from more than one germ layer
- Account for:
  - 53–77% parotid tumours
  - 44–68% submandibular tumours
  - 38–43% minor gland tumours.

Clinical Features

- Common site: Parotid gland
- Unusual sites:
  - Cheek
  - Along Stenson's duct
  - Accessory parotid tissue.
- Salivary gland tissue inclusions within lymph nodes in the neck
- Associated tumors
  - Warthin's tumour
  - Mucoepidermoid carcinoma
  - Adenoid cystic carcinoma
  - Acinic cell carcinoma.
- Age: 30 and 50 years
- Relatively uncommon in children and adolescents
- Mean age: 11.8 years (Ribeiro et al.)
- According to Kessler et al., all benign salivary gland tumour: Pleomorphic adenoma
- Gender predilection: Female > Male; 3:1 or 4:1
- According to Jorge et al. 80% females
- Appears as painless:
  - Slowly growing
  - Firm mass.
- Occurs in lower pole of superficial lobe
- Lies in front of the ear
- Initially movable: Less movable
- About 10% develop within deep lobe
- Recurrent tumors appear multi-nodular
- In submandibular gland, firm discrete masses
- Minor salivary glands site
- Palate > upper lip > buccal mucosa
- Intraoral tumors covered by normal appearing mucosa
- Large lesions covered by erythematous appearing mucosa.

Pathology

- Well circumscribed
- Encapsulated
- Incomplete capsulation: Minor salivary glands
- Smooth or bosselated surfaces
- Cystic degeneration: Long standing cases
- Haemorrhage area: Long standing cases
- Recurrent tumours: Multi-nodular.

Microscopically

Mixed tumor is composed of glandular epithelium, myoepithelial cells and other type of cells.

Epithelial Appearing Component May Form

- Ducts
- Nests
- Solid sheets of cells
- Cords
- Foci of either keratinising squamous cells or spindle cells.

Myoepithelial cells may be:

- Spindle shaped
- Clear
- Plasmacytoid.

Myoepithelial Cells

- Major component:
  - Responsible for chondroid and myxoid stroma
  - Foot and Frazell classified mixed tumour into:
    - Mainly myxoid
    - Myxoid and cellular
    - Mainly cellular
    - Extremely cellular.
- Ductal structures resemble normal ducts
- Lumina lined by ductal epithelium surrounded by myoepithelial cells
- Myoepithelial cells form "collars" around ducts
- Cartilaginous areas present
- Due to accumulation of mucoid material
- Eosinophilic hyaline material seen
- Believed to be basal lamina produced by myoepithelial cells.

Other Cells Seen Are

- Keratinising squamous cells
- Mucus producing cells
- Goblet cells
- Oncocytes
- Sebaceous cells.

Immunohistochemistry

- Myoepithelial cells immunoreactive for:
  - Keratin
  - S: 100 protein
  - Glial fibrillary acidic protein
  - Actin
  - Vimentin.
- Ductal epithelial cells and solid cellular nests reactive for cytokeratin
- Ultrastructurally: Myoepithelial cells show:
  - Desmosomes
  - Actin filaments
  - Remnants of basal lamina.

Differential Diagnosis

- Chondroid syringoma (mixed tumour of skin)
- Monomorphic salivary gland adenomas versus mixed tumour (highly cellular)
- Mixed tumour (stroma rich) versus mesenchymal neoplasms: Immunohistochemical (IHC) analysis
- Spindle/plasmacytoid cell: Diagnosed as latter
- Mixed tumour versus malignant transformation
- Mixed tumour (cellular) versus adenocarcinoma.

Treatment

- Surgical excision
- Conservative enucleation leads to recurrence.

SHORT ESSAYS

Question 1

Write short note on myoepithelioma?

Answer

Myoepithelioma

- Term used by Sheldon (1943)
- Rate <1% of all salivary gland tumours
- Represent one end of spectrum of pleomorphic adenoma
- Also called as mixed tumour with a high content of myoepithelial cells.

Clinical Features

- Same as pleomorphic adenoma
- Occurs in adults
- No sex predilection
- Common site:
  - Parotid gland (51%)
  - Submandibular gland (12%).
- Common intraoral site: Palate
- Other sites.
  - Retromolar gland
  - Upper lip.

Histological Features

- Macroscopically:
  - Well circumscribed
  - Frequently encapsulated (parotid).
- Microscopically:
  - Composed exclusively of myoepithelial cells
  - Three patterns seen.

Spindle Cell Pattern

- Most common
- Spindle shaped cell
- Arranged in sheets/interlacing fascicles
- Little ground substance present.

Plasmacytoid Pattern

- Round cells
- Eccentric nuclei
- Eosinophilic or hyaline appearing cytoplasm
- Also called as hyaline cells
- Arranged in sheets/group of cells
- Loose, myxoid stroma present.

Combination Pattern

- Both cells present
- Spindle cell pattern: Parotid
- Plasmacytoid: Palate.

Immunohistochemistry and Ultrastructure

Show immunoreactivity for:

- Cytokeratin
- S-100 protein
- Vimentin
- Actin
- Glial fibrillary acidic protein.

Ultrastructurally

Myoepithelial cells show:

- Desmosomes
- Cytoplasmic microfilaments
- Basal lamina.

Differential Diagnosis

- Myoepithelioma versus cellular pleomorphic adenoma: Difficulty arises when stromal fragments are seen
- Myoepithelioma versus malignant myoepithelioma: Latter shows:
  - Marked atypical
  - Necrosis
  - Intranuclear/intracytoplasmic inclusions.

Treatment

Complete surgical removal is recommended as there is minimal tendency for recurrence.

- Malignant potential is mild
- Spindle cell differentiation, Well differentiated: Benign course
- Less well differentiated: Aggressive
- Plasmacytoid myoepitheliomas: Benign course.

Question 2

Define oncocytoma/oyphilic adenoma/acidophilic adenoma?

Answer

- Benign salivary gland tumour
- Composed of oncocytes
- Oncocytes term derived from Greek word onkousthai
- Accounts for 1% of salivary tumours
- First described by Schaffer (1897)
- Name derived due to resemblance of tumour cells to normal, called as oncocytes
- Oncocytes are found in:
  - Salivary glands
  - Respiratory tract
  - Thyroid
  - Pancreas
  - Parathyroid
  - Liver
  - Stomach.
- Common finding in old age
- Oncocytes: Large granular acidophilic cells filled with mitochondria.

Clinical Features

- Common site: Parotid gland
- In minor salivary gland:
  - Palate > buccal mucosa > tongue.
- Females > males
- Age: 7th to 8th decades, paediatric cases not reported
- Solid, ovoid encapsulated lesions
- Present in superficial lobe of parotid
- Less than 5 cm in diameter
- Pain generally absent
- Freely movable on palpation
- Rarely seen intraorally
- May be bilateral.

Multi-nodular Oncocytic Hyperplasia (Oncocytosis)

Histopathology

- Macroscopically:
  - White
  - Well encapsulated
  - May be multi-nodular or lobulated
  - Haemorrhagic areas are seen.
- Microscopically
  - Well circumscribed tumour
  - Large polyhedral cells (oncocytes) present
  - Cells contain granular eosinophilic cytoplasm.
- Arranged in sheets
- Nuclei: Centrally placed, hyper-chromatic
- Little stroma present
- Lymphocytic infiltration
- Eosinophilic staining and granularity
- Oncocytes supported by fibrous connective tissue septa.

Immunohistochemistry

- Phosphotungstic acid haematoxylin (PTAH): demonstrates mitochondria
- Periodic acid–Schiff (PAS): stain for glycogen
- Anti-mitochondrial antibodies also used
- Clear cells may be present
- Two types of oncocytes:
  1. Typical oncocytes with uniform mitochondria
  2. Condensed oncocytes with fused and degenerating mitochondria.
- Oncocyte, an epithelial cell:
  - Basement membrane
  - Desmosomes
  - Tonofibrils are seen.
- Oncocyte, a glandular cell:
  - Microvilli
  - Secretory granules.

Differential Diagnosis

- Mixed tumour
- Mucoepidermoid carcinoma with oncocytic features
- Acinic cell carcinoma
- Metastatic carcinoma of adrenal:
  - Thyroid
  - Liver
  - Kidney.
- Oncocytoma versus mucoepidermoid carcinoma:
  - PTAH positive for former
  - Well differentiated.

CHAPTER 8

Disorder of TMJ and MPDS

LONG ESSAYS

Question 1

Describe the anatomy of temporomandibular joint?

Answer

Temporomandibular joint (TMJ) is also called as craniomandibular joint/bilateral diarthrodial joint. It is formed by the articulation of the squamous part of temporal bone with the head of mandibular condyle.

The joint consist of:

- Mandibular/glenoid fossa
- Articular eminence/tubercle
- Condyle
- Articular disc
- Fibrous capsule
- Extra-articular ligaments.

Mandibular/Glenoid Fossa

Anteriorly, it extends up to articular eminence/tubercle and posteriorly it is limited by post-glenoid tubercle.

Articular Eminence

- It is a prominence seen on the zygomatic arch
- It is convex anteroposteriorly and concave mediolaterally.

Post-glenoid Tubercle

It separates the fossa laterally with tympanic plate.

Glenoid Fossa

- It is smooth, oval shaped and hollow with the bone being thin at the depth of the fossa
- Roof separates the middle cranial fossa with the joint
- Posterior wall of the fossa is formed by squamotympanic fissure.

Condyle

- It forms the articular part of the mandible to the cranium
- It has a head and a neck
- The head is ovoid in shape and neck is narrow
- The condyle is broad laterally and narrow medially
- Most of the human condyles (58%) are found to be convex superiorly, while 25% are flat superiorly, 12% being angular or pointed and 3% being bulbous
- The articular part of the condyle is covered with fibrocartilaginous tissue.

Temporomandibular Joint Capsule

- It is a funnel shaped, thin sheet of fibrous tissue investing the joint
- Anteriorly, it is attached to anterior border of articular eminence and posteriorly to the squamotympanic fissure and anterior surface of post-glenoid process.

Ligaments

- Lateral or temporomandibular ligaments
  - Extends downward and backward from articular eminence to the posterior side of condyle neck
  - It limits the anterior excursion of the jaw and prevents posterior dislocation.
- Accessory ligaments
  - Sphenomandibular ligament: It arises from spine of the sphenoid and runs downwards and medial to the TMJ capsule and gets inserted into the lingual of the mandible
  - Stylomandibular ligament: It arises from styloid process and inserts into the angle of mandible.
- Articular disc/meniscus.

Articular disc divides the articular space into two compartments:

1. Lower/inferior compartment: Between condyle and the disc
2. Upper/superior compartment: Between disc and glenoid fossa.

- The disc is biconcave in shape sagitally. The shape also resembles jockey's cap and it overlaps the condylar head
- Medially and laterally it blends into the capsule, anteriorly it is attached to the articular eminence superiorly and inferiorly to the condyle
- Posteriorly the disc is attached to the posterior wall of glenoid fossa above and neck of the condyle below. This area is rich in neurovascular supply and is called as posterior bilaminar zone
- Rees proposed three zones of the disc:
  1. Posterior band
  2. Intermediate zone
  3. Anterior band.

Posterior band is the thickest (3 mm) and widest. Intermediate band is thinnest being only 1 mm while anterior band is moderately thin about 2 mm. The thin band between 2 thick bands gives the disc its flexibility and also the disc is able to change its shape from concave to convex in protrusive movement.

- The disc is designed to promote lubrication, absorb shock and provide the joint a range of motion
- The posterior region of the disc is known as bilaminar zone as it contains two strata of fibres with loose areolar tissues between them.

Blood Supply

- Superficial temporal branch of the external carotid artery supplies the lateral aspect
- Deep auricular, posterior auricular and masseteric branches of maxillary artery supplies the deep and posterior part of capsule.

Nerve Supply

- Auriculotemporal nerve: Posterior, medial and lateral parts of the joint
- Masseteric nerve and branch of posterior deep tem-poral nerve: These supply the anterior parts of joint.

Movements

- Jaw opening (depression): Mainly by digastric muscle contraction assisted by suprahyoid, sternohyoid and geniohyoid muscles along with lateral pterygoid
- Jaw closure (elevation): Simultaneous contraction of masseter, medial pterygoid and temporalis muscle
- Protrusive: Equal and simultaneous contraction of lateral and medial pterygoid muscles
- Retrusion: Posterior fibres of temporalis muscles, along-with middle and deep parts of masseter, digastric and geniohyoid muscles
- Lateral movements: Unilateral contraction of medial and lateral pterygoid muscles.

Question 2

Classify temporomandibular joint disorders. Describe trismus and its causes?

Answer

Classification

- Intrinsic/intra-articular disorders
- Extrinsic/extra-articular disorders.

Extrinsic Disorders

- Masticatory muscle disorders:
  - Protective muscle splinting
  - Masticatory muscle spasm
  - Masticatory muscle inflammation.
- Extrinsic trauma:
  - Traumatic arthritis
  - Tendonitis
  - Fracture
  - Myositis
  - Internal disc derangement
  - Contracture of elevator muscle.

Intrinsic Disorders

- Trauma:
  - Dislocation, subluxation
  - Haematosis
  - Intracapsular fracture, extracapsular fracture.
- Internal disc displacement:
  - Anterior disc displacement with reduction
  - Anterior disc displacement without reduction.
- Arthritis:
  - Osteoarthritis
  - Rheumatoid arthritis
  - Juvenile rheumatoid arthritis
  - Infectious arthritis.
- Developmental defects:
  - Condylar agenesis or aplasia: Unilateral or bilateral
  - Condylar hypoplasia
  - Condylar hyperplasia.
- Ankylosis

- Neoplasms:
  - Benign tumours: Osteoma, osteochondroma, chondroma
  - Malignant tumours: Chondrosarcoma, fibrosarcoma, synovial sarcoma.

Trismus

- It is the inability or restriction to normal oral opening
- It occurs by extra-articular causes and is also called false ankylosis
- It can be defined as "a condition in which muscle spasms or contracture prevents opening of the mouth".

Causes of Trismus

- Infection: Orofacial infection, odontogenic infection, like pericoronitis, Ludwig's angina, space infection, submasseteric, infratemporal infection, etc.
- Trauma: Fracture of zygomatic arch, fracture of mandible
- Inflammation
- Myositis ossificans: Formation of haematoma in the fibres of masticatory muscles, especially masseter, due to trauma which progresses into ossification and stiffness of the muscle
- Tetany
- Tetanus
- Neurological disorders
- Psychosomatic trismus: It is also termed as trismus hystericus. Occurs due to extreme fear, anxiety, etc.
- Drug-induced trismus: Strychnine poisoning
- Mechanical blockage: Elongation, osteoma, osteosarcoma of coronoid process, exostosis can cause mechanical blockage and interfere with mandibular movements.

Question 3

Extra-articular fibrosis. Explain dislocation/subluxation?

Answer

Excursion of condylar heads beyond the articular eminence during excursion movements is termed as dislocation. In such cases, the whole condylar head displaces outside the glenoid fossa beyond articular eminence but stays within the capsule of the joint.

It can be unilateral or bilateral. It can be classified as:

- Acute
- Chronic
- Long standing.

Causes of Acute Dislocation

- Extrinsic or iatrogenic causes: Trauma on the chin in sports, excessive pressure on mandible during dental procedure without adequate support to mandible
- Intrinsic causes: Excessive yawning, vomiting, blowing wind instruments, opening mouth widely, fits, etc.
- Predisposing factors: Laxity of capsule, ligaments and abnormal skeletal form. Flattened eminence, shallow fossa, Parkinson's disease, epilepsy, Ehler Danlos syndrome.

Management

- Overcoming the resistance of the muscle spasm
- Making the patient comfortable to reduce the anxiety by
  - Reassuring the patient
  - Administration of sedative
  - Pressure and massage to the area
  - Manipulation.
- Depending on amount of muscle spasms, manipulation can be done:
  - Without any anesthesia
  - In local anesthesia
  - Under general anesthesia.
- Manipulation:
  - Operator stands in front of the patient and grasps the mandible with both hands on each sid
  - The thumbs should be covered with gauze to prevent accidental trapping into mouth upon reduction
  - The thumbs are placed on the occlusal surface of the mandibular molars with fingertips below the chin
  - Operator exerts full body pressure downwards on the posterior teeth to depress the jaw and at the same time the fingertips below the mandible apply upward pressure
  - Downward pressure is used to overcome spasm of muscles and bring the condyle down below the articular eminence and then a backward force is applied to bring about the movement of mandible posteriorly to place the condyles into the glenoid fossa
  - Once the reduction is done, patient is advised to keep the mouth closed and open mouth with restricted opening
  - Anti-inflammatory analgesic drugs are prescribed.

Chronic Dislocation/Subluxation

- This is characterised by repeated episodes of dislocation, i.e., the condylar heads move beyond the articular eminence, but the patient is able to manipulate it back into the normal position

- This occurs due to:
  - Ligament/capsular flaccidity
  - Eminential erosion
  - Trauma.
- Subluxation can be painful or painless.

Management

- Intermaxillary fixation: Total immobilisation of the jaws for 3–4 weeks. Patient is kept on liquid diet
- Sclerosing solution in joint space: Sodium psylliate, sodium morrhuate, sodium tetradecyl sulphate. The results are temporary
- Surgical procedures: According to Millar and Murphy:
  - Capsule tightening procedure
  - Creating a mechanical obstacle
  - Direct restraint of condyle
  - Creation of new muscle balance
  - Removal of mechanical obstacle.

Capsule Tightening Procedure

- Capsulorrhaphy: It consists of shortening of the capsule by excising a section and suturing to make it tight
- Vertical incision in the capsule and then suturing back the two halves by overlapping them
- Reinforcement of joint capsule can be achieved by suturing a strip of temporal fossa to the capsule.

Creating a Mechanical Obstacle

- Lindermann conducted osteotomy on articular eminence and turned it down thus creating an obstacle in the path of condyle movement
- Mayor advised placing a graft on eminence to increase its size. Placement of silastic block or vitallium mesh implants.

Direct Restraint of Condyle

- Temporal fascia is turned downwards and sutured on lateral surface of capsule
- Piece of fascia lata is threaded through zygomatic arch into the condyle.

Creation of New Muscle Balance

- Medial pterygoid muscle is shortened
- Temporalis tendon is divided and masseter elevated from ramus and then sutured back in horizontal manner
- This brings about scar formation and thus restricts oral opening.

Removal of Mechanical Obstacle

- Removal of torn meniscus
- High condylectomy
- Eminectomy: This involved excision of articular eminence thus allowing condyle to move anteriorly and posteriorly without any hindrance.

Question 4

Describe the surgical approaches to temporomandibular joint/condyle/neck of condyle?

Answer

Surgical access to thymidylate kinase (TMK) requires a thorough knowledge of the anatomy of the area as it is in close proximity to various nerves and vascular supply.

Several approaches to the temporomandibular joint (TMJ) have been proposed.

- Postauricular approach: The incision is done behind the ear near the superior aspect of pinna and extends to the mastoid process. It is a highly aesthetic approach but has many disadvantages:
  - Poor access and visibility
  - Stenosis of the external auditory meatus can occur
  - Infection in external auditory canal may occur
  - Paraesthesia may occur.
- Endaural approach (given my Lamport): Incision begins above the level of zygomatic arch and extends downwards and backwards between tragus and helix extending inwards along the roof of auditory meatus up to 1 cm.
  - Advantages:
    - Highly aesthetic.
  - Disadvantages:
    - Limited access
    - Meatal stenosis and chondritis.
- Submandibular (Risdon) approach:
  - Incision is made 1 cm below the angle of mandible extending forwards, parallel to the lower border of mandible and then it curves backwards slightly behind the angle
  - Approach is achieved by incising pterygomasseteric sling and reflecting the masseter muscle laterally
  - This has poor approach to condyle and articular head and meniscus cannot be approached.
- Postramal approach (Hind):
  - Indication for operating condylar neck and ramus area
  - Incision is placed 1 cm behind the ramus extending 1 cm below the lobe of the ear to angle of mandible
  - Fascia between the sternomastoid muscle, parotid gland and masseter muscle should be separated to expose the posterior border of the ramus
  - Once the ramus is exposed, the pterygomasseteric sling is incised at angle and sternomastoid, parotid and masseter muscle are reflected upwards.

- Advantages:
  - Highly aesthetic approach
  - Good accessibility and visibility.
- Preauricular approach:
  - Initial incision is made in the preauricular fold
  - Oblique incision through the superficial layer of temporalis fascia is made
  - Temporal muscle is reflected to expose the lateral part of zygomatic arch
  - Cut in the capsule is made to approach TMJ
  - Incision through the lateral attachment of disc is made to enter the inferior joint space.

Modifications to the Pre-auricular Incision

- Inverted hockey stick incision (by Blair and Ivy): This incision is made over the zygomatic arch
- Thomas'"angulated vertical incision" is made across the zygomatic arch in the fold, in front of the ear, extending downwards above the ear lobe
- Al Kayat–Bramley incision: This incision is made to avoid damage to the facial nerve
- Incision is made through the temporal fascia and periosteum down to the arch up to 0.8 cm in front of the anterior border of external auditory canal
- Popowich and Crane: Modification off Al Kayat–Bramley incision. Large incision—shaped like a "question mark" is made in the temporal area extending in the pre-auricular area.

Question 5

What is ankylosis of the temporomandibular joint. Describe its etiology, clinical features, diagnosis, and management?

Answer

Ankylosis in Greek means "stiff joint". Hypomobility to immobility of the joint leads to inability to open the mouth. It can be partial or complete.

Classification

- False ankylosis or true ankylosis
- Extra-articular or intra-articular
- Fibrous or bony
- Unilateral or bilateral
- Partial or complete.

Etiology

- Trauma
  - Congenital
  - At birth, forceps delivery
  - Haemarthrosis
  - Condylar fractures: Intracapsular or extracapsular
  - Glenoid fossa fracture.
- Infections
  - Otitis media
  - Parotitis
  - Tonsilitis
  - Furuncle
  - Abscess around the joint
  - Osteomyelitis of the jaw
  - Actinomycosis.
- Inflammation
  - Rheumatoid arthritis
  - Osteoarthritis
  - Septic arthritis.
- Rare causes
  - Polyarthritis
  - Measles.
- Systemic diseases
  - Smallpox
  - Scarlet fever
  - Typhoid
  - Gonococcal arthritis
  - Scleroderma
  - Beriberi
  - Marie–Strumpell diseases.
- Other causes.
  - Bifid condyle
  - Prolonged trismus
  - Prolonged immobilisation
  - Burns.

Clinical Features

- Depends on (1) time of onset of ankylosis, (2) severity of ankylosis, and (3) duration
- Early joint involvement less than 15 years: Severe facial deformity and loss of function
- Later joint involvement after age of 15 years: Facial deformity marginal or nil.

Unilateral Ankylosis

- Facial asymmetry
- Deviation of mandible and chin to the affected side
- Receded chin with hypoplastic mandible on the affected side
- Flatness and elongation of face on unaffected side
- Lower border of mandible of affected side has concavity
- Cross bite
- Class II malocclusion on affected side
- Condylar movement absent on affected side.

Bilateral Ankylosis

- Inability to open mouth
- Bird face deformity with receding chin
- Neck-chin angle completely absent or reduced
- Class II malocclusion
- Anterior open bite with protrusive upper incisors
- Oral opening may be nil in some cases.

Diagnosis

- Orthopantomograph
- Lateral oblique view
- Cephalometric radiograph
- Posteroanterior radiograph
- Computed tomography (CT) scan.

Sawhney Grading of Temporomandibular Joint (TMJ) Ankylosis

- Type I: Condylar head is normal without much distortion. Fibrous adhesions make movement impossible
- Type II: Bony fusion of the distorted condylar head and the articular surface. No involvement of sigmoid notch and coronoid process
- Type III: Bony block across ramus and zygomatic arch. Medially an atrophic dislocated fragment of the former head of the condyle is still found. Elongation of the coronoid process is seen
- Type IV: Normal anatomy of TMJ is completely des-troyed by complete bony block between ramus and skull base.

Management

Ankylosis of TMJ is always treated surgically.

Surgical Techniques

- Condylectomy
- Gap arthroplasty
- Interpositional arthroplasty.

Condylectomy: Advocated in cases of fibrous ankylosis, where the joint space is obliterated with deposition of fibrous bands, but there is not much deformity of the condylar head.

Procedure

- Preauricular incision to expose condylar head
- Sectioning of condylar head
- Breaking the fibrous adhesions
- Condylectomy performed
- Suturing of the capsule
- Skin suturing.

Gap arthroplasty: It is advocated in cases of extensive bony ankylosis. In such cases broad, thick area of bony deposition obliterates the entire joint, sigmoid notch and coronoid process.

Gap arthroplasty is an operation in which level of section is below the previous joint space and in which, no substance is interposed between the two cut bony surfaces. Section consists of two horizontal osteotomy cuts and removal of bony wedges for creation of gap between the roof of glenoid fossa and ramus. Minimum gap of at least 1 cm is created to prevent re-ankylosis.

Interpositional arthroplasty: Interpositional arthroplasty involves insertion of a barrier (autogenous or alloplastic) between the two sections to minimize the risk of recurrence and to maintain the vertical height of ramus.

International Protocol for Management of TMJ Ankylosis (by Kaban, Perrot and Fisher)

- Early surgical intervention
- Aggressive resection: A gap of at least 1–1.5 cm should be created
- Ipsilateral coronoidectomy and temporalis myotomy should be performed along with gap arthroplasty
- If maximum incisal opening of 35 mm is achieved, contralateral coronoidectomy is not performed
- Contralateral coronoidectomy: In cases where 35 mm inter-incisal opening is not achieved, coronoidectomy and temporalis myotomy on the uninvolved site is carried out
- Temporalis fascia is used to create lining for glenoid fossa
- Ramus is reconstructed with costochondral graft
- Early mobilisation and aggressive physiotherapy for at least 6 month postoperatively
- Regular long-term follow-up
- Cosmetic surgery post growth completion.

Question 6

Explain myofascial pain dysfunction syndrome/temporomandibular joint dysfunction syndrome?

Answer

Myofascial pain dysfunction syndrome (MPDS) is a pain disorder in which unilateral pain is referred from the trigger points in myofascial structures, to the muscles of the head and neck.

Pain is constant, dull ache; however, it may range from mild to intolerable.

Etiology

- Muscular hyper-function
- Disuse
- Physical disorders
- Parafunctional habits
- Tissue injury
- Sleep disturbances
- Nutritional problems
- Physiological stress.

Clinical Features

Cardinal Symptoms

- Pain or discomfort (unexplained nature), anywhere in neck or head
- Limitation of movement of the jaw
- Tenderness on palpation of muscles of mastication, without any history of trauma, infection, ear, etc.
- Joint noises: Grating, clicking and snapping.

Additional Symptoms

Neurologic

- Tingling
- Blurred vision
- Twitches
- Numbness
- Lacrimation
- Trembling.

Gastro-intestinal Tract

- Vomiting
- Constipation
- Indigestion
- Nausea
- Dry mouth
- Diarrhoea.

Musculoskeletal

- Fatigue
- Tiredness
- Weakness
- Tension
- Shift joint pains.

Otologic

- Tinnitus
- Dizziness
- Vertigo
- Diminished hearing
- Ear pain.

Diagnosis

Physical Examination

- Amount of oral opening and excursions
- Extent of motion:
  - Range of motion
  - Active range of motion
  - Passive range of motion.
- Palpation of muscles for tenderness
- Grading of click or crepitation
- Occlusal evaluation: Prematurities, interferences, occlusal discrepancies, anterior open bite, deep bite, attrition, wear facets, missing teeth, mobility of teeth, etc.
- Radiographic evaluation: To diagnose intra-articular pathologies, osseous pathologies, soft tissue pathologies.
  - Panoramic radiography
  - Transcranial radiography
  - Temporomandibular joint (TMJ) arthrography
  - Computed radiography
  - CT scan and magnetic resonance imaging (MRI)
  - Bone scintigram-nuclear imaging.

Management

- Auriculotemporal nerve block for TMJ pain
- Counselling of the patient
- Medications
  - Aspirin
  - Piroxicam
  - Ibuprofen
  - Pentazocine
  - Valium/Librium
  - Methocarbamol
  - Amitriptyline
  - Non-steroidal anti-inflammatory drugs
  - Muscle relaxants
  - Ethyl chloride spray.
- Physiotherapy
  - Heat application
  - Ultrasound
  - Cryotherapy
  - Massage with counter-irritants and vibrators
  - Vapocoolant spray, like fluoromethane or ethyl chloride spray
  - Tetanising and sinusoidal currents
  - Electrogalvanic stimulation
  - Transcutaneous electronic nerve stimulator (TENS)
  - Active stretch exercises.

- Intra-articular injections of hydrocortisone +0.5 cc of percent lignocaine
- Occlusal splints.
  - They are given to:
    - Temporarily disengage the teeth
    - To improve/restore the vertical dimension
    - To create balanced joint-tooth stabilisation of the mandible
    - To serve as safety or protective appliance
    - To reduce spasms, contracture and hyperactivity of musculature
    - Occlusal rehabilitation
    - Arthrocentesis: In this lavage or irrigation of the upper joint cavity is performed.

Objective

- Improve the disc mobility
- Eliminate joint inflammation
- Physiotherapy
- Eliminate pain
- Remove resistance of condyle translation.

SHORT ESSAYS

Question 1

Define internal derangement of joint?

Answer

Internal derangement is defined as disruption of the internal aspects of the temporomandibular joint (TMJ), in which an abnormal relationship exists between the disc and the condyle, fossa and articular eminence.

Etiology

- Micro trauma: Overloading due to bruxism or other parafunctional habits
- Macro trauma: Due to trauma.

Symptoms

- Pain during function
- Limited oral opening
- Masticatory and cervical tenderness.

Types

- Type A:
  - Disc displacement
  - Disc displacement with reduction
  - Disc displacement without reduction.
- Type B:
  - Structural incompatibility of the articular surfaces:
  - Adhesions
  - Alterations in the form
  - Due to systemic joint disorders, like rheumatoid arthritis.

Anterior Disc Displacement with Reduction

- Disc is dislocated anteriorly to the condylar head leading to pain during translation
- There is reciprocal clicking in anterior dislocation with reduction, i.e., a click during opening and mild click during closing of the mandible
- During opening: Due to reduction, a clicking sound occurs as the posterior part of the disc interferes with condylar translation
- During closing: Reciprocal click occurs as the condyle returns to the original position, gliding over the posterior part of the disc.

Anterior Disc Displacement without Reduction

In such cases, if the patient is not able to open mouth fully, and if the patient tries to open mouth further, pain in the joint can be elicited alongwith deviation of mandible towards the affected side.

Symptoms of Disc Dislocation without Reduction

- Limited mandibular opening
- Unilaterally mandible cannot translate fully
- Unrestricted ipsilateral eccentric movements
- Loss of joint sounds in case of earlier history of clicking
- Restricted contralateral eccentric movements.

CHAPTER 9

Ionising Radiation and Regressive Alterations of the Oral Cavity

LONG ESSAYS

Question 1

Discuss the complications of radiation of the jaws and its management?

Answer

Complications are as follows

- Radiation mucositis
- Radiation-induced xerostomia
- Radiation caries
- Radiation-induced trismus
- Radiation dysphagia
- Radiation effects on jaw growth and developing teeth.

Complications and their Management

Radiation Mucositis

- It occurs due to acute radiation injury
- There is a diffuse erythema with pain or mucosal ulcerations with a fibrinous exudate
- It may develop in the last 3 weeks of radiotherapy and can extend for about 1 month after radiotherapy
- It is a self-limiting condition
- It is a very painful condition.

Management

- Topical 2% xylocaine/lidocaine gel can be used for pain management
- Systemic analgesics can also be given
- If there is associated lymphadenitis or systemic toxicity, then antibiotics should be given
- To reduce bacterial colonisation of the ulcer, chlorhexidine gluconate can be given if tolerated, by the patient
- Nutritional supplements should also be prescribed
- In extreme cases, IV fluid therapy and nasogastric tube feeding can be provided.

Radiation-induced Xerostomia

- It occurs because of damaging effects of radiation on both major and minor salivary glands located in the path of radiation
- Mouth becomes dry due to loss of salivary gland acini
- Because of loss of sweat and sebaceous glands, the skin becomes dry
- Ductal epithelium is generally radiation resistant.

Management

- 5 mg pilocarpine, orally thrice daily, improves speaking, eating and swallowing
- It is given cautiously in patients with bradycardia, heart block and other medication which slows down the heart rate or conduction.

Radiation Caries

- Teeth which are in dried path of 6,000 cGy or greater than that are at the maximum risk of developing radiation caries
- It is caused because of xerostomia that allows cariogenic bacteria to proliferate
- This caries is black in colour and hard. It occurs mostly at the gingival margin, cusp tips and incisal surfaces
- Enamel is lost because of dentinoenamel junction destruction and dentinal dehydration.

Management

- Maintenance of a good oral hygiene
- Should be treated promptly using restorative techniques appropriate for the degree of lost and involved tooth substance.

Radiation-induced Trismus

- It is generally accompanied by osteoradionecrosis in the posterior body and ramus region of the mandible

- It occurs due to radiation fibrosis within the masseter and medial pterygoid muscles or because of restrictive fibrosis in the mucosa of the anterior tonsillar pillar and the retromolar areas.

Management

- It is generally improved with the successful treatment of the osteoradionecrosis
- Tissues can be excised and replaced with a viable skin paddle from either a myocutaneous or a free microvascular flap
- This would lead significant increase in mouth opening
- Bilateral coronoidectomies or partial excisions of the fibrosis in the massetor or medial pterygoid muscles can also lead to modest gains
- Jaw opening exercises, such as by tongue blade exercises, or by the chewing of soft, sugarless gum.

Radiation Dysphagia

- Patient complains of difficulty in swallowing food or complains of food getting stuck in the hypopharynx
- It occurs due to radiation fibrosis within the pharyngeal constrictors.

Management

- Swallowing therapies are helpful
- Mouth moisture should be improved by increasing the liquid content in the diet.

Radiation Effects on Jaw Growth and Developing Teeth

- During growth and development years, radiation can create a dose-related hypoplasia of the mandible
- It can also lead to partial or complete agenesis of teeth
- These effects can be manifested as an anteroposterior deficiency of the mandible that is retrognathism
- There will be a reduction in the size of the ramus and body of the mandible, which leads to deficiency in the appearance of chin
- Within the radiated bone, the teeth appear smaller and generally exhibit arrested root development
- Few teeth would fail to form altogether
- This is referred to as agenesis.

Management

- For missing teeth, they should be replaced with removable partial dentures or with implant supported fixed dental appliances
- Osteotomies can be done using bone grafts
- Patients should undergo 20/10 hyperbaric oxygen (HBO) protocol (20 sessions at 2.4 ATA for 90 minutes on 100% oxygen prior to surgery and 10 sessions after surgery)
- Distraction osteogenesis can also be done in a young patient who has undergone the 20/10 HBO protocol.

Question 2

What is the classification of regressive alterations of teeth?

Answer

- Tooth wear
  - Attrition
  - Abrasion
  - Erosion (corrosion)
  - Abfraction.
- Teeth resorption
  - External
  - Internal.
- Dentinal changes
  - Reparative dentin
  - Secondary dentin
  - Dead tracts.
- Cemental changes
  - Cementicles
  - Hypercementosis.
- Pulpal changes.
  - Reticular atrophy of pulp
  - Pulp calcifications.

Tooth Wear

- Attrition: It is the physiologic wearing of tooth material
- Abrasion
  - It is the pathological wearing of tooth material, occurring generally at exposed root surface of the tooth
  - Seen as a wedge-shaped ditch near the CEJ.
- Erosion
  - It is the chemical loss of tooth material due to acidic substances
  - It appears as smooth, highly polished scooped out depression near CEJ.
- Abfraction.
  - It is the loss of tooth material due to repeated tooth flexure by occlusal stresses.

Teeth Resorption

- External resorption
  - It occurs because of periapical granuloma or by pressure due to any cyst, commonly the apical periodontal cyst and tumours of heavy orthodontic forces.

- Internal resorption.
  - It is also called as odontoclastoma or pink tooth of mummery
  - It occurs mainly because of inflammatory hyperplasia of the pulp.

Dentinal Changes

- Reparative dentin
  - Also referred to as transparent dentin/dental sclerosis
  - Due to trauma, caries, etc. there is calcification of dentinal tubules.
- Secondary dentin
  - It is an irregular dentin, also referred to as adventitious dentin, which is deposited after the completion of primary dentin and is associated with normal ageing process
  - It is also called as irritation dentin since it can also be stimulated by trauma, caries, attrition, etc.
  - Tertiary dentin is localised, adjacent to the irritated zone, tubules are less in number, very irregular.
- Dead tracts.
  - They are permeable to penetration of dyes and they are not calcified.

Cemental Changes

- Cementicles
  - There are foci of calcified tissue which are free in periodontal ligament
  - They are formed by calcification of nests of epithelial cell rests in PDL.
- Hypercementosis/cementum hyperplasia.
  - It is due to deposition of secondary cementum (cellular), on the root surface
  - It occurs more commonly in non-functional teeth.

Pulpal Changes

- Reticular atrophy of pulp
  - Atrophy of pulp tissue and there is a decrease in the size of pulp chamber because of increase in age.
- Pulp calcifications.
  - Various types of denticles are:
    - True denticles
    - False denticles
    - Free denticles
    - Attached denticles
    - Diffuse calcification.

SHORT NOTES

Question 1

What are the reasons of resorption of roots?

Answer

There are Two Types of Resorptions

1. External resorption
2. Internal resorption.

Causes of External Resorption are as Follows

- Tumours and cysts
- Periapical inflammation
- Excessive mechanical or occlusal forces, like orthodontic treatment
- Reimplantation
- Impacted teeth
- Hormonal disturbances
- Trauma
- Idiopathic.

Causes of Internal Resorption are as follows

- Odontoclastoma/internal granuloma
- Pink tooth of mummery
- Inflammatory hyperplasia of pulp
- Idiopathic.

CHAPTER 10 Odontogenic and Non-odontogenic Tumours

LONG ESSAYS

Question 1

Explain ameloblastoma and its management?

Answer

According to WHO, "Ameloblastoma can be defined as a true neoplasm of enamel orgal type tissue, which does not undergo differentiation to a point of enamel formation."

Etiology

- Cell rests of enamel organ
- Remnants of dental lamina or epithelian cell rests of Malassez
- Remnants of Hertwig's sheath
- Disturbances of developing tooth bud, dental lamina, enamel organ
- Basal cell of the surface epithelium of the oral mucosa
- Epithelium of primordial cyst, dentigerous cyst, odontoma and lateral periodontal cyst
- Epithelium of pituitary gland
- Incidence: Comprises 18% of all odontogenic tumours and 1% of all oral tumours
- Age: Can occur at any age
- Site: Mandible:maxilla in the ratio of 5:1
- Most common in molar: Ramas region in mandible and in posterior region in maxilla.

Classification

- Central or intraosseous
- Peripheral or extraosseous.

Clinical Features

- Generally asymptomatic in early stages
- Intraoral or extraoral jaw swelling once it becomes larger in size
- Occlusal disturbances
- Slow growing, painless, hard, nontender, ovoid swelling
- Mobility of teeth
- Ill-fitting dentures
- Nasal obstructions
- Pain may occur in case of secondary infection
- Large lesion exhibits fluctuation and egg shell crackling
- Size: 1–16 cm in diameter.

Radiographic Finding

- Unilocular (monocytic) or multilocular (multicystic) radiolucency in different shapes and sizes
- Honey comb or soap-bubble appearance
- May contain a teeth and mimic dentigerous cyst
- Maxillary sinus is often involved in maxillary lesions.

Histopathology

- Follicular type: Resembles a tooth follicle. Consists of small to large odontogenic epithelial nests and ameloblastomatous island of various shapes and sizes
- Plexiform type: Consists of interlacing strands of odontogenic epithelial trabeculae which resemble dental lamina.

Both these types can be seen in same tumour.

Subtypes

- Acanthomatous type
- Basal cell type
- Desmoplastic type
- Granular cell type
- Mural ameloblastoma
- Peripheral ameloblastoma.

Management

The treatment modality is determined based on the age and general health of the patient.

- Complete excision of the lesion
- Reconstruction of the resultant defect.

Note: Curettage should never be done as the recurrence rate of the lesion is high.

The characteristic feature of this tumour is that it infiltrates bone beyond the bone–tumour interface. A safe margin of 2 cm of uninvolved bone for solid and multicystic lesion is taken.

For Intraosseous Solid / Multicystic Ameloblastoma

- En bloc resection or marginal resection without continuity defects
- Segmental resection with continuity defect:
  - If cortical bone is resorbed and penetrated, periosteum layer is included in resection
  - If only 1 cm of bone is left in mandible after resection, a reconstruction plate (only when complete removal of tumour has been ascertained) should be used or a second surgical procedure should be considered
  - Immediate reconstruction can be done using autogenous bone graft (iliac graft or a rib graft)
  - In maxilla following guidelines should be followed (by Jackson and Callon Forte):
    - Tumour confined to maxilla without orbital floor involvement: Partial maxillectomy
    - Tumours involving orbital floor but not peri-orbital area: Total maxillectomy
    - Tumour involving the skull bone alongwith skull base: Neurosurgical procedure.

Question 2

Classify odontogenic and non-odontogenic tumours of the jaws?

Answer

- Benign odontogenic tumours of the jaws (Kramer, Pindborg and Shear classification):
  - Odontogenic epithelium without odontogenic ectomesenchyme
  - Ameloblastoma
    - Calcifying epithelial odontogenic tumour (CEOT), Pindborg's tumour
    - Clear cell odontogenic tumour
    - Squamous odontogenic tumour.
  - Odontogenic epithelium with odontogenic ectomesenchyme, with or without dental hard tissue formation:
    - Ameloblastic fibroma
    - Ameloblastic fibrodentinoma
    - Odontoameloblastoma
    - Adenomatoid odontogenic tumour (AOT)
    - Complex odontoma
    - Compound odontoma.
  - Odontogenic ectomesenchyme with or without included odontogenic epithelium.
    - Odontogenic fibroma
    - Myxoma (odontogenic myxoma, myxofibroma)
    - Benign cementoblastoma (true cementoma).
- Classification of odontogenic tumours (Gorlin, Chaudhry, Pindborg)
  - Epithelial odontogenic tumours
    - Minimal inductive change in connective tissue (Ectodermal origin)
      - Ameloblastoma
      - Adenomatoid odontogenic tumour
      - Calcifying epithelial odontogenic tumour (CEOT).
    - Marked inductive change in connective tissue (mixed agents).
      - Ameloblastic fibroma
      - Ameloblastic odontoma
      - Odontoma
      - Complex odontoma
      - Compound odontoma.
  - Mesodermal odontogenic tumours.
    - Odontogenic myxoma
    - Odontogenic fibroma
    - Cementoma.
      - Periapical cemental dysplasia
      - Benign cementoblastoma
      - Cementifying fibroma
      - Familial multiple (gigantiform) cementoma [florid osseous dysplasia (FOD)].
- Non-odontogenic tumours and fibro-osseous lesions of the jaw bones:
  - Non-odontogenic tumours:
    - Central fibroma
    - Myxofibroma
    - Ossifying fibroma
    - Osteoma
    - Osteoid osteoma
    - Benign osteoclastoma
    - Chondroma
    - Giant cell granuloma
    - Central haemangioma
    - Benign tumours of nerve tissues.
  - Fibro-osseous lesions:
    - Fibrous dysplasia of bone
    - Cherubism (inherited fibro-osseous bone disease)
    - Ossifying fibroma
    - Central giant cell granuloma.

- World Health Organization (WHO) classification of non-odontogenic tumours of the jaws (Kramer, Pindborg, and Shear):
  - Osteogenic neoplasms:
    - Cemento-ossifying fibroma.
  - Non-neoplastic bone lesions:
    - Fibrous dysplasia of the jaws
    - Cemento-osseous dysplasia:
      - Periapical cemento-osseous dysplasia
      - Focal cemento-osseous dysplasia
      - Florid cemento-osseous dysplasia (gigantiform).
  - Other cemento-osseous dysplasias:
    - Cherubism
    - Central giant cell granuloma.

Question 3

Define fibrous dysplasia of the jaws?

Answer

It is a self-limiting lesion in which the medullary bone is slowly replaced by the abnormal fibrous connective tissue proliferation. The mesenchymal tissue consists of variable amount of osseous matrix consisting of only woven bone.

Types

- Solitary monostotic lesion: Involves a single bone. 80–85% more common
- Multifocal or polyostotic lesion: Involves several bones. Uncommon.
  - In Jaffe type: 3/4th of the entire skeleton may be involved
  - Mazabraud's syndrome: Fibrous dysplasia is associated with soft tissue myxoma
  - Lichtenstein syndrome: Entire skeleton is involved alongwith cutaneous melanotic pigmentation
  - McCune–Albright syndrome: More in females. Multiple areas of cutaneous melanotic pigmentation (café-au-lait macules) and hyper-function of one or more endocrine glands.

Etiology

Unknown. Multiple hypotheses have been proposed:

- Focal bone expression of endocrine disturbance
- Inherited basis
- From altered mesenchymal cell activity.

Monostotic Fibrous Dysplasia of the Jaws

- 10–20 years of age
- Insidious, painless, asymptomatic, slow-growing lesion
- Both male and females are equally affected
- Maxilla more commonly affected than mandible
- Slow-growing enlargement may be seen due to expansion of the buccal cortical plate (lingual cortex is rarely involved)
- Teeth involved in lesion are generally firm but may be displaced.

Radiographic Feature

Four pictures generally are seen:

- Ground glass appearance in mature stage
- Unilocular or multilocular radiolucencies in early stage
- Radiolucency with patchy, irregular opacities similar to Paget's disease in intermediate stage
- Finger print bone pattern can be seen
- Superior displacement of mandibular canal is seen frequently
- In maxilla, maxillary sinus gets obliterated by the lesion tissue
- Characteristic feature is poorly defined clinical and radiological demarcating margins of the lesion

Polyostotic Fibrous Dysplasia (McCune– Albright Syndrome)

- Skull and jaws both get affected leading to facial asymmetry. Both jaws along with long bones get infected simultaneously
- "Hockey stick" deformity of the femur can be seen
- Café-au-lait pigmentation is seen on trunk, thighs and oral mucosa. Margins of these spots are irregular in contrast to smooth border of café-au-lait spots of neurofibromatosis.

Management

- The treatment plan depends on extent of involvement, functional disability, danger to function, neurologic symptoms and aesthetic consideration
- Differentiation between monostotic and polyostotic can be done using bone scintigraphy
- Treatment can vary from minor lesion to radical resection
- Resection with reconstruction is not done as complete excision is not possible rather recontouring of the bone is done.

SHORT ESSAYS

Question 1

Calcify epithelial odontogenic tumour (CEOT)/Pindborg tumour?

Answer

First described by Pindborg:

- Origin: Arises from epithelial elements of enamel organ
- Incidence: 1% of all odontogenic tumours
- No sex predilection
- Age: 3–50 years of age
- Site: Mandible most commonly involved in molar region.

Clinical Features

- Painless
- Slow growing tumour
- If it approaches nasal cavity, produces nasal symptoms, like stuffiness, epistaxis, etc.

Radiographic Features

- Unilocular or multilocular radiolucency with a well-circumscribed border
- Multilocular honey comb appearance
- Driven snow appearance: Scattered flakes of calcification
- Lesion may be associated with a tooth.

Histopathology

- Amyloid-like nature which calcifies and is liberated as cells break down
- The areas of calcification form concentric rings called as "Liesegang rings".

Management

Complete excision of tumour with normal tissue margins.

Question 2

Explain TNM staging?

Answer

TNM classification/staging of malignant tumours is a notation system that gives codes in order to identify the stage, malignancy and spread of the tumour.

- T describes the size of the original (primary) tumour and whether it has invaded nearby tissue
- N describes nearby (regional) lymph nodes that are involved
- M describes distant metastasis (spread of cancer from one part of the body to another).

T: Size or direct extent of the primary tumour:

- Tx: Tumour cannot be evaluated
- Tis: Carcinoma in situ
- T0: No signs of tumour
- T1, T2, T3, T4: Size and/or extension of the primary tumour.

N: Degree of spread to regional lymph nodes:

- Nx: Lymph nodes cannot be evaluated
- N0: Tumour cells absent from regional lymph nodes
- N1: Regional lymph node metastasis present (at some sites: Tumour spread to closest or small number of regional lymph nodes)
- N2: Tumour spread to an extent between N1 and N3 (N2 is not used at all sites)
- N3: Tumour spread to more distant or numerous regional lymph nodes (N3 is not used at all sites).

M: Presence of distant metastasis:

- M0: No distant metastasis
- M1: Metastasis to distant organs (beyond regional lymph nodes).

Question 3

Explain adenomatoid odontogenic tumour (AOT)?

Answer

It is a haematoma first described by Stafne.

- Incidence: 3–7% of odontogenic tumour
- Age: 10–20 years. Rarely above 30 years
- Sex: More in females (65%)
- Site: Maxilla (65% usually in anterior region).

Clinical Features

- Associated with impacted permanent teeth, commonly with impacted canine
- Painless swelling.

Radiographic Features

- Unilocular radiolucency around associated tooth crown
- Resembles a dentigerous cyst
- Snowflake appearance due to fine calcification in the lesion
- Well defined and sclerotic margins.

Histopathology

- Thick, fibrous capsule surrounds the lesion
- Epithelial cells are polyhedral or spindle shaped
- Cells are arranged in sheets, cords or whorled masses forming a rosette-like structure
- Calcification is seen in several forms:
  - Laminated or ring like
  - Irregular dystrophic bodies
  - Large globular masses.

Management

- Surgical excision is done conservatively or enucleation is done
- Recurrence is rare .

Question 4

Explain odontoma?

Answer

Odontomas are tumours in which both epithelial cell and ectomesenchymal cells exhibit partial or complete differentiation of tooth formation. These are of two types:

1. Compound odontoma: It consists of formed calcified tooth-like structures
2. Complex odontoma: In this all the dental tissues are formed but are arranged in disordered pattern.

- Age: 10–20 years of age
- Sex: Equal predilection in both males and females
- Site: Occurs in both jaws
- Complex odontoma is more common in mandible (about 67%) and in posterior region
- Compound odontoma is more common in maxilla and in anterior region
- Clinically, they are asymptomatic.

Radiographic Features

- Compound odontoma:
  - Radiographic opacity is seen resembling normal tooth structure surrounded by a narrow radiolucent zone
  - Commonly seen alongside an unerupted tooth or between deciduous teeth roots.
- Complex odontoma:
  - May be small, large or huge, irregular or smooth, densely radiopaque surrounded by a radiolucent zone
  - Commonly seen overlying an unerupted tooth.

Clinical Features

- Asymptomatic
- No expansion of bone and facial asymmetry
- May show association with unerupted or impacted tooth.

Management

- They can be left untouched as they are biologically inert. Excised in case of:
  - Patient may be psychologically affected upon diagnosis
  - To remove blockage of unerupted tooth
  - To obtain definite diagnosis between complex odontoma and cementoblastoma or CEOT, etc.

Compound odontoma can be enucleated if capsule is intact; however, if the capsule is disrupted, individual tooth are removed carefully.

CHAPTER 11 Orofacial Pain

LONG ESSAYS

Question 1

Describe and classify nerve injuries?

Answer

Nerve injuries are injury to nervous tissue. These include total or partial transection of the nerve from cutting or laceration, shearing, crushing, compression or stretching injuries.

Etiology

- Accidents
- Acute trauma
- Carpel tunnel syndrome
- During or after surgery from traction
- Iatrogenic
- Some sports activity.

Incidence and Prevalence

- 95% of nerve injuries that occurs with fractures are located in the upper extremity
- 48% with shoulder dislocations
- 18% with knee dislocations
- 13% with hip dislocations.

Classification of nerve injury aids the clinician in making a diagnosis, developing a rational plan of management and determining whether surgical intervention is required.

Seddon's Classification

- Grade 1: Mildest or neuropraxia
- Grade 2: Severe or axonotmesis
- Grade 3: Most severe or neurotmesis.

Grade 1: Neuropraxia

- These are the least severe among nerve injuries
- Almost complete recovery can be achieved
- In these injuries the actual structure of the nerve is not damaged
- Interruption in the conduction of the impulse in the nerve fibre is seen in this type of nerve injury
- These injuries occurs due to compression of the nerve fibre or due to disruption of the blood supply
- The temporary loss of function is recovered within few hours to few months of injury
- These types of injuries are generally characterised by the involvement of motor function of the nerve while the sensory function remains intact.

Etiology

- Concussion or shock-like injury to the fibre
- Compression or relatively mild blunt blows.

Diagnosis

Electrodiagnostic testing with nerve conduction studies, there is a normal compound motor action potential amplitude distal to the lesion at day 10.

Grade 2: Axonotmesis

- More severe
- Disruption of the neuronal axon
- Myelin sheath maintained
- Wallerian degeneration: In this, the loss of continuity of the axon and myelin covering is seen
- However, the connective tissue is unharmed
- It leads to paralysis of autonomic, sensory, and motor function
- If the force that lead to the nerve damage is removed early, complete recovery of function can be achieved
- The nerve elicits rapid and complete degeneration with loss of voluntary motor units.

Etiology

- More severe crush injury than neuropraxia
- Contusion
- Also when the nerve is stretched (without damage to the perineurium).

Diagnosis

- Fibrillations and denervation potentials in musculature distal to the injury site can be seen when electromyography is done after 2–3 weeks
- Recovery take a long time as it occurs only through the regenerations of the axons.

Grade 3: Neurotmesis

These are most severe and damaging injury with least potential of recovering.

Etiology

- Local anaesthesia toxicity
- Stretch
- Laceration
- Severe contusion.

In this type of injury, involvement of complete axon alongwith the loss in continuity of the entire encapsulating connective tissue is seen.

Diagnosis

- Electromyography shows denervation changes similar to axonotmesis injury
- Complete loss of autonomic, sensory and motor function is seen
- In cases where the nerve gets completely divided, axonal regeneration causes a neuroma to form a proximal stump.

Sunderland's Classification

- 1st degree: Seddon's neuropraxia
- 2nd degree: Seddon's axonotmesis
- 3rd degree: Endoneurium disrupted, epineurium and perineurium intact
- 4th degree: Interruption of all neural and supporting elements
- 5th degree: Complete disruption with loss of continuity.

Question 2

Define trigeminal neuralgia and its management?

Answer

Definition

Trigeminal neuralgia is defined as sudden, usually unilateral, severe, brief, stabbing, lancinating, recurring pain in the distribution of one or more branches of fifth cranial nerve. Nicholaus Andre in 1756 coined the term "tic douloureux".

Etiology

- Dental etiology: According to Westrum and Black differentiation from loss of teeth and degeneration of nerve is not restricted to peripheral parts of ganglia, but proceeds proximally to involve areas of spinal nucleus
- Infections: Various granulomatous and non-granulomatous infections involving fifth nerve
- Ratner's jaw bone cavities: Cavities found in the alveolar and jaw bones are the causative factors
- Multiple sclerosis: Olfson suggested the presence of sclerotic plaque located at the root entry zone of trigeminal nerve
- Petrous ridge compression: Lee suggested trigeminal neuralgia maybe caused by compression of nerve at the dural foramen
- Post-traumatic neuralgia: Following traumas those resulting from some dental procedures may lead towards neuralgic pain
- Intracranial tumours: Many lesions, such as epidermoid tumours, meningiomas of cerebellopontine angle and Meckel's cave, arteriovenous malformations, aneurysms and vascular compression have been suggested as causes
- Intracranial vascular abnormalities: Compression at pons by an arterial loop of superior cerebellar artery or by venous compression by arteriovenous malformations. Aneurysm of internal carotid artery may cause trigeminal neuralgia
- Viral etiology: History of previous episode of infection by varicella zoster virus. Viral lesions of ganglion can be etiological factor.

Clinical Features

- It manifests as a sudden, intermittent, paroxysmal, unilateral, sharp shooting, lancinating, shock-like pain, which is elicited by slight touching of superficial "trigger points," which radiates from that points across the distribution of one or more branches of trigeminal nerve
- Pain is generally confined to one part of one division of trigeminal neuralgia
- Pain rarely crosses the midline
- Short duration pain lasting for few seconds
- Patient with pain clutches his hands over the effected side of the face and holds or rubs his face which may redden or the eye water until the attack subsides
- The paroxysms occur in episodes, each episode lasting for weeks or months and with time the cycle appears closer and closer

- Presence of intraoral or extraoral trigger points provocable by obvious stimuli is seen
- Locations of trigger points (**Fig. 11.1**):
  - In v2 (infra orbital commonly): On the skin of upper lip, ala nasi or cheeks or on upper gums
  - In v3 (inferior alveolar commonly): Over the lower lip, teeth or gums of the lower jaw, tongue is rarely involved
  - In v1: Over the supraorbital ridge.
- Attacks do not occur during sleep
- It is very common for these patient to undergo dental extractions on the effected side without any relief from pain
- More than 50% of the patients experience early remissions of greater than 6 months before return of active pain.

Diagnosis

- Well-recorded history
- Clinical examination
- Magnetic resonance imaging (MRI) scanning
- Computed tomography (CT) scan for localisation of compressive vessels
- Response to treatment with carbamazepine
- Diagnostic injections of local anesthesia into trigger zone should temporarily eliminate all pain.

Treatment

Medicinal treatment (modification of paroxysmal pain at cortical level):
- I/m morphine
- Trichloroethylene
- Diphenylhydantoin sodium
- Carbamazepine.

Carbamazepine: 100–400 mg tds

- For 1–5 weeks
- Maximum dose: 1200 mg/day
- Side effects: Visual blurring, dizziness, skin rashes, ataxia and rarely liver dysfunction, leukopenia and thrombocytopenia.

Clonazepam

- Maximum dose: 1.5 mg/day
- Side effects: Drowsiness, fatigue, lethargy.

Gabapentin: 100–300 mg tds

- Maximum dose: 900 mg/day
- Side effects: Ataxia, fatigue, headache, nausea, dizziness, tremor, diplopia and nystagmus.

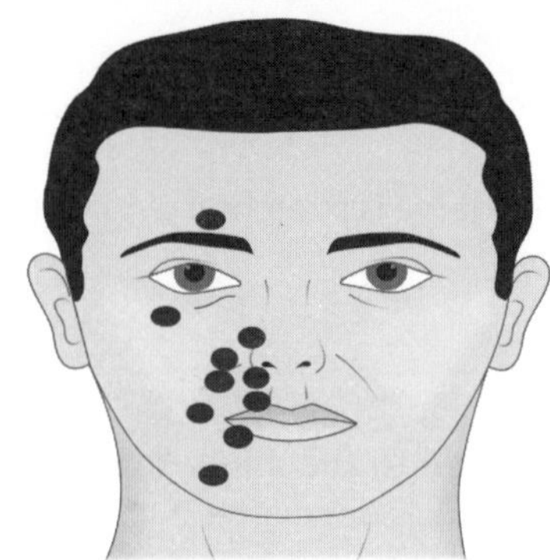

Fig. 11.1: Trigger points

Phenytoin: 100 mg tds

Side effects: Slurred speech, abnormal movements, swelling of lymph glands, gingival hypertrophy, hirsutism.

Oxcarbazepine

- Maximum dose: 1200 mg/day
- Side effects: Hyponatremia, double vision.

Valproic Acid

- Maximum dose: 600 mg/day
- Sideeffects: Irritability, tremors, confusion, hepatotoxicity, weight gain.

Mephenesin Carbamate (Tolceram)

Maximum dose: 5–15 mL/5 times a day to every 3 hours.

Surgical Management

- Extracranial management
- Intracranial management.

Extracranial

- Alcohol block in peripheral nerves
- Peripheral neurectomy
  - Supraorbital
  - Infraorbital
  - Lingual
  - Inferior alveolar.
- Electrosurgery
- Cryosurgery
- Radio frequency thermocoagulation.

Alcohol Block

- Injection of destructive substances into peripheral branches of trigeminal neuralgia helps to relieve pain

- Effect is short-lived
- Injection can be repeated if pain recurs
- Long anaesthetic agents: Bupivacaine without adrenaline with/without corticosteroids
- Alcohol injections: 95% absolute alcohol.

Disadvantages

- Repeated injections causes local tissue toxicity, inflammation and fibrosis
- Burning alcohol neuritis.

Peripheral Neurectomy

- Acts by interrupting the flow of a significant number of afferent impulses to central trigeminal apparatus
- Infraorbital nerve
  - Two approaches:
    - Intra oral conventional approach: U-shaped Caldwell–Luc incision
    - Braun's transantral approach: Provides direct access and visualisation.
- Lingual nerve
  - Vertical incision at the inner border of the ramus
  - In the region of the floor of the mouth, the nerve lies even more superficially and it can be easily found between the anterior pillars of the fauces at the root of the tongue.
- Inferior alveolar nerve.
  - Two approaches:
    - Extraoral approach: Risdon's incision
    - Intraoral approach: via Dr Ginwalla's incision.
  - Two incisions:
    - Inverted Y-incision
    - In buccal vestibule overlying mental foramen.

Cryosurgery

- Cryotherapy probe (nitrous oxide probe) at less than –60° C
- Applied for 1–2 minutes followed by 3 minutes thaw. To be repeated 3 times
- Regeneration of axon is expected.

Radio Frequency Thermocoagulation

- Radio frequency electrode with a capacity to destroy pain fibres is used
- 22 gauge lesion probe
- 65–75°C for 1–2 minutes.

Advantage

Low morbidity.

Disadvantages

- Patient cooperation
- Needs specific electric armamentarium.

Intracranial

- Gasserian ganglion procedures
- Medullary tractotomy
- Nerve decompression.

Gasserian ganglion Procedures

Three main percutaneous Gasserian ganglion procedures are:

- Glycerol injections
- Thermocoagulation
- Balloon compression
- Anaesthesia protocol:
  - Patient is admitted on the day of surgery
  - Nil by mouth 4 hours prior to surgery
  - Injection atropine (0.6 mg IM) 1 hour before surgery
  - Injection methahexitone: 1–2 mg/kg IV
  - Pulse oximeter, oxygen (O_2) saturation and vital signs continuously monitored
  - Intranasal O_2 and intravenous (IV) fluids to be given
  - Duration of procedure is 1 hour.
- Glycerol injections:
  - Glycerol or absolute alcohol is used
  - Causes low grade damage to nerve cells, presumably through dehydration
  - Induces pain relief in 80% cases
  - Spares the important ophthalmic division and motor root
  - 16 gauge spinal needle is used
  - Contrast medium is injected to check the position of the needle
  - 0.5–0.75 mL of pure glycerol or 0.5 mL of absolute alcohol.
- Radio frequency thermocoagulation: When an alternating current of high frequency is passed through the electrode, it produces ionisation in biological tissues. Heat results from ionic friction which leads to coagulation of tissues.
  - Indications:
    - Toxicity of drugs
    - Failure of other modalities
    - Dependence of drug for lifetime
    - Elderly patient
    - Medically compromised patients
    - Recurrence cases.

- Lesion production: Thermal lesions of 30–90 seconds duration are made at 65–75o C using RF generator of microwave energies
- Power: 25 watts, 40–45 volts. Current: 120–140 mAH
- A 5 mm bare tip electrode with 2 mm diameter will produce a lesion of 10 x 6 mm within the trigeminal root at 75o C.

- Balloon compression:
  - Done under general anesthesia
  - Mechanical technique to destroy root fibres partially
  - Done by advancing 4 FG Fogarty catheter 1–2 cm within Meckel's cave and inflating the balloon at the ventral aspect of the ganglion root
  - 12 gauge spinal needle
  - Balloon takes up pear shape of the Meckel's cave and it should remain inflated for 1 minute.

Nerve Decompression

- Most commonly performed intracranial open procedure
- Open craniotomy approach is used to gain access to the root entry zone of trigeminal nerve
- A compressing branch of the superior cerebellar artery will be seen medial to the nerve at the root entry zone
- The artery is carefully separated from the nerve and interpositioned by using sponge or Teflon wool
- Mortality rate: 2%
- Contraindicated in elderly and medically compromised patients.

Question 3

Define pain pathway?

Answer

Pain can be defined as"An unpleasant emotional experience usually initiated by a noxious stimulus and transmitted over a specialised neural network to the central nervous system where it is interpreted as such."

- Pain generally starts with a physical stimulus, like a cut, burn, tear or bump. Inhibitory effects are achieved by descending pathways, which send signals from conscious brain down to the subconscious brain and the spinal cord
- The pain system has a set of ascending pathways that convey nociceptive information from peripheral nociceptors to the central nervous system, as well as to descending pathways that modulate that information
- The body has mechanical peripheral nociceptors (first order neurons), which project to second order neurons in the spinal cord and medulla, from where the sensory information is carried (in the form of electrical impulse) to the thalamus, where it synapses with third order neurons that transmit the impulse to the cortex
- Second order neurons send their sensory inputs to the thalamus via two ascending pathways (**Fig. 11.2**):
  - Dorsal column medial: Lemniscal system
  - Anterolateral system (includes the spinothalamic, spinoreticular, and spinotectal fibers)
  - The lemniscal system transmits impulse involving position sense, touch, and pressure. The anterolateral pathway is involved in pain transmission
  - The spinal cord is the centre concourse along which all pain messages travel to and from the brain.

Chemical Mediators of Pain

- Nociceptors are specialised nerve endings in skin and deeper tissues. They activate only at high thresholds which are in the range of potentially damaging stimuli: Chemical, thermal, electrical or mechanical
- Nociceptors are activated by a variety of chemical mediators which are also associated with the redness and swelling of inflammation. They are as follows:

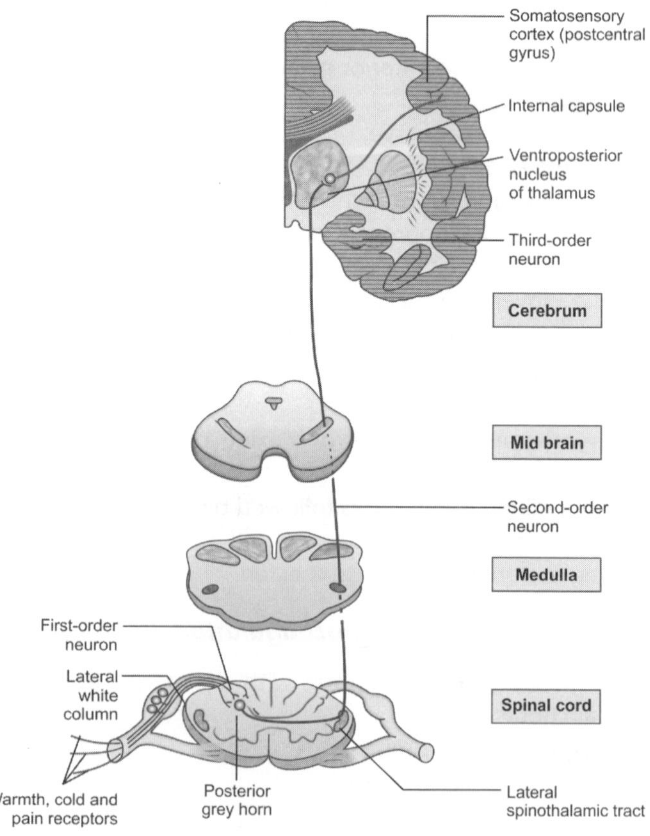

Fig. 11.2: Sensory pathway for pain and temperature— the lateral spinothalamic pathway

- Potassium (from damaged cells)
- Histamine (released from mast cells)
- Leukotrienes (released from damaged tissue)
- Serotonin (from platelets)
- Bradykinin (a peptide activated from a precursor in plasma)
- Prostaglandins
- Substance P (released from active nociceptors ending).

Question 4

Define Bell's palsy?

Answer

Bell's palsy is defined as an idiopathic paresis or paralysis of the facial nerve of sudden onset when there is unilateral lower motor neuron paralysis of sudden onset, not related to any other disease.

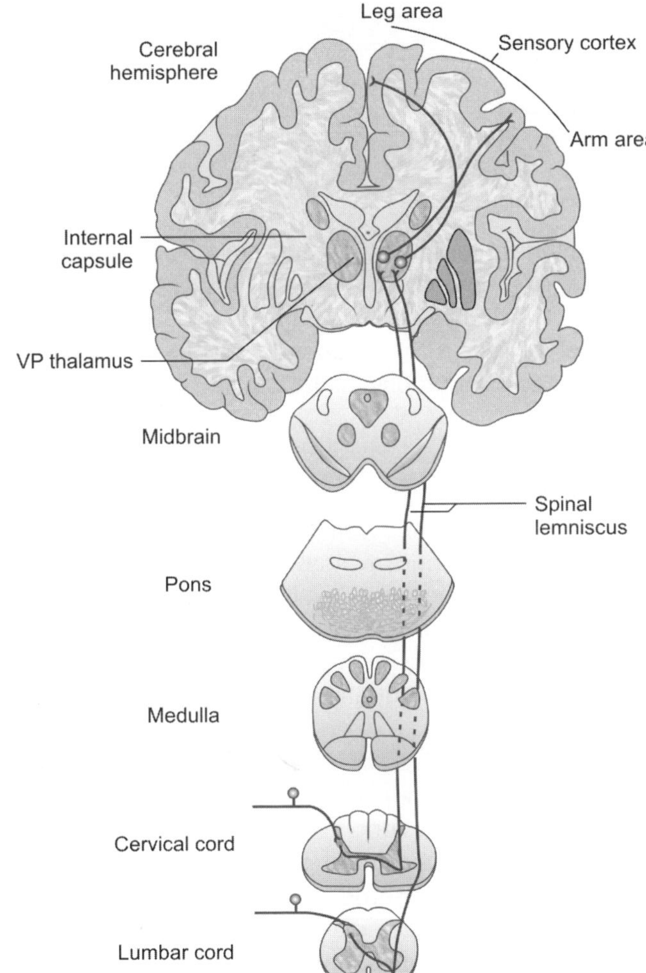

Fig. 11.3: The spinothalamic track system. The central pathways for pain, temperature, touch and pressure are illustrated

Sex Predilection

Women more affected than man especially pregnant women.

Age

At any age, but more common in middle-age people.

Etiology

Five hypotheses have been proposed, and a combination of these is considered to the cause.

- Rheumatic hypothesis: Rheumatic swelling may press the nerve against the walls of the fallopian canal. Obsolete theory
- Cold hypothesis: Caused due to exposure to extreme cold or cold draught
- Ischaemic hypothesis: Ischaemia because disturbed circulation in the vasoneurosum cause facial paralysis. The factors causing vasospasm are:
  - Cold
  - Anoxia
  - Carbon dioxide (CO_2) excess
  - Vasomotor instability
  - Injury
  - Allergy or hormonal imbalances.
- Immunological hypothesis: In vivo sensitisation of lymphocytes to peripheral nerve myelin gives rise to a cell-mediated immune response
- Viral hypothesis: This proposes that Bell's palsy occurs due to herpes zoster or herpes simplex infection.

Clinical Features

- Sudden onset, history generally elicits that occurrence after waking in early morning
- Unilateral involvement of the entire side of the face
- Whistling is impossible
- Abrupt loss of muscular control of one-half of the face
- Corner of mouth droop leading to drooling of saliva
- Inability to wrinkle the forehead
- When an attempt is made to close the eyelids, the eyeball rolls upwards with pupil being covered and only the sclera being visible
- This is called as Bell's sign
- Eye waters due to inability to close
- Widening of palpebral fissure and loss of blink reflex
- Speech becomes slurred
- Occasionally loss of taste also have been seen
- Slurred speech.

Management

- Physiotherapy: It is advised to maintain muscle tone and should be instituted as early as possible
- Medication: Patients with Bell's palsy who report within 3 days of the onset of symptoms should be prescribed a 7-day course of oral acyclovir/valacyclovir with a tapering course of oral prednisone
  - Acyclovir:
    - Adults: 400 mg 5 times daily for 7 days
    - Children older than 2 years: 80 mg/kg daily divided every 6 hours for 5 days, with a maximal dose of 3,200 mg daily.
  - Valacyclovir:
    - Adults and children older than 12 years: 1 g 3 times daily for 7 days.
  - Prednisone or prednisolone:
    - Adults: 60 mg daily for 5 days, then 40 mg daily for 5 days
    - Children: 2 mg/kg daily for 7–10 days.

Patients who do not improve in 2 weeks after above medication should be referred to an otolaryngologist for evaluation of other possible causes of the facial nerve palsy. Patients should be prescribed eye lubrication as eye irritation is a common feature in such cases. Patients with corneal abrasions should be immediately referred to an ophthalmologist for treatment.

Surgical decompression within 3 weeks of onset has been recommended for patients who have persistent loss of function (greater than 90% loss on electroneurography) at 2 weeks. The most common complication of surgery is postoperative hearing loss.

SHORT ESSAYS

Question 1

Define atypical facial pain?

Answer

Atypical facial pain is a pain disorder which resembles trigeminal neuralgia but is a different entity.

The symptoms are more persistent, localised to one side of the face, and can be presented as sharp, dull, crushing, burning, aching, squeezing or pulling type.

Etiology

- Dental infection
- Sinus infection
- Temporal tendinitis
- Ernest syndrome
- Vagus nerve tumors
- Trigeminal ganglia compression
- Trigeminal nerve trauma
- Cervical spine disorder
- Facial trauma.

Risk Factors

- Facial injury
- Adult age
- Infections
- Inflammation
- Extensive dental work.

Diagnosis

- Neurological examination and ruling out trigeminal neuralgia, temporomandibular joint (TMJ) disorders, cluster headaches, and migraine
- X-rays of the skull. Magnetic resonance imaging/computed tomography (MRI/CT) scan.

Treatment

- Medications:
  - Amitriptyline (antidepressant)
  - Gabapentin (anticonvulsant)
  - Carbamazepine (anticonvulsant)
  - Baclofen (muscle relaxant/antispasmodic)
  - Clonazepam (muscle relaxant/anticonvulsant)
  - Valproic (anticonvulsant).
- Invasive procedures:
  - Microvascular decompression
  - Glycerol injection
  - Balloon compression
  - Peripheral nerve stimulation
  - Stereotactic radiosurgery
  - Percutaneous trigeminal tractotomy
  - Motor cortex stimulation.

SHORT NOTES

Question 1

Define Tinel's sign?

Answer

Tinel's sign is elicited by percussion over the divided nerve, which results in a tingling sensation in the part supplied by the peripheral section.

This method was earlier used as an indication of the start of nerve regeneration. Now electroneurography diagnostic studies are carried out serially for evidence of reinnervation.

Question 2

Define trigger zones?

Answer

Trigger zone is a characteristic feature of trigeminal neuralgia patient. This is a small area in the central part of the face, generally on cheek, nose or lips, which when stimulated, triggers a sharp burst of pain.

The stimulant can be:

- A light touch or vibration
- Gust of air striking the face
- Striking of water while washing of face
- Eating
- Chewing
- Shaving
- Talking.

Many people avoid food and drink rather than experience the severe pain. People generally remain pain free between attacks.

However, few patients experience a dull ache between attacks, suggesting physical compression of the affected nerve, either by a blood vessel or some other structure.

CHAPTER 12 Aids, Bacterial and Viral Infections

LONG ESSAYS

Question 1

What are the oral manifestations of HIV infection? Explain in detail?

Answer

Oral lesions in HIV infected patients are very common. Commonly associated oral manifestation seen in HIV infected patients are:

- Oral hairy leukoplakia
- Oral candidiasis
- Kaposi sarcoma
- Bacillary (epithelioid) angiomatosis
- Oral hype pigmentation
- Atypical ulcers and delayed healing.

Oral Hairy Leukoplakia

Commonly seen in patients with HIV infection:

- Site of infection is generally lateral borders of tongue, commonly bilaterally distributed and sometimes may extend to the ventrum
- Sometimes, it also affects dorsum of tongue, buccal mucosa, floor of mouth, retromolar area and soft palate
- Characterised clinically by asymptomatic, poorly demarcated keratotic areas ranging from few millimetres to several centimetres. Often, vertical striations are seen which give it a corrugated appearance. Sometimes, surface is shaggy and gives a hairy appearance
  - The lesion does not rub off and resembles other keratotic oral lesions
  - Candidal infections are secondary to this and colonies can be seen on surface of the lesion.
- Microscopically, hyperkeratotic surface with projection that resemble hair
  - Below parakeratotic surface, acanthosis and balloon cells resembling koilocytes are seen
  - These cells contain virus particles of herpes group and Epstein–Barr virus.
- Differential diagnosis: Dysplasia, lichen planus, carcinoma, tobacco-related leukoplakia, frictional and idiopathic keratosis, psoriasiform lesions and hyperplastic candidiasis
- Microscopic confirmation of oral hairy leukoplakia serves as an indicator that patient will develop AIDS
- Severity of lesion is not correlated with chances of developing AIDS, thus, small as well as extensive lesions are diagnostically significant.

Oral Candidiasis

- It is a fungal infection, which is associated with Candida albicans
- It is the most common oral lesion and is seen in 90% of AIDS patients
- It is of four types:
  1. Pseudomembranous candidiasis: It is also known as oral thrush. It is a white lesion that can be easily scraped and removed from oral mucosa. Commonly seen on hard and soft palate and buccal and labial mucosa
  2. Erythematous candidiasis: It is a pseudomembranous type lesion. Appears as red patches on buccal and palatal mucosa. May be associated with depapillation of the tongue
  3. Hyperplastic candidiasis: Least common form. Seen on tongue and buccal mucosa. It is resistant to removal
  4. Angular cheilitis: Commissures are erythematous with crusting and fissuring of surface.
- Microscopically, smear of lesion is obtained by scraping the lesion and viewed in a microscope. The lesion shows hyphae and yeast forms of organisms
- Candidiasis in HIV infected patients respond to antifungal treatment but is refractory and recurs within 4 weeks to 3 months due to the decreased immunocompetency of the individual.

Kaposi Sarcoma

- Kaposi sarcoma is generally a rare, multifocal, slow growing malignant vascular neoplasm
- However, in AIDS patient, it is an aggressive lesion and is reported in almost 70% of the patients affecting oral mucosa mainly palate and gingiva
- In early stages, the oral lesions are painless, reddish purple macules of the oral mucosa
- As the lesion progresses, they become nodular
- It manifests as modules, papules, or non-elevated macules generally brown, blue or purple in colour
- Microscopically, formed of four components, endothelial cell proliferation with atypical vascular channels, extravascular haemorrhage with hemosiderin deposition, spindle cell proliferation with atypical vessels and mononuclear inflammatory infiltrate formed mainly of plasma cells
- Differential diagnosis: Pyogenic granuloma, atypical hyper-pigmentation, sarcoidosis, angiosarcoma, haemangioma, bacillary angiomatosis, pigmented nevi and cat scratch disease.

Bacillary (Epithelioid) Angiomatosis

- Bacillary angiomatosis (BA) is an infectious vascular proliferative disease similar to Kaposi sarcoma clinically and histologically
- Aetiology: Rickettsia-like organisms, Bartonella henselae, Bartonella quintana, etc.
- Clinically, BA appears as red, purple or blue oedematous soft tissue lesion, which causes destruction of periodontal ligament and bone
- Differentiation of BA from Kaposi sarcoma is done by biopsy, which shows an epitheloid proliferation of angiogenic cells with acute inflammatory cell infiltrate
- Warthin–Starry silver stain reacts with causative organisms in the biopsy specimen.

Oral Hyperpigmentation

- There is an increased incidence of oral hyperpigmentation in HIV-affected individuals
- Pigmented areas appear as spots or striations on buccal mucosa, gingiva, palate or tongue
- Pigmentation can be due to prolonged use of drugs as zidovudine, ketoconazole or clofazimine.

Atypical Ulcers and Delayed Healing

- Atypical ulcers in HIV infected individual are commonly associated with neoplasms, lymphoma, Kaposi sarcoma, squamous cell carcinoma and neutropenia
- Klebsiella pneumoniae, Enterobacter cloacae and Escherichia coli have been seen causing ulcers in oral mucosa
- Herpes simplex virus, varicella zoster virus, Epstein–Barr virus or cytomegalovirus have been retrieved from oral ulcers
- Management: Neutropenia can be treated with recombinant human granulocyte colony stimulating factor
- Prolonged oral ulcers can be managed using prednisone or thalidomide
- Viral infection can be treated with zidovudine, trimethoprim-sulfamethoxazole or ganciclovir.

Question 2

Discuss in detail about the aetiology, clinical features, differential diagnosis and treatment options for acute necrotizing ulcerative gingivitis?

Answer

It is also referred to as Vincent's infection.

- Acute necrotizing ulcerative gingivitis (ANUG) is rapid in onset, painful microbial disease of the gingiva
- Its main causative microorganism is fusobacterium species, along with spirochetes
- ANUG has been renamed as NUG (necrotizing ulcerative gingivitis)
- It is also referred to as trench mouth, because of its prevalence in the soldiers working in trenches in World War I
- Disease is also known as Vincent angina because this disease was first described by Vincent.

Aetiology

- It is mainly caused by fusobacterium and spirochetes
- The consular of microorganisms consists of following bacteria—Treponema microdentium, intermediate spiro-chetes, Vibrios, fusiform bacilli and filament airs organism Borrelia species.

Predisposing Factors

It can be divided into three:

1. Local factors
2. .Systemic factors
3. Psychosomatic factor.

Local Factors

- Smoking and use of tobacco
- Preexisting gingivitis, deep periodontal pockets and pericoronal flaps which favour the proliferation of anaerobic fusiform bacilli and spirochetes.

Systemic Predisposing Factors

- Immunodeficient patients
- Nutritional deficiencies like vitamin C and B2 deficiencies
- Chronic sleep deficiency leading to fatigue
- Habits, like alcohol or drug abuse
- Systemic disease like diabetes
- Other desalinating diseases like syphilis, cancer, severe GIT disorders, anaemia, leukaemia and AIDS.

Psychosomatic Factor

This disease is attributed to stressful situations like patients with depression or any emotional disturbances, patients feeling inadequate at handling life situations.

Clinical Features

- It presents as an acute disease and symptoms are under in onset
- In some cases, it can resolve on its own and shows milder symptoms which lead to absolute stage
- Some common predisposing factor cause be debilitating disease or acute respiratory tract infection, psychological stress, nutritional deficiencies, use of tobacco, smoking and continuous work without rest.

Characteristics Clinical Signs are as follows

- This infection shows punched-out, crater-like depression at the curst of the interdental papillae and it might involve the marginal gingiva
- Attached gingiva and oral mucosa are rarely involved
- As lough, which is grey in colour and pseudomembranous in nature, covers the gingival craters
- It can be demarcated from the healthy gingiva by a pronounced linear erythema
- In some cases, lesions may be divided of the pseudo-membranous, imposing red, shiny and haemorrhagic gingival surface
- Lesion bleeds even on slightest provocations
- Fetid odour
- Increased salivation
- Pasty silver
- Metallic foul texts
- Generally, patient complains of a constant radiating, graving pain that aggravate upon taking hot and spicy food and upon churning
- Extra-oral and systemic sign and symptoms are local lymphadenopathy and mild fever
- In severe cases, following sign can occur: High fever, increased pulse rate, leukocytosis, loss of appetite and general lassitude
- These signs and symptoms are more severe in children.

Clinical Courses

If NUG is undertaken, it may progress to necrotizing ulcerative periodontitis.

The staging of NUG given by Horning and Cohen is as follows:

- Stage 1: Necrosis of the tip of the interdental papilla (NUG)
- Stage 2: Necrosis of the inertia papilla (either NUG or NUP)
- Stage 3: Necrosis of the marginal gingiva (NUP)
- Stage 4: Necrosis intending to the marginal gingiva (NUP)
- Stage 5: Necrosis involving the buccal and labial mucosa (necrotizing stomatitis)
- Stage 6: Necrosis imposing alveolar bone (necrotizing stomatitis)
- Stage 7: Necrosis perforating skin of cheek (NOMA).

Various zones of the Lesion

Various zones in the lesion, described by Listgarten, may overlap one another, and all zones may not be present at the same time.

Zone I (Bacterial Zone)

This is the most superficial zone. It consists of various bacteria and fuel spirochetes, which can be of small medium and large types.

Zone 2 (Neutrophil-rich Zone)

This zone contains numerous leukocytes, mainly leukocyte with bacteria, including spirochetes of various types interspersed in between the leukocytes.

Zone 3 (Necrotic Zone)

It consists of disintegrate torsos cells, fibular material, remnant of collagen fibres, and many intermediate and large types of spirochetes, with few other bacteria.

Zone 4 (Zone of Spirochetes Infiltration)

This zone contains well-preserved tissues infiltrated with intermediate and large spirochetes without other organisms.

Diagnosis

- Diagnosis can be made by clinical picture of the patient, which includes gingival pain, bleeding and ulceration
- Biopsy specimen, or a microscopic examination of a bacterial smear would not give a clear diagnosis
- NUG can be differentiated from other infections, such as tuberculosis through a biopsy specimen.

Treatment for NUG

Treatment objectives of NUG are as follows:

- Resolution of acute phase
- Treatment of chronic disease either underlying the acute involvement or in the oral cavity
- Alleviation of generalized symptoms, such as fever and malaria
- Correction of systemic aetiological factors, such as smoking and stress
- NUG can be treated in three clinical visits.

First Visit

- Primary goal of this visit is the treatment of acute lesion
- Complete medical history and history of present illness should be recorded
- Dietary history and smoking history should be taken
- HIV risk factor and psychological factors should be evaluated
- Vitals signs should be recorded, along with palpation of lymph nodes, mainly submaxillary and segmental lymph nodes
- Any skin lesion present should be evaluated
- After all these basic evaluations and recordings, the pseudomembrane and surface debris should be gently removed with a most action and a topical anaesthetic should be applied over the affected area
- Supragingival scaling, using an ultrasonic instrument should be done
- Subgingival scaling is contraindicated at this stage, since it can lead to extension of the infection and bacteraemia
- Any kind of periodontal surgery or extractions are postponed, until the patient becomes symptom-free. And, it usually takes about 4 weeks, for a patient to become symptom-free
- Patient should be prescribed the following antibiotics:
  - Amoxicillin 500 mg rarely every 6 hours for 10 days
  - If patient is allergic to penicillin, then in that case, erythromycin 500 mg every 6 hours, or metronidazole 500 mg twice daily for 7 days.

Analgesics, such as NSAIDS, can be prescribed to the patient, so as to get relief from pain. Instructions to be given to the patient on first visit are as follows:

- Patient should avoid habits, such as tobacco, smoking, alcohol and condiments
- Patients are advised to rinse with 3% hydrogen peroxide mixed with equal amount of warm water every 2 hours, or twice daily with 0.2% chlorhexidine mouthwash
- Overzealous tooth brushing and interdental cleaning device should be avoided
- For tooth brushing, an ultra soft toothbrush should be used
- Adequate rest should be taken by the patient.

Second Visit

- 1–2 days after the first visit, the second visit should be scheduled
- All the systemic signs and symptoms should be checked if they have or not resolved
- The lesion would be still present but with marked reduction of necrotic tissue
- Scaling can be performed during their visit
- All the instruction given during the first visit should be followed by the patient.

Third Visit

- Patient is evaluated after a period of 5 days after the second visit, to check for resolution of the symptoms
- Complete protocol for the periodontal management is planned during this visit
- Patient avoids to discontinue the hydrogen peroxide rinse and continue with chlorhexidine mouthwash for 2 or 3 times
- Scaling and root planning can be repeated if required
- Patient should be reinterred to following proper plaque control measurements
- The patients are counselled on nutrition, smoking cessation and other associated habits, to present further possible recurrence
- All the local irritants like faulty restorations should be removed. Chronic gingivitis, periodontal pockets, should be treated well
- After a period of one month, the patient to re-evaluated for oral hygiene maintenance, habits, psychosocial factors and determination of the need for reconstructive or aesthetic surgery
- Other than their treatment, some additional treatment should also be given to the patient such as:
  - Contouring of gingival margin (gingivoplasty)
  - Nutritional and supplements
  - Contouring of gingival margin.

The normal gingival architecture is applied in cases of NUG because there is severe loss of interdental gingiva and bone. This can be removed by a procedure known as gingivoplasty or gingivectomy in which normal gingival architecture is obtained.

Nutritional Supplements

- Patient is unable to take food because of pain, therefore nutritional supplement should be indicated with the local treatment

- A standard multivitamin preparation should be given to the patient, along with therapeutic dose of vitamins B and C.

Question 3

Describe in detail about the aetiology, clinical features, histopathology and differential diagnosis of acute herpetic gingivostomatitis?

Answer

- Acute herpetic gingivostomatitis is an infection of the mouth mostly affecting infants and children younger than 6 years of age
- The causative organisms is HSV-1 (herpes simplex virus type 1)
- Clinical Features
- This infection is mostly seen in children and young adult
- Males and females are equally affected
- There are vesicular lesions, which are painful and develop on all mucosal surfaces and rupture to produce foul smelling ulcers
- Patient is usually febrile, drools, and has significant malaria and will have tender cervical lymphadenopathy
- Acute illness and lesions last about 10 days and resolve with scar formation
- HSV-1 has access to the patient through direct or airborne water droplet transmission from an infected individual
- The mucous membrane lesions represent direct viral infection at the sites of inoculation
- After primary infection, the virus ascends through nursery and autonomic nerves and persists as latent HSV in the neuronal ganglia that innervates the sites
- HSV-1 mostly resides in the trigeminal ganglion
- Various sources, such as sunlight, trauma, fever and stress can result in secondary manifestation.

Oral Signs

- Gingiva and oral mucosa, both are involved
- In the initial stage, the characteristic feature is the presence of discrete, spherical grey vesicles on the gingiva, labial and buccal mucosa, soft palate, pharynx, sublingual mucosa and the tongue
- The vesicles rupture in 24 hours and form painful, small ulcers with a red, elevated, hole-like margin and a depressed, whitish or greyish white contra portion
- The ulcers may occur in dust as or can be widely separated
- In a few cases, the lesion may be diffuse, erythematous, shiny discoloration and oedematous enlargement of the gingiva with a tendency to bleed
- The lesion wound resolve by 7–10 days on its own
- It heals without scarring.

Symptoms

- Slowness of the mouth associated with difficulty in drinking and eating food
- Lesions are painful and sensitive to touch.

Constitutional Signs and Symptoms are as follows

- High grade fever
- Generalized malaria
- Cervical adenitis.

Diagnosis

- Diagnosis is made mainly by taking a detailed history and performing a proper clinical examination
- Virus culture and immunologic tests should be performed using monoclonal antibodies or DNA hybridisation techniques to confirm the diagnosis.

Differential Diagnosis

- Necrotizing ulcerative gingivitis
- Recurrent aphthous stomatitis
- Erythema multiforme
- Stevens–Johnson syndrome
- Bullous lichen planus.

Treatment

- Earlier the treatment only consisted of supportive care but recently on antiviral therapy with 15 mg/kg of an acyclovir suspension is given 5 times daily for 7 days
- But, this therapy is affective only if the patient reports or is being diagnosed within 3 days of onset
- Patients reporting after 3 days of onset should be given a palliative care, which includes removal of plaque and food debris, administration of NSAIDS and nutritional supplements
- Periodontal theory should be postponed until the acute symptoms subside.

SHORT ESSAYS

Question 1

What are the periodontal manifestations of HIV infection?

Answer

Periodontal manifestation of HIV infections are:

Linear Gingival Erythema

- This is characterised by persistent, linear, easily bleeding erythematous gingivitis
- May serve as precursor to rapidly progressing necrotizing ulcerative periodontitis
- May be localized or generalized
- May be limited to marginal tissue
- Extends into attached gingiva in a punctuate or diffuse erythema
- Extends into alveolar mucosa.

Necrotizing Ulcerative Gingivitis (NUG)

Some reports have shown increase in incidence of NUG in HIV infected patients.

Necrotizing Ulcerative Stomatitis (NUS)

- NUS is characterized by necrosis of oral soft tissue and underlying bone
- It can occur alone or in conjunction with necrotizing ulcerative periodontitis
- Severe depression of CD4 immune cells is seen.

Necrotizing Ulcerative Periodontitis

- Characterized by soft tissue necrosis, rapid periodontal destruction and interproximal bone loss
- Lesions are seen anywhere in dental arches and are generally localized to a few teeth
- Generalized NUP can be seen after marked CD4+ cell depletion
- Exposed bone undergoes necrosis and subsequent sequestration
- It is a severely painful condition and requires immediate treatment.

Question 2

What are the periodontal findings of AIDS?

Answer

All HIV infected patients may not know that they are infected when they report for dental treatment. Individuals with known HIV infection may not admit their status on the medical history.

- Thus, every patient receiving dental treatment should be managed as a potentially infected person, using universal precautions for all therapy
- Extensive periodontal treatment plans must be considered in regard to the patients systemic health, prognosis and survival time
- Large variations in progression of HIV disease exist among individuals, and selection of an appropriate treatment plan depends on the state of the patients overall health
- Although there appears to be few contraindications to routine dental treatment for many HIV infected patients, the periodontal treatment plan is influenced by the patients overall systemic health and coincident oral infections or diseases
- Anawareness of oral disorders associated with HIV infection allows the clinician to recognize previously undiagnosed disease or to modify treatment protocols appropriately.

SHORT NOTES

Question 1

What is necrotizing gingivostomatitis?

Answer

The three conditions, i.e., linear gingival erythema, necrotizing ulcerative gingivitis and necrotizing ulcerative periodontitis, all these conditions may be collectively referred to as necrotizing gingivostomatitis.

Staging of Necrotizing Gingivostomatitis

Staging of necrotizing infections was proposed by Pindborg, who described four stages:

1. Only the tip of the interdental papilla is affected
2. Marginal gingiva was affected with punched out papilla
3. Attached gingiva is also affected
4. Exposure of bone.

CHAPTER 13

Metabolic Disorders

LONG ESSAYS

Question 1

Classify vitamins and what are the causes of vitamin deficiency? Discuss vitamin B complex?

Answer

Classification of vitamins is shown in the following **Flowchart 13.1**:

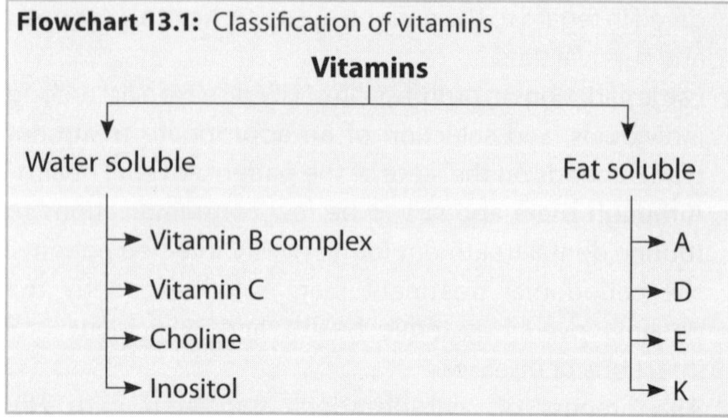

Flowchart 13.1: Classification of vitamins

Causes of Vitamin Deficiency

- Decreased amount of intake of essential nutrients
- Impaired absorption from the alimentary tract
- Increased metabolism due to rapid growth
- Inadequate storage, fever and pregnancy.

Vitamin B Complex

- Most of vitamin B complex occurs in nature in the bound form within the cells of vegetables or animal tissues
- Vitamin B complex is not stored in appreciable amounts in the body tissues except vitamin B_{12}
- Excretion of vitamins occur in the kidneys
- Vitamin B complex has:
  - Vitamin B_1 (Thiamine)
  - Vitamin B_2 (Riboflavin)
  - Vitamin B_3 (Niacin)
  - Vitamin B_5 (Pantothenic acid)
  - Vitamin B_6 (Pyridoxine)
  - Vitamin B_8 (Biotin)
  - Vitamin B_9 (Folic acid)
  - Vitamin B_{12} (Cyanocobalamin).

Vitamin B_1 (Thiamine)

- Also known as aneurin
- It is readily absorbed from both small and large intestine
- It is phosphorylated by liver and kidney
- Excess thiamine is excreted in the urine.

Sources

Cereals, pulses, vegetable, nuts, oilseeds, fruits, milk and meat.

Daily Requirements

- Men: 1.3 mg daily
- Women: 1.0 mg daily
- Children: 1.1 mg daily
- Pregnancy and lactation: 2 mg daily.

Functions

- Promotes growth, stimulates brain action and protects heart muscle
- Helps in normal functioning of nervous system
- Helps in digestion
- It is a mild diuretic and increases urine formation
- It improves peristalsis
- Maintains the normal blood count and improves circulation.

Deficiency Symptoms

- Digestive symptoms: Patient complains of loss of appetite, poor digestion, chronic constipation and weight loss

- Nervous disorders: Mental depression, nervous exhaustion and insomnia
- Heart: Hypertrophy of heart can take place
- Beri-beri: Prolonged deficiency can cause beri-beri. There are three types of beri-beri:
  1. Wet beri-beri
  2. Dry beri-beri
  3. Infantile beri-beri.
- Other diseases associated with it are:
  - Wernicke's encephalopathy
  - Peripheral neuritis
  - Korsakoff's psychosis.

Beri-Beri

Wet Beri-Beri

There is cardiac dilation with pallor, flabbiness of myocardium and four chamber enlargements.

Aetiology:

- Diet: It can be due to intake of polished rice
- Seen in chronic alcoholics
- Can be precipitated by infection, pregnancy and lactation
- Pathogenesis (**Flowchart 13.2**).

Flowchart 13.2: Pathogenesis of wet beri-beri

Thiamine deficiency
↓
Incomplete metabolism of glucose
↓
Accumulation of pyruvic acid and lactic acid in tissue and body fluid
↓
Dilation of peripheral blood vessels
↓
Fluid may leak out through capillaries, producing oedema
↓
High cardiac output
↓
Heart dilation

Clinical features:

- Pain in legs
- Tachycardia, increased blood pressure, cardiomegaly, increased JVP and palpitations
- Presence of sinus tachycardia and inverted T-waves
- Skin becomes warm due to vasodilation
- Oedema may be there involving leg, face and trunk. Management
- Complete rest
- 50 mg thiamine i.m. for 3 days and then 10 mg 3 times daily orally
- Infantile beri-beri is treated by mother's milk.

Dry Beri-Beri

Clinical features:

- It is a peripheral neuropathy
- Demyelination and degeneration of both sensory and motor nerve fibres resulting in severe wasting of muscles.

Oral manifestation:

- Oral mucosa becomes hypersensitive
- Pain in teeth, jaw, tongue and face.

Vitamin B_2 (Riboflavin)

- Also referred to as beauty vitamin
- Absorbedreadilyfromtheintestineandisphosphorylated in the wall of the intestine
- Stored in liver, kidneys and heart
- Riboflavin is excreted primarily in the urine and bile and sweat.

Sources

Cereals, pulses, legumes, vegetables, milk and fruits.

Daily Requirements

- Infants: 60 mcg value per kg of body weight daily
- Men: 1.5 mg daily
- Women: 1.2 mg daily
- Children: 1.3 mg daily
- Pregnancy and lactation: 2–2.3 mg daily.

Functions

- It is important for growth and general wealth
- Involved in metabolism of carbohydrates, fats and proteins
- Helps in proper functioning of nervous system
- Promotes healthy skin, nails and hair and alleviates eye strain.

Reasons for Deficiency

- Primary deficiency: Due to inadequate diet
- Secondary deficiency:
  - It can occur because of the intestinal tract

- Can occur due to prolonged use of drug, like psychological drugs which interfere with production of flavin monophosphate
- Burns, trauma and chronic alcoholism.

Deficiency Symptoms

- Nasolabial fold and ala of the nose exhibits a scaly gray dermatitis
- There is corneal vasodilation, photophobia and superficial and interstitial keratitis
- Increase burning and itching of eyes can be there
- Can lead to dull hair and oily skin, premature wrinkles
- There can be malfunctioning of adrenal glands, anaemia, vaginal itching and cataract.

Oral Manifestation

- Glossitis
- Filiform papillae becomes atrophic
- In several cases, tongue may become glazed and smooth because of complete atrophy of the papillae and exhibits a magenta colour
- Lips become red and shiny due to desquamation of epithelium
- Lips can also turn pale and cheilitis can be seen as maceration and fissuring at the angle of the mouth
- Angular cheilitis may spread to the cheek as the disease advances, the tissues bleed easily and are painful if secondarily infected.

Management

Riboflavin 25,000–50,000 mcg daily in divided doses.

Vitamin B_3 (Niacin)

Also called as nicotinic acid.

- It is essential for formation of co-enzyme NAD and NADP that are essential pyridine nucleotides, which are important for redox reactions involving carbohydrate, protein and lipid metabolism
- Its deficiency leads to pellagra which causes the skin to be dry and rough
- It can be absorbed from stomach and intestine and stored in all tissues
- Excreted in the urine. Sources
- Cereals, pulses, legumes, vegetables, nuts, oilseeds, fruits and milk and tryptophan.

Daily Requirements

- Men: 17 mg daily
- Women: 13 mg daily
- Children: 15 mg daily
- Pregnancy and lactation: 12–15 mg daily.

Functions of B_3

- Helps in proper blood circulation
- Helps in proper functioning of nervous system
- Important for metabolism of proteins and carbohydrates
- Increases the flow of blood to the peripheral capillary system
- Necessary for the synthesis of sex hormone, oestrogen, progesterone and testosterone
- Helps in skin maintenance.

Pellagra

Caused due to deficiency of vitamin B_3.

Reasons for Deficiency

- In cases of deficient tryptophan which is important for synthesis of niacin
- Deficiency of diet of niacin
- Diarrhoea, carcinoid syndrome and chronic alcoholism.

Clinical Features

- Prodromal symptoms can develop in 3 weeks which are decrease of appetite, vague gastrointestinal disturbances and numbness or burning in various sites. It is known as 3-Ds:
  - Dermatitis
  - Diarrhoea
  - Dementia.
- Skin shows erythema
- Acute cases may have skin lesions producing vesicles, cracking, exudation, crusting with ulceration and secondary infection
- Dermatitis can occur in chronic cases
- Anorexia, nausea, dysphagia
- Diarrhoea is due to atrophy of gastric epithelium formed by sub-mucosal inflammation, which is followed by ulceration
- Delirium occurs in acute cases and dementia in chronic form
- Loss of appetite, irritability and burning sensation in different areas of the body.

Oral Manifestation

- Oral mucosa becomes fiery red and painful
- There is profuse salivation
- Filiform papillae are lost first as they are most sensitive
- Fungiform papillae becomes enlarged

- Tongue becomes beefy red and swollen, and may lead to black tongue in animals
- Sore mouth is there and shows angular stomatitis
- At the interdental papillae, pain, tenderness and ulceration begins which spreads rapidly
- Superimposed acute necrotizing ulcerative gingivitis (ANUG) is commonly seen.

Management

- Niacin: 10 mg or 10,000 mcg per day
- Vitamin-B complex
- Alcohol should be avoided.

Vitamin B_5 (Pantothenic Acid)

- It plays a vital role in the metabolism of carbohydrate, fats and proteins, and in the synthesis of amino acids and fatty acids
- Important for formation of porphyris.

Deficiency Symptoms

- Chronic fatigue, muscle cramps, painful and burning feet
- Mental depression, irritability, dizziness and insomnia
- Can lead to gastric distress and constipation.

Management

Given in dose of 1000 mg daily for 6 weeks.

Vitamin B_6 (Pyridoxine)

It is an essential co-enzyme in the intramedullary metabolism of amino acids and complex glycolipids.

Deficiency Symptoms

- Peripheral neuropathy, mental retardation, irritability, mental confusion and nervousness
- Anaemia, albuminuria and leukopenia
- Dermatitis and eczema.

Oral Manifestation

Cheilosis, glossitis, angular stomatitis, tooth decay and halitosis.

Management

10–50 mg daily in divided doses.

Vitamin B_8 (Biotin)

It acts as a co-enzyme for four carbohydrates involved in fatty acid and amino acid metabolism.

Functions

- Helps in metabolism of carbohydrates, fats and proteins
- Important for the growth and health of the hair
- Prevents premature greying of the hair
- Helps to maintain skin and nervous system.

Deficiency Symptoms

- Scaly dermatitis, eczema, prickling of the skin and eczema
- Alopecia and dandruff
- Confusion, mental depression and drowsiness
- Muscular weakness, extreme fatigue and lassitude.

Management

- 20 mg of biotin for 10 days i.m. for skin lesion
- Oral biotin can be taken 400 mcg daily for 8–12 weeks.

Vitamin B_9 (Folic Acid)

- Also called as folacin or folate
- Absorbed along the entire length of the intestine
- Small amount excreted in the faeces and urine, and additional amount is presumed to be metabolised and lost by cells coming off in the form of scales, from the body surface.

Dietary Lower

Cereals, pulses, legumes, nuts, oilseeds, vegetables and meat.

Daily Requirements

- Men and women: 100 mcg
- Children: 80 mcg
- Infants: 25 mcg
- Pregnant women: 400 mcg
- Lactating women: 150 mcg.

Functions

- Folic acid along with vitamin B_{12} is essential for the formation, maturation and multiplication of red blood cells
- Important for growth and division of all body cells, including nerve cell and for manufacturing a number of nerve transmitters
- Important for the health of skin and hair, and helps to prevent premature greying of hair.

Clinical Features

- Anaemia
- Skin becomes pigmented and loss of hair

- Difficulty during labour
- Loss of libido can occur in males
- Dementia, mental depression and fatigue.

Oral Manifestation

- Disappearance of filliform papillae and fungiform papillae remain prominent
- Small ulcerative stomatitis
- Smelling and redness of lips and lateral margin of tongue.

Management

Daily dose of 500 mcg to 10,000 mcg of folic acid is sufficient and a maintenance dose of 500 mcg once in week is given in cases of megaloblastic anaemia.

Vitamin B_{12} (Cyanocobalamin)

- It is a complex organomatrix compound known as cobalamin which is cobalt containing porphyrin
- Stored in liver
- Excreted in normal urine, stools and breast milk
- Absorption is through intestine.

Sources

Foods of animal origin, fish, meat, poultry, milk and milk products.

Daily Requirements

- Men and women: 1 mcg
- Children: 0.2–1 mcg
- Infants: 0.2 mcg.

Function

- Improves concentration, memory, balance, and relieve irritability
- Production and regeneration of red blood cells (RBCs)
- Helps in proper utilisation of fats, carbohydrates and proteins
- Deficiency Symptoms
- Vitamin B12 deficiency leads to megaloblastic anaemia or pernicious anaemia
- Occurs in 5th to 8th decades of life
- More seen in men than females.

Symptoms

- Generalised weakness, numbness and tingling of the extremities
- Fatigue, headache, dizziness, nausea, vomiting, diarrhoea pallar, loss of appetite and abdominal pain.

Oral Manifestation

- Sore painful tongue, glossitis and glossodynia
- Tongue is inflamed and beefy red
- Burning and pain in the lingual region
- Atrophy of papillae with a loss of normal muscle tone, known as Hunter's glossitis.

Management

- Oral: Dose from 6–150 mcg
- Parenteral: 1000 mcg of vitamin, given twice weekly in case of anaemia.

SHORT ESSAYS

Question 1

Discuss vitamin C. Discuss scurvy in detail?

Answer

- It is also referred to as ascorbic acid or antibiotic vitamin
- Absorption of vitamin C takes place in the upper part of small intestine
- It gets excreted out by the kidney through urine.

Sources

Cereals, pulses, legumes, vegetables, nuts, fruits, fish and meat, milk and milk products.

Daily Requirements

- Men and women: 40 mg
- Infants: 25 mg
- Children: 40 mg
- Pregnant and lactating women: 80 mg.

Functions of Vitamin C

- It helps in the formation of collagen chondroitin sulphate and neurotransmitter
- It helps in the maintenance of phagocytic activity of neutrophils
- Important for proper functioning of adrenal and thyroid glands and maintenance of bones

- Important for maintaining the folate pool
- Helps in absorption of iron in the body
- Vitamin C is required for the metabolism of tryptophan, norepinephrine and tyrosine
- Helps is wound healing and provides protection against all forms of stresses.

Deficiency Symptom

- Slight deficiency can lead to lassitude, fatigue, muscular pain, anaemia and increased susceptibility to infection
- Scurvy results in cases of prolonged deficiency.

Scurvy

Scurvy results from prolonged deficiency of vitamin C.

General Characteristics

- Wound healing is impaired
- Blood vessels become weak
- Due to impaired collagen synthesis, there is defective synthesis of osteoid
- Pathogenesis **(Flowchart 13.3)**.

Flowchart 13.3: Pathogenesis of scurvy

Failure of hydroxylation of proline to hydroxyproline

↓

Defective formation of collagen in the connective tissue

↓

Increased permeability of capillary (haemorrhage)

↓

Anaemia because of erythropoiesis and defective collagen formation

Clinical Features

- Infantile scurvy: There is general lassitude, anaemia, limbs become painful and enlargement of costochondral junction
- Folliculosis: Hair follicle rises above skin and there are perifollicular haemorrhages
- Haemorrhage: Seen in joint, into the nerve sheath under nails or conjunctiva
- Petechiae haemorrhage can be seen in abdomen, legs, arm, ankle, buttocks and nail beds
- Epistasis, anaemia and delayed wound healing
- Oedema of face and limb
- Can lead to premature aging, thyroid insufficiency and decreased resistance to infection.

Oral Manifestation

- Commonly seen in gingival and periodontal region
- Marginal and interdental gingiva are bright red in colour, swollen and smooth, shiny surface and produces an appearance which is called as scurvy bed
- In severe cases, the gingiva becomes baggy, ulcerated and easily bleeds
- Colour changes to violaceous red
- There is a typical fetid breath along with fusospirochetal stomatitis
- Haemorrhage and swelling of periodontal ligament membrane occurs
- There is a severe bone loss and teeth becomes loose and exfoliated.

Histopathological Features

- There is a failure to form osteoid
- Cartilage cells of epiphyseal plate continue to proliferate in normal fashion and salts are deposited in the matrix between the columns of cartilage cells
- There is no destruction of calcified matrix, therefore the wide zone of calcified but non-ossified matrix, known as scorbutic lattice develops is the metaphysis.

Management

Patient should be given vitamin C 250 mg 3 times a day.

Question 2

Discuss vitamin D and discuss rickets in detail?

Answer

- Vitamin D is also known as sunshine vitamin
- Scientific name for vitamin D is 1,25-dihydroxyche-mcalciferol.

Forms

- D_1: It is present in fish liver oils and animal fats. It is called as cholecalciferol
- D_2: It is obtained artificially by irradiation of ergosterol and known as ergocalciferol.

Absorption

- Bile is important for the absorption of vitamin D
- Fat also helps in absorption
- It is absorbed from the jejunum of the small intestine and is transported in the lymph chylomicrons to the bloodstream
- Vitamin D excretion and its metabolites occur primarily in the faeces with the help of bile salts.

Functions

- It helps in the maintenance of normal plasma levels of calcium and phosphorous
- It is essential for the proper formation of teeth and bones
- It also helps in the prevention of dental caries
- It is essential for healthy functioning of parathyroid gland, which regulated the calcium levels in the blood.

Requirements

- Infants and children: 0.01 mg
- Men and women: 0.01 mg
- Pregnancy and lactating women: 0.01 mg.

Sources

Fish, eggs, shark oil, ghee, butter, sunlight.

Rickets

- It is a disorder in vitamin D calcium phosphorous axis which results in hypomineralised bone matrix that is failure of endochondral calcification
- It is seen in areas where there is deficient sunlight.

Pathogenesis

- There is overgrowth of epiphyseal cartilage because of inadequate provisional calcification and failure of cartilage cells to form a matrix and disintegrates
- Because of persistence of distorted, irregular masses of cartilage
- Due to osteoid matrix deposition on inadequately mineralised cartilaginous remnants
- There is abnormal growth of capillaries and fibroblasts in the disorganised zone due to microstructure and stresses on inadequately mineralised and poorly formed bone.

Clinical Features

- Seen in infants and children
- Common manifestations because of hypocalcaemia
- Ankles and wrist are swollen
- Craniotabes: There is presence of a localised area of thinning such that a finger can produce indentations
- Patients have short stature and deformed extremities
- There is bowing of legs
- Frontal bowing which gives a square appearance to the head
- There is deformation of chest
- There is weakening of metaphyseal areas of the ribs
- Deformation of pelvis.

Oral Manifestation

- There is developmental abnormalities of enamel and dentin
- Malalingned teeth
- Eruption is delayed
- High caries index
- Hypoplasia of enamel
- Large pulp chambers
- Displacing of teeth.

Radiographic Features

- Widening and fraying of epiphysis of long bones
- Green stick fracture
- Thinning of cortical bone
- There is reduction in trabecular bone
- Enamel hypoplasia
- Enlargement of pulp chamber
- Density of dentin remains normal
- Periodontal ligament space becomes narrow.

Chapter 14 Haematological Disorders

LONG ESSAYS

Question 1

Classify anaemia. Describe aetiology, clinical features, oral manifestation, investigation and management of (a) iron (Fe) deficiency anaemia, (b) megaloblastic anaemia, (c) pernicious anaemia?

Answer

Anaemia is an abnormal decrease in the red blood cells or haemoglobin in blood circulation in a given unit of blood.

Aetiological Classification of Anaemia

- Loss of blood
  - Acute post-haemorrhagic anaemia
  - Chronic post-haemorrhagic anaemia.
- Excessive destruction of RBCs
  - Extra-corpuscular causes:
    - Antibodies
    - Infections like malaria
    - Splenic sequestration and destruction
    - Associated diseases like lymphomas
    - Drugs, chemical and physical agents
    - Trauma to RBC.
  - Intra-corpuscular haemolytic diseases:
    - Hereditary:
      - Disorders of glycolysis
      - Erythropoietic purpura
      - Faulty synthesis or maintenance of reduced glutathione
      - Qualitative or quantitative abnormalities in the synthesis of globulin
      - Abnormalities in RBC membrane.
  - Acquired:
    - Paroxysmal nocturnal haemoglobinuria
    - Lead poisoning.
- Impaired blood production resulting from deficiency of substances essential for erythropoiesis:
  - Iron deficiency
  - Deficiency of Vit. B12, folic acid
  - Pyridoxine responsive anaemia
  - Protein deficiency
  - Ascorbic acid deficiency.
- Inadequate production of immature erythrocytes:
  - Deficiency of erythroblast
    - Aplastic anaemia
      - Chemical or physical agents
      - Hereditary
      - Idiopathic.
    - Pure red cell aplasia.
      - Thymoma
      - Chemical agents
      - Antibodies.
  - Infiltration of bone marrow
    - Leukaemia
    - Multiple myeloma
    - Carcinoma
    - Sarcoma
    - Myelofibrosis.
  - Endocrine abnormalities
    - Myxoedema
    - Addison's diseases
    - Pituitary insufficiency
    - Hyperthyroidism.
  - Chronic renal failure
  - Chronic inflammatory diseases
    - Infectious
    - Non-infectious.
  - Cirrhosis of liver.

Morphologic Classification

- Macrocytic anaemia: Increased mean corpuscular volume (MCV), mean corpuscular haemoglobin (MCH) and normal MCH concentration
- Normocytic anaemia: Reduction in RBC membrane, normal MCV, MCH and MCH concentration
- Simple microcytic: Reduced MCV, MCH and MCH concentration
- Hypochromic microcytic: Reduced MCV, MCH and MCH concentration.

Iron Deficiency Anaemia

Causes

- Inadequate consumption of iron
- During pregnancy and in growing child when iron requirement is more
- Due to malabsorption of iron (in hypochlorhydria and diarrhoea)
- Blood loss due to injury, epistaxis, peptic ulcer
- In chronic blood loss.

Clinical Features

- Seen more in females
- 40–60 years of age
- Tiredness, headaches, loss of concentration, paraesthesia
- Koilonychias: Nails are brittle, flattened and become spoon shaped
- Neuropathy recognized by tingling and pin and needle sensation in extremities
- Dysphagia.

Oral Manifestation

- Pallor of oral mucosa: Pink colour of the oral mucosa is lost due to lack of oxygenated blood
- Oral mucosa gets atrophied
- Changes in tongue:
  - Tongue is red, sore and has burning sensation
  - Filiform papillae get atrophied
  - In severe cases, the fungiform papillae also get atrophied causing the tongue to appear waxy and glistening.
- Angular cheilitis: Cracking and fissuring of the corner of the mouth. Pain is felt during opening and closing of mouth along with bleeding from ulcers
- Aphthous ulcers and candida lesions
- Patients exhibit slow healing characteristics.

Haematological Findings

- Anaemia is microcytic and hypochromic
- Reduced haemoglobin levels
- Normal or mildly reduced RBC count
- Reduced MCH, MCV, MCHC.

Management

- Iron supplements: Oral supplement of iron as ferrous fumarate or ferrous sulphate, 300 mg thrice daily for 6 months
- Patients who are unable to take supplements orally are administered parenterally
- Iron sorbitol 1.5 mg of iron per kg body weight daily
- Plummer-Vinson syndrome: Characterized by dysphagia, iron deficiency anaemia, koilonychias and glossitis.

Megaloblastic Anaemia

This occurs due to deficiency of Vitamin B12 and folate or both leading to disorganized proliferation of cells.

Aetiology

Folate-deficiency megaloblastic anaemia:

- More prevalent in pregnant or lactating women
- Deficiency of folate in diet
- Prolonged cooking of food
- Malabsorption syndrome (tropical sprue)
- Malaria.

Vitamin B12 deficiency megaloblastic anaemia:

- Elimination of Vitamin B12 from the gut by parasites or bacteria
- Dietary deficiency.

Clinical Features

- Weakness, palpitations and loss of appetite. Periodic diarrhoea
- Skin shows lemon yellow tint in severe cases
- Paraesthesia of finger and toes
- Spleen can be palpated in severe cases
- Dementia.

Oral Manifestations

- Burning sensation, hypersensitivity, paraesthesia and dryness in tongue
- Atrophied fungiform and filiform papillae causing atrophic fiery red surface of tongue (Hunter's glossitis)
- Angular cheilitis
- Yellow-brown pigmentation of oral mucosa due to increased bile pigments in circulation.

Haematological Findings

- Macrocytic blood picture with abnormal forms of RBCs
- Leukopenia
- Thrombocytopenia
- Bone marrow exhibits presence of megaloblasts.

Management

- Education about food habits
- Blood transfusion
- Oral administration of Vitamin B12
- Folic acid supplement.

Pernicious Anaemia

Occurs due to deficiency of Vitamin B12 secondary to deficiency of intrinsic factor.

Aetiology

Due to atrophy of gastric mucosa leading to failure of secretion of intrinsic factor.

Clinical Features

- Males more affected then females
- Symptoms: Generalized weakness, sore painful tongue, numbness and tingling of extremities
- Fatigue, headache, nausea, dizziness, loss of appetite, vomiting, loss of weight, shortness of breath, pallor and abdominal pain
- Weakness, stiffness in walking, paraesthesia of extremities, irritability, depression, tingling sensation in fingers and toes
- Epigastric discomfort.

Oral Manifestation

- Inflamed tongue (beefy red in colour) entirely or in patches
- Gradual atrophy of tongue causing smooth and bald tongue (hunters glossitis)
- Oral mucosa shows greenish-yellow colour at junction of hard and soft palate.

Haematological Findings

- RBC count decreased to 3 or less per cubic mm
- Many cells show macrocytosis while some show poikilocytosis
- Reduced WBS count
- In advanced cases, polychromatic cells, stipples cells, nucleated cells, Howell Jolly bodies, Cabot rings are seen.

Management

Vitamin B12 administered parenterally, 100 mg IM every 30 days.

Question 2

Describe in detail about aplastic anaemia?

Answer

It is a rare disorder characterized by anaemia, leucopoenia and thrombocytopenia due to bone marrow suppression.

Types

- Primary: Idiopathic
  - Generally seen in young adults
  - Rapid onset and is fatal.
- Secondary: Known aetiology.
  - Any age
  - Better prognosis than primary.

Aetiology

- Drugs and chemicals: Three ways
  1. Myelosuppressive effects of cancer chemotherapeutic agents
  2. Some drugs like benzene derivatives, amidoprine, colloidal silver, chloramphenicol, bismuth, penicillin, anticancer drugs, sulphonamides, mercury, etc.
  3. Idiosyncratic or hypersensitivity induced.
- Infections: Tuberculosis, hepatitis, infectious mononucleosis
- Radiation.

Clinical Features

- Any age
- Weakness, pallor of skin
- Breathlessness, headache, ankle oedema
- Numbness and tingling of extremities
- Anginal pain
- Congestive cardiac failure
- Bleeding from nose, vagina, GIT
- Fever due to infection.

Oral Manifestation

- Oral mucosa shows pallor
- Spontaneous haemorrhage in gingiva
- Petechiae on soft palate
- Submucosal ecchymosis
- Large ragged ulcers covered by grey or black necrotic membrane.

Haematological Findings

- RBC count is diminished to 1 million cell/cubic mm
- WBC count reduced to 2000/cubic mm
- Platelet count below 20000/cubic mm
- Pancytopenia along with reduction of absolute reticulocyte count
- Prolonged bleeding time
- Normal clotting time
- Anaemia is normocytic with some macrocytosis
- Bone marrow is fatty.

Management

- Removal of etiologic agent
- Administration of antibiotics and transfusion
- Administration of androgens for stimulation of haemopoiesis
- Bone marrow transplantation
- Anti-fibrinolytic agents to reduce gingival bleeding, e.g., aminocaproic acid or tranexamic acid.

Question 3

Define and classify leukaemia. Explain in detail acute leukaemia?

Answer

It is defined as the neoplastic proliferation of WBC in bone marrow, usually in circulating blood and sometime in other organs like liver, spleen and lymph nodes.

Classification

Acute

- Acute lymphoblastic leukaemia
  - L1: Acute lymphoblastic (principally paediatric)—in it, small cells predominate and nuclei are round
  - L2: Acute lymphoblastic (principally adults)—in it, cells are heterogeneous in size and sharp in features, nuclei often show cleft
  - L3: Burkitt's—there is homogeneous population of large cells. Nuclei are round to oval and have prominent nucleoli.
- Acute non-lymphoblastic or myeloid leukaemia.
  - M1: Myeloblastic (without maturation)—myeloblasts predominate with distant nucleoli, few granules are present
  - M2: Myeloblastic (with maturation)—myeloblasts and promyelocytes predominate and Auer rods can be seen
  - M3: Promyelocytic—hypergranular promyelocytes often with Auer rods are seen
  - M4: Myelomonocytic—myelocytic and monocytic differentiation is evident, myeloid elements resemble peripheral monocytosis
  - M5: Monocytic—promonocytes or undifferentiated blasts
  - M6: Erythroleukaemia—bizarre, multinucleated, megablastoid erythroblast predominate
  - M7: Megakaryocytic—pleomorphic undifferentiated blast cells with anti-platelet antibodies, myelofibrosis is seen.

Chronic

- Chronic lymphatic leukaemia
- Chronic myeloid leukaemia.

Acute Leukaemia

- Acute leukaemia is characterized by the failure of maturation of leucocytes leading to accumulation of immature cells in the bone marrow and eventually in blood
- Most common type of leukaemia in adults.

Pathophysiology

- The differentiation of leucocytes and stem cells does not occur and leucoblasts have prolonged generation time
- As leukaemic cells accumulate in bone marrow, they began to suppress the normal hematopoietic stem cells.

Clinical Features

- More common in children and young adults between ages of 15–40 years
- Male: Female ratio is 3:2
- Sudden onset accompanied with pyrexia and enlargement of spleen
- Bone marrow suppression and infiltration of organs with leukaemic cells
- Weakness, headache, fever, swelling of lymph nodes, petechiae, haemorrhage in skin and mucous membrane
- Pain and tenderness of bones due to bone marrow expansion and infiltration of subperiosteum
- CNS manifestation like vomiting, headache, nerve palsies is also seen
- Pallor, dyspnoea, fatigue, ecchymosis, petechiae epistaxis and melena are seen due to anaemia and thrombocytopenia
- Hepatosplenomegaly occurs in advanced stages
- Intracranial and subarachnoid haemorrhages result from thrombocytopenia and leukostasis
- Recurrent infection of urinary tract, oral cavity, skin, upper respiratory tract and rectum are commonly seen.

Oral Manifestations

- Cervical, pre- and post-auricular, and submental lymph nodes are enlarged and tender
- Paraesthesia of chin and lower lip
- Oral mucous membrane shows pallor, ulceration with necrosis, ecchymosis, petechiae
- Massive necrosis of lingual mucosa accompanied by sloughing
- Gingiva is hypertrophic and shows cyanotic discoloration
- Oral infections like candidiasis, viral and bacterial infections are common.

Haematological Findings

- Total WBC count varies from 1×10^6/cu mm to 5000×10^6/cu mm
- Peripheral smear layer shows increased number of immature granulocytes or precursor cells
- Bone marrow is hypercellular.

Management

- Induction phase: Vincristine(1.4 mg/sq m) every week of 1 month + L-asparaginase (600 units/sq m) twice weekly for 1 month + prednisone (40mg/sq m) orally daily for 1 month
- Consolidation phase: Daunorubicin, mercaptopurine. Cytarabine, and methotrexate along with intrathecal therapy using methotrexate and cytarabine together with irradiation
- Maintenance phase: Patient receives repeated cycles of above drugs for 2–3 years
- Non-lymphocytic leukaemia is treated with daunorubicin, cytarabine and 6-thioguanine
- Catabolic products of leukaemic cell cause uric acid accumulation and hyperuricemia
- This is prevented by using the drug allopurinol
- Supportive phase: Transfusion of RBC and platelets. Combination of antibiotics like aminoglycosides with cephalosporin
- Topical treatment to stop gingival bleeding includes application of direct pressure along with absorbable gelatine
- Povidone iodine, chlorhexidine rinses, tetracycline rinses to treat oral ulcers.

SHORT ESSAYS

Question 1

Explain in detail about polycythaemia vera?

Answer

It is an abnormal increase in the number of red blood cells in the peripheral blood.

- Also known as Osler's disease
- Characterized by uncontrolled proliferation of erythroid stem cells leading to excess of RBCs
- It is accompanied by increase in the granulocyte and megakaryocytes.

Clinical Features

- More common in middle-aged males
- Common symptoms are lack of concentration, headache, dizziness, pruritus and slurred speech
- Paraesthesia involving cranial nerves
- Skin is flushed
- Spleen in palpable
- Superficial veins are dark, enlarged and distended
- Fingertips are cyanotic
- Purplish-red discoloration of head and neck.

Oral Manifestation

- Purplish discoloration of ears, oral mucosa, tongue and gingiva
- Gingiva is swollen and bleeds spontaneously
- Petechiae in oral mucosa.

Haematological Findings

- Haemoglobin levels are greater than 18 g/dL
- Elevation of WBC and platelet count
- Bone marrow is hypercellular.

Management

- Venesection at periodic intervals to remove 500–600 mL of blood
- Radioactive phosphorus once diagnosis is certain
- Oral administration of 30 mg triethylenemelamine (TEM) with remission of 8–9 months
- Busulfan 2–4 mg/day orally.

Question 2

Explain in detail about cyclic neutropenia?

Answer

It is a blood disorder characterised by periodic diminishing levels of neutrophils in the blood stream because of failure of stem cell in bone marrow.

- It is an autosomal dominant trait
- Patient is healthy between the drops when the neutrophils levels can fall up to 500/cubic mm
- In some cases, the count has dropped to zero as well.

Clinical Features

- In infancy or childhood, affecting both males and females
- Once in 2–4 weeks drop of neutrophil is seen lasting up to 3–5 days
- Sore throat, stomatitis, and regional lymphadenopathy, headache, arthritis, conjunctivitis, sometimes urinary tract infections
- Amyloidosis has also been seen in some cases.

Oral Manifestations

- Severe gingivitis
- Ragged ulcers, which have core-like centre found on lip, buccal mucosa, tongue, gums and palate which spontaneously heal in two weeks but lead to scarring
- Radiologically, mild to severe loss of superficial alveolar bone is seen.

Haematological Findings

- Decline of neutrophils in blood is seen which is compensated by increase in monocytes and lymphocytes
- Neutrophils completely disappear during peak days.

Management

- Early management of infections
- Oral hygiene should be maintained and patient should be recalled every 2–3 months.

Question 3

Explain about infectious mononucleosis?

Answer

It is an acute infectious disease cause by Epstein–Barr virus affecting the B-lymphocytes.

It is also called as glandular fever.

Clinical Features

- In children and young adults
- Cervical and anterior lymph nodes are enlarged and tender on palpation
- Patient complains of high fever (101–103 °F) along with extreme fatigue ability
- Headache, vomiting, nausea, diarrhoea and erythematous macular rash are seen
- On examination, enlarged palatine tonsils along with filled with cheesy yellow exudate tonsillar crypt
- Splenomegaly is commonly seen
- Can lead to complications like progressive neurological involvement, airway obstruction and haemolytic anaemia.

Oral Manifestations

- Small petechiae on soft palate, buccal mucosa and labial mucosa
- Acute gingivitis and stomatitis persisting from 3 to 11 days
- Enlargement and inflammation of tonsils covered with white/greyish pseudomembrane
- Some patients show haemorrhagic tendency through nose and gums
- Oral ulcers and lymphadenopathy is also seen.

Haematological Findings

- Increase in mononuclear cell count exhibiting pleomorphism with an oval or kidney-shaped nucleus
- Haemoglobin and platelet counts are normal
- Increase in WBC count and positive Paul Bunnel test.

Diagnosis

- Mono spot test
- Leucocyte count between 4000 and 5000/dL
- Positive heterophile antibody test
- Atypical lymphocytes.

Management

- Antiviral drugs: Ganciclovir and alpha interferon
- Corticosteroids in complication like airway obstruction, etc.
- Anaesthetics for oral lesions.

Question 4

Explain about thrombocytopenic purpura?

Answer

Purpura is defined as purplish discoloration of the skin and mucus membrane due to subcutaneous and submucous extravasation of blood.

Clinical Features

- Characterised by spontaneous appearance of purpuric haemorrhagic lesion of skin of various sizes, i.e., from tiny red pinpoint petechiae too large purplish ecchymosis
- Bruising tendency
- Epistaxis, haematuria and melena
- Rarely intracranial haemorrhage has also been seen especially in children.

Oral Manifestation

- Excessive bleeding post tooth extraction
- Petechiae and ecchymosis are the junction of hard palate and soft palate
- Appear as numerous, tiny clusters of red spots
- Petechiae do not blanch on stretching differing it from telangiectasia
- In severe case, extensive spontaneous gingival bleeding is seen.

Haematological Findings

- Platelet count below 60,000/cu mm
- Prolonged bleeding time
- Clotting time is normal
- Bone marrow reveals megakaryocytic hyperplasia.

Management

- In children, treatment is not necessary unless intracranial bleeding is seen
- In adults, prednisone 60 mg/dL until platelet count is in normal range
- In case of no improvement upon administration of prednisone in 3–4 days, splenectomy is indicated
- Platelet transfusion
- Local haemostatic is administered from sites of bleeding.

Question 5

Explain about haemophilia A?

Answer

It is a hereditary disorder characterized by excessive haemorrhage tendencies due to prolonged coagulation time.

- Caused due to deficiency of factor VIII (anti-haemophilic factor)
- It is an X-linked recessive character trait
- Males are clinically affected while females are carriers.

Clinical Features

- Bleeding tendencies begin at an early age when the child sustains some injury
- Most common bleeding tendency is seen in joints, which is generally spontaneous and is usually associated with warmth and muscular spasms
- Repeated bleeding episodes in joint lead to damage along with wasting of muscle, which eventually causes deformity or crippling
- Haemorrhage is seen subcutaneously in internal organs and in musculature
- Any trauma causes uncontrolled bleeding.

Oral Manifestation

- Most common sites of bleeding in oral cavity are fraenum, lips and tongue
- Tooth extraction in such cases is associated with prolonged bleeding
- Haematoma from floor of mouth can spread to larynx leading to respiratory complications
- Normal process of tooth exfoliation and eruption is associated with sever and prolonged bleeding.

Haematological Findings

Clotting time is prolonged, although bleeding time, platelet count and prothrombin time are all normal.

Management

- Replacement therapy to raise factor VIII by plasma, cryoprecipitate and factor VIII concentrates
- Factor VIII concentrate dosage and duration depends on the site and type of bleeding
- Administration of fresh frozen plasmas is generally associated with complications like hypovolaemia, allergy, transfusion hepatitis, haemolytic anaemia and development of factor VIII antibodies
- To reduce the above complications various drugs can be administered especially before dental extractions like anti-diuretic 1-deamino (8-D-arginine) vasopressin (DDVAP) in combination with tranexamic acid and epsilon-aminocaproic acid.

Question 6

Explain about Christmas disease/haemophilia B?

Answer

It is caused due to the deficiency of factor IX.
It is an X-linked recessive character.

Clinical Features

- Bleeding tendencies begin at an early age when the child sustains some injury
- Most common bleeding tendency is seen in joints, which is generally spontaneous and is usually associated with warmth and muscular spasms
- Repeated bleeding episodes in joint lead to damage along with wasting of muscle, which eventually causes deformity or crippling
- Haemorrhage is seen subcutaneously in internal organs and in musculature
- Any trauma causes uncontrolled bleeding.

Oral Manifestation

- Most common sites of bleeding in oral cavity are fraenum, lips and tongue
- Tooth extraction in such cases is associated with prolonged bleeding
- Haematoma from floor of mouth can spread to larynx leading to respiratory complications
- Normal process of tooth exfoliation and eruption is associated with severe and prolonged bleeding.

Question 7

Explain in detail about dental management of haemophilia A and B?

Answer

- Anaesthesia: Local anaesthesia is contraindicated
  - If required it should be administered intrapulpally, in periodontal ligament and papillary injection
  - Sedation with diazepam or nitrous oxide should be used.
- Endodontic therapy: Haemorrhage in canal can be controlled using 1:1000 aq. epinephrine
- Restorative: Rubber dam should be used to prevent injury to oral soft tissue during restorative procedures
- Prosthodontics therapy: Complete dentures and partial dentures are well tolerated. The patient is told to maintain good oral hygiene and have regular check-up
- Periodontics therapy: Conservative treatment protocol is recommended. Osseous surgery and gingival surgery require hospitalization and extensive replacement therapy
- Oral surgery procedures: Pressure surgical packs, oxidized cellulose saturated with bovine thrombin solution, vasoconstrictors, sutures, absorbable haemostatics, and topical thrombin are used as local haemostatic agents
- Post-operative use of anti-fibrinolytic agent and adherence to soft diet is advised
- Aspirin and NSAIDs are avoided in patients with bleeding disorders
- Pre-operative levels of factors should be 30–40% of normal activity
- Electro surgery is avoided to avoid tissue necrosis and subsequent haematoma formation
- Intramuscular injections should not be administered to avoid haematoma formation.

Question 8

Explain about chronic myeloid leukaemia?

Answer

Associated with presence of chromosomal abnormality, i.e., Philadelphia chromosome.

Clinical Features

- 30–70 years of age
- Slowly advancing anaemia with loss of weight, prominence of abdomen, and splenomegaly
- Sudden acute left upper abdominal pain may occur due to infarction of spleen
- Weakness, fatigue and dyspnoea on exertion
- Thrombocytopenia leads to petechiae, ecchymosis, and haemorrhages from skin and mucous membrane
- Liver enlarged
- Lymph nodes are normal.

Haematological Findings

- Normocytic and normochromic anaemia
- WBC count increased and is between 50×10^6 to 500×10^6/cu mm
- Peripheral smear layer shows mature leucocytes along with a few immature cells
- Platelet count is high.

Management

- Chemotherapy using busulphan orally 4 mg daily, large doses of 50–100 mg spaced between 2–3 weeks apart
- Treatment is continued for 12–18 weeks and should be stopped once WBC count is between 10×10^6 to 20×10^6 /cu mm
- Combination therapy of busulphan 2 mg daily along with mercaptopurine 50 mg daily or thioguanine 80 mg daily
- Radiotherapy and splenectomy may be advised.

CHAPTER 15 Diagnostic Laboratory Procedure

LONG ESSAYS

Question 1

What is sialography? Discuss its technique in detail. How can a sialolith be removed from parotid gland duct?

Answer

Sialography is a specialized radiographic technique done for the detection of the major salivary glands (generally parotid and submandibular glands)

- Cannulation is done with filing with a radiopaque contrast agent so that it becomes visible on the radiograph
- This procedure indicates any kind of changes in the internal structure of the salivary glands.

Indications

- In cases of any swelling of the salivary glands
- Detection of any calculi
- Sialadenitis
- Xerostomia
- Detection of residual stones
- Pain of unknown aetiology.

Contraindications

- Patients who are sensitive to iodine-containing compounds
- Acute infection of salivary glands
- Presence of calculus at the entrance of the duct.

Contrast Media

There are two types of contrast media available:

1. Water soluble
2. Fat soluble.

Water-soluble Contrast Media

- They are iodinated benzene, or pyridine derivatives
- They have a low surface tension and low viscosity
- They are easily miscible with salivary secretions
- These properties of water-soluble contrast media allow the filling of the finer ductal system under low pressure and also facilitate prompt drainage.

Fat-soluble Media

They are present as two types:

1. Iodized oil
2. Water insoluble organic iodine compounds. Examples of iodized oil are iodized poppy seed oil (lipiodol) and ethiodized poppy seed oil (ethiodol).

Ethiodol has a low viscosity and a low irritational factor, as compared to other oil-based media, therefore it is the medium of choice. It consists of 37% iodine and has a very high radiographic density, therefore it can generate an excellent acinar opacification and a clear ductogram.

Technique

It is divided into three phases:

1. Preliminary phase: In this, film is evaluated to rule out any obvious radiopaque pathosis
2. Filling or injection phase: In this phase, a contrast media is injected so as to outline the ductal system
3. Parenchymal phase (if water-soluble medium is used) or evacuation phase (if fat-soluble medium is used).

In the presence of any obstruction or inflammation, evacuation and postevacuation phase are most helpful Processes, which cause parenchymal destruction, such as autoimmune disorders, irradiation or chronic infections, are generally responsible for delayed or incomplete evacuation. By observing the clearance of the contrast media during sialography, amount of secretion and the functioning capacity of the gland can be determined.

Armamentarium

- Polyethylene tubing with a special blunt metallic tip with side-holes for parotid injection
- Similar tubing for injection into submandibular gland with an end terminal hole
- A 5–10 mL syringe
- Lacrimal dilator
- Contrast medium
- Lemon slices or artificial lemon extracts

Procedure

Identification of the location of duct orifices:

- The parotid duct is situated at the base of the papilla in the buccal mucosa, opposite maxillary first and second molar teeth
- Using a small piece of gauze, the mucosal area around the orifice is dried
- Exploring the duct using a lacrimal probe: Parotid duct has a tortuous course, patients' cheek should be lifted upwards before the insertion of probe into the duct
- The probe should slide easily back and forth inside the duct and also rotate fully without dragging.

Cannulation of the Parotid Duct

- The orifice of the parotid duct is located on the buccal mucosa, opposite the maxillary second molar
- The duct passes posteriorly and laterally through the buccinators muscle
- Cannulation procedure is facilitated by pulling the cheek forward, thereby straightening the right angle bend in the parotid duct
- A syringe is used to inject the contrast media with gentle pressure, once the duct is cannulated
- 0.5–0.75 mL of contrast material can be accommodated painlessly in the parotid duct system
- Most commonly, views taken for parotid are antero-posterior, anteroposterior with open jaw, antero-posterior with cheek in blowout position, lateral and orthopantomogram (OPG).

Question 2

What are the various diagnostic methods of investigating salivary gland tumour?

Answer

Various imaging modalities used are:

- Conventional radiography
- Sialography
- Ultrasonography
- Computerized tomography
- Radionuclide imaging
- Magnetic resonance imaging (MRI).

Conventional Radiography

- It can be used to detect the calcification within the glands to determine the presence of metastasis to the salivary glands
- Radiographs have a limitation that they cannot determine the extent of rapid, destructive and invasive lesion, as the changes appear only after 30% of the mineral content is lost
- Most commonly used radiographs of salivary glands is posterioranterior, lateral, lateral oblique and frontal views.

Sialography

Refer question 1.

Ultrasonography

Ultrasounds can differentiate between intraglandular and extraglandular masses. They can determine the presence of solid, cystic, complex masses and sialoliths.

CT and MRI

They demonstrate excellent soft tissue details.

- They can show lesions, as well as their involvement in the adjacent structures
- MRI is beneficial in demonstrating early extension along the neuromuscular pathways.

Radionuclide Salivary Imaging

- It is useful for major salivary glands
- It is helpful in evaluating pathology as well as physiology
- Patients who have obstructed sialadenitis in whom, contrast sialography is contraindicated or cannot be done due to technical on anatomical reason, are more suited for this technique
- It can detect the parenchymal masses of greater than 1 cm in diameter and can identify specific types of tumour.

SHORT ESSAYS

Question 1

What is exfoliative cytology?

Answer

- It is the study of cells that exfoliate or shed from the body surfaces
- This technique is used for the diagnosis of the oral mucosal lesions.

Technique

- Firstly, the surface which has to be studied should be cleaned properly and then the entire surface should be scraped vigorously using a metal cement spatula, a moistened tongue blade or a cytobrush
- Then, a microscopic slide is taken, over which the collected scrapings is spread evenly and is fixed before the smear dries
- Fixative used for fixing the material can be commercial preparations, like spray-cyte, 95% alcohol, or equal parts of alcohol and ether
- After using the fixative, the slide should be allowed to stand for 30 minutes to air dry
- It is important to repeat the procedure and a second smear should be prepared
- Separate scraping should be taken in the preparation of duplicate slide.

There are five classes of the reports given by the cytologist:

- Class I: Normal—normal cells are observed
- Class II: Atypical—there is presence of minor atypia, but no evidence of malignant changes
- Class III: Intermediate—it separates cancer from non-cancer diagnosis
- Class IV: Suggestive of cancer—few cells with malignancy are detected. Biopsy is essential
- Class V: Positive for cancer—cells are malignant. Biopsy is essential.

Question 2

What is the definition of biopsy? What are its various types, indications and technique?

Answer

It is a procedure which is done by removing a sample of tissue from patient.

Various types of biopsies are as follows:

- Aspiration biopsy
- Cone biopsy
- Endoscopic biopsy
- Core needle biopsy
- Punch biopsy
- Suction assisted core biopsy
- Surface biopsy
- Excisional biopsy.

Indications

- For diagnosis of lesions that interfere with oral functions, like fibrous hyperplasia and osseous lumps
- Lesions that do not have any specific aetiology
- For assessment of any unexplained oral mucosal abnormalities, which persist even after the treatment.

Technique

- The site from where the sample is to be collected should be cleaned properly and local anaesthesia should be given
- A needle is taken which is passed into the site of a cyst or a tumour, and a vacuum is created with the syringe and multiple in and out motions are performed
- The cells are sucked into the syringe through the fine needle
- Before the microscopic examination, the sample of fluid and cells is centrifuged at high speed and then a small amount is placed on the slide and covered with a plastic slip
- Then a smear is prepared by spreading the sample of the fluid and cells on the slides
- The slides are then fixed and stained
- Bunsen burner is used for heating so as to do preservation
- Should be conservative or radical.

SECTION 2

RADIOLOGY

CHAPTER 16 Radiation Physics

LONG ESSAYS

Question 1

Describe the principle, construction and working of an X-ray tube, along with significance of each component.

Answer

Principle

The fundamental principle behind the production of X-ray is that X-rays are produced by the sudden deceleration or stoppage of rapidly moving electrons towards a positively charged metal target in a high vacuum tank.

Construction of X-ray Tubes

- X-ray tube is a very essential part of the X-ray generating system and is very important to the production of X-rays
- X-ray tube components are as follows:
  - Leaded-glass housing
  - Cathode (–ve)
  - Anode (+ve)
  - Circuits used in the production of X-rays
  - Transformers
  - Timer
  - Tube rating
  - Duty cycle.

Leaded-glass Housing

- It is a leaded-glass vacuum tube, which prevents the X-rays from escaping in all direction
- One of the central areas of the leaded-glass tube has a window, which allows the X-ray beam to escape out of the tube and direct it towards the aluminium discs, lead collimator and the position indicating device (PID)
- It is also used for the purpose of earthing

Negatively Charged Cathode

- It consists of two parts:
  1. Filament: It is tungsten-made coiled wire, which when heated produces electrons
  2. Focusing cup: It is a holder, which is in shape of a cup, made up of molybdenum. It houses the filament. It focuses the electron into a narrow beam and direct the beam across the tube towards the tungsten target of the anode.
- Function of cathode is to provide electrons required to generate X-rays
- In the X-ray tube, negatively charged cathode produces electrons which accelerate towards the positively charged anode.

Positively Charged Anode

- Anodes are of two categories:
  - Stationary or fixed
  - Rotating: These types of anode help in dissipating heat and are most commonly used in extraoral or cephalometric machines.
- The anode helps in converting electrons into X-ray photons
- It consists of:
  - Tungsten target.
    - It is an extremely thin plate made up of tungsten which is embedded in a copper stem
    - It functions as a focal spot and produces X-rays by converting bombarding electrons
    - It is placed at an angle of 20° to the central electron ray to make the effective focal spot smaller (1 × 1 mm) as compared to the actual focal size (1 × 3 mm)
    - This is referred to as "Line Focus Principle."

Circuits used in the Production of X-rays

- Filament circuit: Low voltage (3–5 V)
  - It is controlled by current (mA) setting in control panel.
- It controls and regulates the flow of current to filament
- High voltage circuit: Uses 65,000 – 1,00,000 V.
  - Controlled by kVp setting in control panel
  - Its function is to Accelerate electrons.

Transformers

- It is a device used for controlling voltage in the electrical circuit
- Different types of transformers used in the generation of X-rays are:
  - Step down transformer
  - Step up transformer
  - Auto transformer.

Timer

A timer helps in completing the circuit with high-voltage transformer and also controls the time for which high voltage is applied to the tube.

Tube Rating

It is the maximum safe intervals (seconds) the tube may be energized at a given range of voltage (kVp) and the tube current (A) values.

Duty Cycle

Duty cycle refers to the frequency in which successive exposure can be made.

Working of X-ray Tube and Production of X-rays

Following steps are involved in the production of X-rays:

- Upon turning on the X-ray machine, the control panel receives the electrical current from the wall outlet and sends it to the tube head via electrical wires in the extension arm
- In the tube head, the electrical current is then directed to the filament circuit into the step down transformer, which minimizes the 110–220 entering line voltage to 3–5 volts
- The tungsten filament is heated by this voltage (3-5 V) by the filament circuit, in the cathode portion of the X-ray tube
  - Once the tungsten filament is heated to incandescence or red hot, thermionic emission occurs
  - Thermionic emission: It is the release of electrons from the tungsten filament when the filament gets heated to red hot by the passing electrical current
- This heat energizes the outer shell electrons of the tungsten atom which allows them to move away from the filament surface and they form an electron cloud around the filament
- The electrons that are produced at the cathode (negatively charged) get accelerated across the X-ray tube to the positively charged anode
- The molybdenum cup in the cathode provides direction to the emitted electrons towards the cathode
- Kinetic energy of electron when they hit the tungsten target is converted to X-rays and heat
- 99% of the energy is lost as heat while less than 1% is converted to X-rays
- This heat is carried away from the copper stem and absorbed by insulating oil in the tube head
- The X-rays are emitted in all direction
- The leaded housing prevents the X-rays from escaping and only a small number of X-rays travel through the unleaded glass window, tube head seal and the aluminium disc
- The aluminium disc filters the long wavelength X-rays from the beam
- The X-ray beam is restricted by lead collimator
- X-ray beam then travel through the position indicating device and then exits the tube head
- Exposure time is about 8–9 seconds
- X-rays are emitted in a series of impulses of radiation
- In a 60-second cycle of AC, there are 60 pulses of X-rays per second
- A full wave rectified X-ray machine produced 120 bursts of X-ray photons per second.

Bremsstrahlung Radiation (Breaking Radiation)

- It is defined as X-ray radiation produced when high-speed electrons are suddenly stopped at the target
- This process of rapidly decelerating high speed electron gives rise to Bremsstrahlung radiation or breaking radiation
- These are produced by:
  - When an electron directly hits the nucleus of an atom of the target material
  - When an electron passes by the side or near the nucleus leading to deflection or deceleration of the electron.
- The striking the nucleus directly by the electron leads to conversion of entire kinetic energy into a single X-ray photon
- When the electrons passes near the nucleus, the negatively charged electron gets attracted towards the

positively charged nucleus and therefore it decelerate and loses some kinetic energy

- This lost kinetic energy leads to formation of the X- ray photon
- The electron that misses the nucleus strikes the tungsten atom leading to production of many low-energy X-ray photons
- Bremsstrahlung radiation thus, consists of X-rays of different energies and wavelengths and hence is known as continuous spectrum.

Characteristic Radiation

- When a high-speed electron hits the tungsten atom, in the inner shell, it causes dislodgement of an electron leading to ionization of atom
- When the electron is dislodged the other orbiting electron, rearrange themselves to fill the vacancy created by dislodged electron
- This rearrangement leads to loss of energy that causes the generation to X-ray photon with energy equal to the difference in the two orbital energy states
- This is termed as characteristic radiation
- The radiation emitted, constitutes the line spectrum.

Question 2

What are the factors that affect the X-ray beam?

Answer

The factors affecting the X-ray beam are:

- Tube current
- Voltage
- Exposure time
- Filtration
- Collimation
- Inverse square law
- Quality of X-ray beam
- Quantity of X-ray beam
- Half value layer.

Tube Current (mA)

- Tube current determines the number of X-ray photons generated
- Upon increasing the mA, more number of electrons are generated at the cathode which strike the target to produce more number of X-ray photon
- X-ray are produced by the number of electron striking the target
- The number of electron produced is directly proportional to tube current
- The number of X-ray photon produced depends on both mA and the duration of the time of X-ray tube operation.

Tube Voltage

- Voltage is the potential difference between two electrical charges
- The voltage determines the speed at which the electron moves from negative cathode to positive anode
- Tube voltage controls the energy of the electron, as kilo voltage peak (kVp) is increased, the energy of each electron striking the target increases, thus increasing the number of X-ray photons produced
- kVp is directly proportional to number of photons generated
- kVp α mean energy of the photon
- kVp α maximum energy of the photon.

Exposure Time

- Keeping mA and kVp constant, if exposure time is doubled, then number of X-ray photons generated also doubles
- The quantity of X-ray photons can be controlled by increasing or decreasing the exposure time.

Filtration

- By this process, X-ray photons of less penetrating power are removed by placing a filter in the path of primary beam
- This filter only allows the photon with sufficient energy to pass through
- Filter is made up of an aluminium disc
- Filtration of 3 types:
  1. Inherent filtration
  2. Added filtration
  3. Total filtration.
  - **Inherent filtration**: It is produced by materials, which are present in the X-ray tube
    - Example: Glass wall of X-ray tube, insulating oil and barrier material
    - This provides 5–2 mm filtration provided by the aluminium disc filter.
  - **Added filtration**: Obtained by placing the aluminium disc in the path of primary beam
  - **Total filtration**:
    - It is the sum of inherent filtration and added filtration
    - It should be 1.5 mm of aluminium up to 70 kVp and aluminium above 70 kVp
    - Use of filters determines the contrast and quality of the film.

Collimation

- The size of X-ray beam striking the patient tissue can be shaped or restricted by the helps of Collimator
- It is made up of materials, which can absorb radiation, e.g., Lead.

Inverse Square Law

It states that the intensity of an X-ray beam is inversely proportional to the square of the distance from the source of the radiation.

Quality of the X-ray Beam

- It refers to the mean energy or the penetration power of the X-ray beam
- X-ray beam with short wavelength have more penetrating power and vice-versa
- The quality of the X-ray beam is determined by the kVp, i.e., when the kVp increases, the energy of the photons increases thus they have a better penetration power.

Quantity of the X-ray Beam

- It refers to the number of the X-ray photons produced
- It depends on the product of mA and exposure time in seconds.

Half Value Layer

- It refers to the thickness of specified materials like aluminium which are required to reduce the intensity of an X-ray beam by half
- Quality of the X-ray beam can be determined by determining its half value layer.

SHORT NOTES

Question 1

What is position indicating device?

Answer

There are three types of position indicating devices (PIDs)

1. Rectangular PID
2. Cone PID
3. Round PID.

The use of rectangular PID with an exit orifice of 3.58 × 40.4 cm will reduce the area of patient skin surface exposed by 60% as compared to a round PID.

Question 2

What is electromagnetic spectrum?

Answer

Electromagnetic spectrum is a band of electromagnetic radiation arranged according to their energies, e.g., gamma rays, X-rays, cosmic rays, UV rays, visible light, Infrared light, radio waves and microwaves.

- The electromagnetic spectrum is far below the infrared and far above the ultraviolet radiation
- Electromagnetic radiations move through space as both particle and wave therefore a dualistic theory describes the electromagnetic radiation characteristics.

Question 3

Describe inverse square law.

Answer

It states that the intensity of an X-ray beam at a given point is inversely proportional to the square of the distance from the source of radiation.

For the calculation of inverse square law, there is a formula:

$$\frac{\text{Original intensity } (I_1)}{\text{New intensity } (I_2)} = \frac{\text{New distance}^2\ (D2)2}{\text{Original distance}^2\ (D1)2}$$

- This decrease in the intensity of X-ray beam is because X-rays are divergent in nature
- If the distance from the source to the object is increased, the X-ray beam intensity decreases, which changes the Image quality, for e.g., if the distance from the source to the film is doubled, say from 8 inch to 16 inch, it results in a beam that is one fourth as intense.

CHAPTER 17

Radiation Biology

LONG ESSAYS

Question 1

What are the biologic effects of ionizing radiations/X-rays?

Answer

Initial interaction between ionizing radiation and matter occurs within first 10^{-13} seconds after exposure. Molecular changes lead to alterations in cells and organism (persist for hours, decades and even generations).

Biological effect of ionizing radiation is divided into:

- Deterministic effect
- Stochastic effect.

Deterministic Effect

Deterministic effects are those in which:

- Severity of response is proportional to dose
- Usually cause cell death
- Occur in all people in high doses, e.g.,—oral changes after radiation therapy.

Stochastic Effect

- Stochastic effects are those for which probability of the occurrence of a change, rather than its severity, is dose-dependent
- Individual has or does not have the condition (all or none response), e.g., radiation-induced cancer because greater exposure to ionizing radiation increase the probability of cancer but not its severity.

Effect of Ionizing Radiation May Be

- Direct effect
- Indirect effect.

Direct Effect

- When the energy of photon or secondary electron ionizes biologic macromolecule, the effect is termed as direct
- About 1/3rd of the biological effect of ionization result from direct effect
- Begin within 10^{-10} seconds after the passage of photon
- Direct alteration of biologic molecule (RH, where R is molecule and H is hydrogen atom) by ionizing radiation begins with absorption of energy and forming free radical
- Fate of free radicals:
  Dissociation: $R^{\cdot}$ $X + Y^{\cdot}$ stable but altered
  Cross-linking: $R^0 + S^0$ RS molecule.

Radiolysis of Water

Water is predominant molecule in biologic system.

It frequently participates in interactions between X-ray photon and biological molecule of an organism.

First step: Ionization of water due to absorption of photon or interaction with photoelectron or Compton electron.

Displacement of electron from water result in positively charged water molecule and displace electron.

$$\text{Photon} + H_2O \longrightarrow e^- + H_2O^+$$
$$\text{Photoelectron } e^- + H_2O \longrightarrow 2e^- + H_2O^+$$

Displace electron captured by water and form negatively charged water molecule.

$$e^- + H_2O \longrightarrow H_2O^-$$

not stable ↓ and dissociate

$$H_2O^- \longrightarrow OH^- + H^{\cdot}$$

Positively charged water molecule react with another molecule and form hydroxyl free radical—

$$H_2O^+ + H_2O \longrightarrow H_3O^+ + OH^{\cdot}$$

Water may also be excited and dissociate directly into hydrogen and hydroxyl free radical—

$$\text{photon} + H_2O \longrightarrow H_2O^* \longrightarrow OH^{\cdot} + H^{\cdot}$$

When dissolved with molecular oxygen (O_2) present in irradia-ted water, hydroperoxyl free radicals may also form—

$$H^{\cdot} + O_2 \longrightarrow HO_2^{\cdot}$$

Hydroperoxyl (HO_2) free radical also may contribute to formation of hydrogen peroxide in tissues—

$$HO_2^{\cdot} + H^{\cdot} \longrightarrow H_2O_2$$
$$HO_2^{\cdot} + HO_2^{\cdot} \longrightarrow O_2 + H_2O_2$$

HO_2 and H_2O_2 are oxidizing agent, can alter biological molecules and cause cell destruction.

Indirect Effect

- Photon may get absorbed by H_2O in an individual, ionizing the H_2O molecule
- Resulting ions form free radicals which intern interacts and produces changes in biological molecules, the effects is termed as indirect
- About 2/3rd of biologic effects of ionizing radiation exposure result from indirect effect
- The photon may be absorbed by HO_2, form H and OH free radicals, which interact with organic molecule forming organic free radicals
- OH^0 free radical is more important in producing the damage:

$$RH + OH^{\cdot} \longrightarrow R^{\cdot} + HO_2$$
$$RH + H^{\cdot} \longrightarrow R^{\cdot} + H_2$$

- Organic free radicals are unstable and transform into stable altered molecule
- These altered molecules have different chemical and biological properties than original molecules
- Fate of free radicals—

$$\left.\begin{array}{ll}\text{Dissociation:} & R^{\cdot} \longrightarrow X + Y^{\cdot} \\ \text{Cross-linking:} & R^0 + S^{\cdot} \longrightarrow RS\end{array}\right\} \begin{array}{l}\text{stable but} \\ \text{altered molecule}\end{array}$$

Effect on Biologic Molecules

Nucleic Acids

Radiation-induced cell death, mutation and carcinogenesis actually occur due to damage to DNA **(Figs. 17.1 and 17.2)**.

Effect of ionizing radiation on DNA includes:

- Breakage of one or both strands of DNA
- Cross-linking of DNA strands within the helix to other DNA strands
- Change or loss of base
- Disruption of hydrogen bonds between DNA strands.

Proteins

Radiations does not significantly alter the primary structure of the protein but changes the secondary or tertiary structures by disrupting the side chains or due to the breakage of H or – S – S bonds.

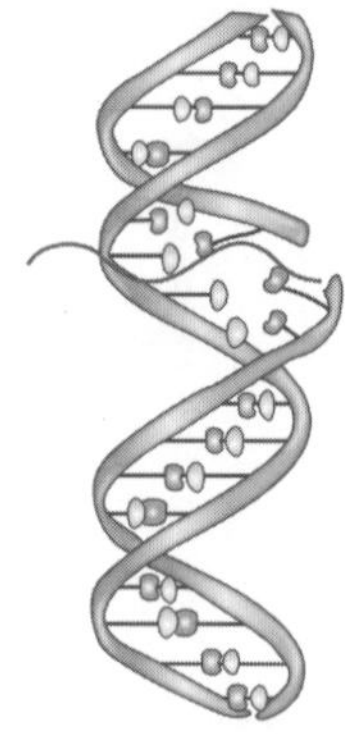

Fig. 17.1: DNA single-strand break

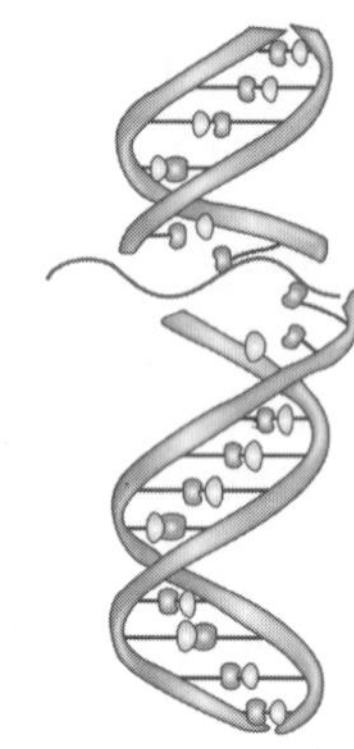

Fig. 17.2: DNA double-strand break

Thus, protein gets denatured. The effect is more severe when an enzyme gets irradiated because it leads to inactivation of an enzyme. The dose of radiation for denaturation of proteins or inactivation of enzyme is much higher than that required for inducing gross cellular changes or cell death. Dose required is more than 4 Gy.

Question 2

What are the effects of radiation on biological structures?

Answer

Effect on Intracellular Structures

The initial molecular changes starts with fraction of second after exposure but it may take minimum hours for cellular changes to become apparent after moderate exposures.

The changes include:

- Structural changes
- Functional changes and cell death.

Effect on Nucleus

The nucleus is more radiosensitive than cytoplasm especially in dividing cells.

Chromosome Aberrations

- Chromosomal aberrations are observed in the irradiated cells at the time of mitosis when DNA condenses to form the chromosomes
- The type of damage depends on the stage of the cell cycle at the time of irradiation, **(Fig. 17.3)** e.g., if irradiation occurs after DNA synthesis only one arm of the affected chromosome is broken **(Fig. 17.4)**
- But, if irradiation occurs before DNA has replicated then both arm of the chromosome may be broken at next mitosis **(Fig. 17.5)**
- Most simple breaks are repaired by biologic processes and go unrecognized
- Radiation-induced aberrations may result in unequal distribution of chromatin material to daughter cells or prevent completion of a subsequent mitosis **(Fig. 17.6)**.

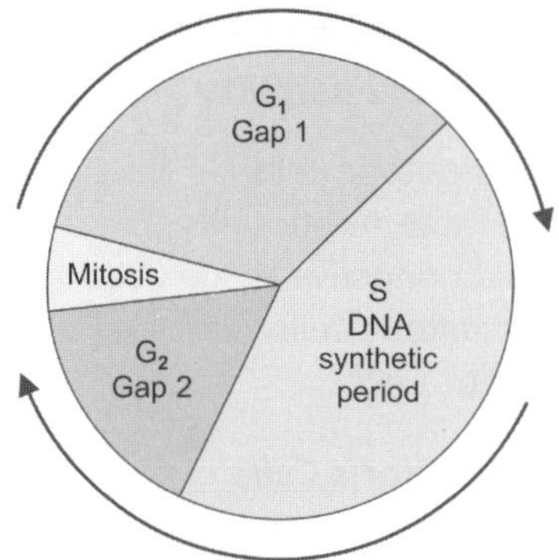

Fig. 17.3: Stages of cell cycle

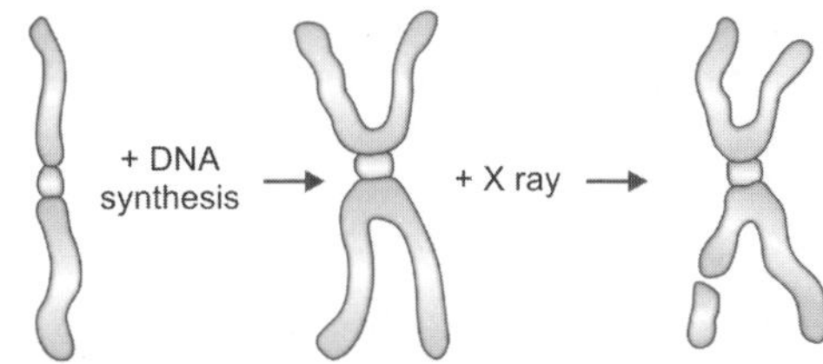

Fig. 17.4: Effect of irradiation after DNA synthesis

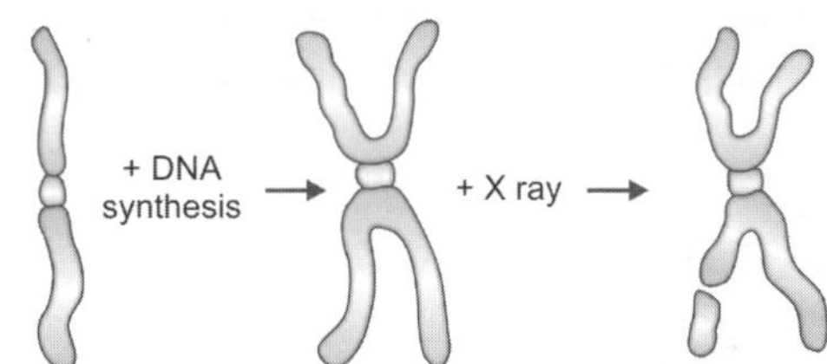

Fig. 17.5: Effect of irradiation before DNA has replicated

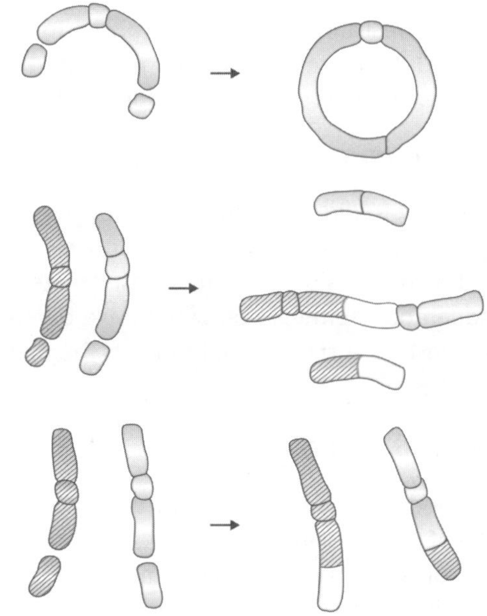

Fig. 17.6: Radiation induced chromosomal aberrations

Effect on Cytoplasm

At doses larger than 30–50 Gy, mitochondrias show increased permeability, swelling and disorganization of internal cristae.

Effect on Mitosis

- Low doses–Mild delay of mitosis in G_2 cells
- Moderate doses–Longer mitotic delay (G_2 block)
- Larger doses–Profound mitotic delay with incomplete recovery.

Cell Death

- Means loss of capacity of cell for mitotic division
- The cell death is caused by the damage to the nucleus that leads to chromosomal aberrations
- This damage causes the cell to die, usually during an attempt to complete the first few mitosis after irradiation
- Reproductive death occurs in dividing cell populations after exposure to moderate dose of irradiation
- Larger doses and longer time intervals are required for inducing interphase death to a population of non-dividing cells.

Radiosensitivity and Cell Type

Most radiosensitive cells are those that:
- Have a high mitotic rate
- Undergo many future mitoses
- Are most primitive in differentiation.

Mammalian Cells may be Divided into Five Categories of Radiosensitivity

1. Vegetative Inter-mitotic Cells
2. Differentiating Inter-mitotic Cells
3. Multi Potential Connective Tissue Cells
4. Reverting Post-mitotic Cells
5. Fixed Post-mitotic Cells.

Vegetative Inter-mitotic Cells

- Most radiosensitive
- They divide regularly, have long mitotic futures and do not undergo differentiation between mitoses, e.g., early precursor cells, such as those in spermatogenic or erythroblastic series and basal cells of oral mucous membrane.

Differentiating Inter-mitotic Cells

- Less radiosensitive because they divide less often
- Examples include intermediate dividing and replicating cells of the inner enamel epithelium of developing teeth, cells of haematopoietic series that are in the intermediate stages of differentiation, spermatocytes and oocytes.

Multi Potential Connective Tissue Cells

- Intermediately radiosensitive
- Divide irregularly, e.g., vascular endothelial cells, fibroblasts and mesenchymal cells.

Reverting Post-mitotic Cells

Generally radio-resistant because they divide infrequently, e.g., acinar and ductal cells of salivary glands and pancreas as well as parenchymal cells of liver, kidney and thyroid.

Fixed Post-mitotic Cells

- Most resistant to direct action of radiation
- Most highly differentiated cells and once mature are in capable of division, e.g., neurons, striated muscle cells, squamous epithelial cells that have differentiated and are close to surface of oral mucous membrane and erythrocytes.

Effect at Tissue and Organ Level

- Loss of moderate number of cells does not affect the function of most organs
- But, loss of large number of cells may lead to changes and severity of this change depends upon the dose of radiation and thus amount of cell loss
- Moderate doses to localized area may lead to a repairable damage
- But, comparable doses to a whole organism may lead to death from damage to most sensitive systems of the body.

Short-term Effect

- If continuously proliferating tissues, e.g., bone marrow, oral mucous membranes, etc. with moderate doses, cells are lost by mitosis-linked death
- Tissues composed of cells that rarely or never divide (e.g., nucleus) show little or no radiation-induced hypoxia over short term
- The extend of cell loss depends on the damage to the stem cell pools and on the proliferative rate of the cell population
- The effects of irradiation of such tissues become apparent relatively quickly as a reduction in the number of mature cells in the series.

Long-term Effect

- The long-term effects depends primarily on the extend of the damage to the fine vasculature (capillaries)
- Irradiation of capillaries causes swelling, degeneration and necrosis resulting in increased capillary permeability and initiating slow fibrosis around the vessels
- Leads to premature narrowing and eventual obliteration of vascular lumens
- As a result, transport of oxygen, nutrients and waste products are impaired and result in death of all cell types
- Such progressive atrophic changes lead to loss of cell function and decrease the resistance of irradiated tissues to infection and trauma.

Question 3

What are the effects of radiation on oral tissues?

Answer

The effects of radiation on various oral tissues are as follows:

Oral Mucous Membrane

Basal layer contains radio sensitive, vegetative and differentiating inter-mitotic cells.

- First week: No changes seen
- End of second week: Mucositis (Redness and inflammation of mucosa)
- As therapy continues: Mucosa breaks down and form white-to-yellow pseudomembrane (Desquamated epithelial cell layer)

- At the end of therapy: Severe mucositis, maximum discomfort, and food intake difficulties
- Secondary infection with *C. albicans* becomes common
- After completion of radiation, mucosa begins to heal rapidly and gets completed by about 2 months
- After months to years, the mucosa tends to become atrophic, thin, avascular due to the progressive obliteration of fine vascular and fibrosis of underlying connective tissue
- These atrophic changes: Denture wearing gets complicated as oral ulcers may be formed from denture sore, radiation necrosis or tumour recurrence.

Taste Buds

Taste buds are sensitive to radiation. Doses in therapeutic range:

- Extensive degeneration of normal histologic architecture of taste buds
- Loss of taste acuity (during 2nd or 3rd week) (acuity decreased by a factor of 1,000 to 10,000 during the full course of radiotherapy)
- Bitter and acidic flavours severely affected (irradiation of posterior 2/3rd)
- Salty and sweet flavours are more severely affected (irradiation of anterior 1/3rd)
- Recovery occurs within 2–4 months after irradiation.

Salivary Glands

Parenchymal component of glands is more radio sensitive (parotid > submandibular > sublingual salivary glands).

- Marked loss of salivary secretion during first week
- May reach to 0 at 60 Gy
- Mouth become dry (xerostomia) and tender
- Swallowing difficult and painful (residual saliva loses its normal lubricating properties)
- Dry mouth more severe if parotids are irradiated bilaterally
- pH of irradiated saliva 5.5 (Normal pH—6.5)
- Decalcification of normal enamel (due to low pH)
- Buffering capacity of saliva falls by 44%
- Radiation caries (oral microflora becomes more acidogenic, *S. mutans*, Lactobacillus and Candida count increased)
- If some portion of major salivary gland spared dryness of mouth usually subsides in 6–12 months because of compensatory hypertrophy of residual salivary gland tissue
- The reduced salivary flow, if persist beyond a year is unlikely to show significant recovery.

Teeth

- Destruction of tooth bud (irradiation before calcification)
- Inhibition of cellular differentiation causing malformations and arresting general growth (irradiation after calcification)
- Retarded root development, dwarfed teeth or failure to form one or more teeth (permanent dentition), irradiation of jaws in children
- Pulpul tissue shows long-term fibroatrophy after irradiation
- Eruptive mechanism of teeth is relatively radiation resistant
- Adult teeth are very resistant to direct effect of radiations
- Radiation has no severe effect on crystalline structure of enamel, dentine and cementum and also does not increase their solubility.

Bone

- Irradiation of mandible occurs during treatment of cancer in oral region
- Damage to mature bone due to damage to the vasculature of periosteum and cortical bone
- Destruction of osteoblasts, osteoclasts to a lesser extent
- Subsequent to irradiation, normal marrow gets replaced by fatty marrow and fibrous connective tissue
- Marrow spaces become hypovascular, hypocellular and hypoxic
- Endosteum becomes atrophic, shows lack of osteoblastic and osteoclastic activity, some lacunae of compact bone are empty (indicative of necrosis)
- Degree of mineralization altered or reduced leading to brittleness
- When these changes become severe, osteoradionecrosis occurs (death of bone due to irradiation).

Question 4

Explain acute radiation syndrome (ARS).

Answer

When the whole body is exposed to low or moderate doses of radiations, characteristic changes (ARS) develop. Acute radiation syndrome is collection of signs and symptoms experienced by persons after acute whole body exposure to radiations.

Doses (Gy)	Manifestations
– 2	Prodromal symptoms
– 4	Mild haematopoietic symptoms
4 – 7	Severe haematopoietic symptoms
7 – 15	Gastrointestinal symptoms
50	Cardiovascular system (CVS) and central nervous system (CNS) symptoms

Prodromal Period

Within first minute to few hours after exposure to whole-body irradiation about 1.5 Gy gastrointestinal tract (GIT) disturbances may occur.

GIT disturbances, i.e.,
- Nausea
- Vomiting
- Diarrhoea
- Weakness
- Fatigue.

The severity and time of onset of prodromal symptoms are dose related. So, higher the dose, the more rapid the onset and greater the severity of symptoms.

Latent Period

- It is period of apparent wellbeing after radiations during which no signs or symptoms of radiation sickness occurs
- The extent of latent period is also dose related, e.g., latent period is of few weeks at sublethal doses of less than 2 Gy
- But, at supralethal doses of more than 5 Gy, the latent period extends from few hours to few days only.

Haematopoietic Symptoms (2–7 Gy)

- Injury to haematopoietic stem cells of bone marrow and spleen occurs
- They are highly sensitive because their mitotic activity is high and presence of many differentiating cells
- Falls in the number of circulating granulocytes, platelets and finally erythrocytes. They as such are very resistant but their decreasing count in peripheral blood after irradiation shows the radiosensitivity of their precursors
- The differential changes in blood count do not all appear at same time but it depends on the life span of that cell in the peripheral blood
- Granulocytes with short life span, fall off in a matter of days where as RBC with their long life spans falls off slowly
- The clinical picture becomes evident only as the circulating cellular elements show decline
- Hence, in a week after radiation, first there is
  - Infection (lymphopenia, granulocytopenia)
  - Haemorrhage (thrombocytopenia)
  - Anaemia (erythrocytopenia).
- Death may occur within 10–30 days after irradiation at doses on higher range side
- Since, periodontitis is a likely source of entry for micro-organisms into blood stream, dentist has sufficient time of about 7–10 days (before clinically significant leukopenia develops) in preventing periodontal or pulpal infection in haemopoietic syndrome
- The removal of sources of infection, vigorous administration of antibiotics and transplantation of bone marrow have saved the lives of several irradiated individual from ARS.

Gastrointestinal Symptoms (7–15 Gy)

- Extensively damages the GIT in addition to the haematopoietic damage
- Prodromal symptoms of nausea, vomiting, diarrhoea, weakness and fatigue start within few hours of exposure
- Followed by latent period of about 5th day
- During this period, injury to rapidly proliferating basal epithelial cells of intestinal villi, leads to loss of epithelial layer of intestinal mucosa (denudation of mucosa)
- Due of denudation, plasma and erythrocytes are lost, impaired intestinal absorption, etc.
- Ulceration and haemorrhages of intestines
- Septicaemia (because of invasion of denuded mucosal surface by endogenous intestinal flora)
- By the time, the developing damage to gastrointestinal reaches a maximum, the effect of bone marrow depression is just beginning to be manifested
- Death generally occurs within 2 weeks due to:
  - Destruction of rapidly proliferating cells of intestine
  - Lowered body's defence against bacterial infections
  - Decreased effectiveness of clotting mechanisms
  - Fluid and electrolyte loss
  - Nutritional impairment.

Cardiovascular and Central Nervous System

Exposure in excess of 50 Gy. Usually cause death in 1–2 days.
- Collapse of circulating system due to precipitous fall in blood pressure
- Intermittent stupors, in coordination, disorientation and convulsions (suggestive of severe damage to CNS)
- Symptoms are more likely to be due to the radiation-induced damage to the neurons and fine vasculature of the brain
- CVS, CNS syndrome is irreversible with the clinical course of few minutes to about 48 hours before death occurs
- Patient may die even before the effects to bone marrow and GIT can develop.

Management of Acute Radiation Syndrome

- Antibiotic (during infections or leucopenias)
- Fluid and electrolyte replacement
- Administration of platelets (to arrest haemorrhage)

- Whole blood transfusion (to treat anaemia)
- Bone marrow graft indicated between identical twins (as, there is no risk for graft v/s host disease).

Question 5

What are the measures used for radiation protection?

Answer

Principles of Radiation Protection

The current radiation protection standards are based on three general principles:

- Justification of a practice, i.e., no practice involving exposures to radiation should be adopted unless it provides sufficient benefit to offset the detrimental effects of radiation
- Protection should be optimized in relation to the magnitude of doses, number of people exposed and also to optimize it for all social and economic strata of patients
- Dose limitation, on the other hand, deals with the idea of establishing annual dose limits for occupational exposures, public exposures and exposures to the embryo and foetus.

Methods of Exposure and Dose Reduction

Selection of Patient

- Prescribing dental radiographs should be justified in order to minimize the unwanted exposure
- Diagnostic radiography should be used only after clinical examination, consideration of patient history and consideration of both dental and general health needs of patient.

Choice of Equipment

It includes:

- Image receptor selection
- Use of intensifying screens
- Focal spot to film distance
- X–ray beam collimation and filtration
- Use of lead apron and collars.

Intraoral Image Receptors

- Films with faster speed (sensitivity) should be used
- Faster the speed, more sensitive the image receptor and less time required for its exposure
- Regular dental X–ray film was in 1920 (but so slow speed requires 9 sec for maxillary molars)
- Currently, intraoral films are available in three speed D, E and F
- Clinically, film speed of E is about twice as fast as film of group D and about 50 times as fast as regular film
- F–speed film requires only 75% of exposure of E film and 40% for that of D–speed films
- This means that the 9 sec exposure required for regular film has been reduced to 0.2 sec for E-speed films and to 0.12 sec for F-speed films.

However, the possible decrease in image quality associated with increased speed obtained by increasing the size and shape of silver halide crystals must be considered.

It has been found that F–speed films had the same useful density range, latitude, contrast and image quality as D and E–speed film when processed in automatic processors.

Using digital intraoral radiography patient dose reduction is about 75% compared with D–speed films, about 50% compared with E–speed films and about 40% compared with F–speed films.

Intensifying Screens

- Used for extraoral radiography
- Contains rare earth elements gadolinium and lanthanum, which decreases patient exposure by as much as 55% as compared to older tungstate screens.

Further, reduction in patient exposure is achieved by using T grain film, which contains tabular or flat silver halide crystals rather than pebble like.

These grains present a greater cross-section, which increases their capacity to gather light from intensifying screens.

The Ultravision and Ektavision films should be used, which minimize the cross over because it contains phosphors that emit UV light, which is less able to pass through the film to expose the opposite emulsion. This also reduces patients' exposure.

Focal Spot to Film Distance (FSFD)

- Extended FSFD reduces the amount of radiations to the patient
- Two standard FSFDs have evolved for use in intraoral radiography, i.e., 20 cm (8 inch) and 4 cm (16 inch)
- The X-ray source—skin distance should not be less than 17.5 cm (7 inch) assuming 2.5 cm (1 inch) distance from the skin surface to the film
- Use of long FSFDs result in 32% reduction in exposed tissue volume because at greater distance, the X-ray beam is less divergent
- Use of longer FSFD also results in smaller apparent focal spot size, which thereby increases the resolution of the radiograph.

Collimation

- It is the process of reducing the size of the X-ray beam so as to reduce the area exposed
- The X-ray beam used in intraoral radiography be collimated so that the field of radiation at the patients skin surface is "contained in a circle having a diameter of no more than 7 cm at or above 50 kVp, which is more than sufficient to expose the no 2 intraoral film"
- Limiting the size of the X-ray beam also increases the qual- ity of image by decreasing the amount of scattered radiation production and hence, decreases the chances of film fogging.

Methods of decreasing the size of X-ray beam (collimation):

- Rectangular position indicating device (PID) may be attached to the tube housing having an exit opening of 3.5 × 4.4 cm, which reduces the patients skin surface exposure by about 60% than an round (7 cm) PID. Reducing the beam, however, makes aiming the beam difficult
- So, to avoid cone cuts, a film-holding device that centres the beam over the film is recommended
- Film holders with rectangular collimators may be used with round PIDs. It reduces the patients' exposure to the same degree as rectangular PIDs.

Filtration

- The filtration is the process of removing low-energy photons, which do not have any diagnostic value but only adds to the patients' exposure
- When an X-ray beam is filtered with 3 mm of aluminium, the surface exposure is reduced to about 20% of that with no filtration
- Patients' exposure may further be reduced by filter of both very high-energy and low-energy photons from the beam leaving the mid-range photons for exposing the film (between 35 and 55 kev)
- Use of aluminium filter along with the rare earth elements (samarium, erbium, yttrium, gadolinium, etc.) further reduces the patients' exposure by 20%–80% of that done with aluminium filtration.

Lead Aprons and Collars

- Leaded thyroid collars are strongly recommended
- Although scattered radiation to the patients' abdomen is extremely low, leaded aprons should be used to minimize patients' exposure to radiations
- Thyroid shield reduces the exposure of this gland by as much as 92%, while lead aprons reduce the exposure to gonads by as much as 98% (by attenuating the beam)
- As per the ALARA principle, no matter how small the dose is, some adverse effects may result
- Therefore, any dose that can be reduced without any difficulty, great expense or inconvenience should be reduced
- However, use of faster speed films and rectangular collimation are far more important means of protecting the patient.

Choice of Intraoral Technique (Operating the Equipment)

- Paralleling long cone technique preferred
- Film holder to be used instead of patients manual support (reduces the number of unacceptable periapical films)
- Precision instrument with rectangular field of collimation reduces patients' exposure even more.

Kilo Voltage (kVp)

- Range of 70–100 kVp is suitable for most purposes
- When kVp is decreased, effective energy of the beam is decreased with an increase in the image contrast
- When kVp is increased, effective energy of beam is also increased, with a decrease in the image contrast
- High kilo voltage technique, which produces images of low contrast, also reduces the effective dose delivered per intraoral examination
- An increase in kVp from 70 to 90, reduces the effective dose by as much as 23%.

MilliAmpere—Seconds (mAs)

- The exposure time is shown to be the most crucial factor in influencing diagnostic quality which means that the radiograph is of diagnostic density neither overexposed (too dark) or underexposed (too light)
- Both over/under exposed films result in repeated exposures adding to needless further patient exposure
- Image density is controlled by the quantity of X-rays produced which itself depends upon the combination of milliampere (mA) and exposure time in seconds termed as milliampere seconds (mAs)
- Patient exposure is directly related to mAs
- The use of a photo timer measures the quality of radiation reaching the film and automatically terminates the exposure when enough radiations have reached the film to provide optimal density
- This also reduces the unnecessary prolonged exposure.

Protection of Personal Taking Radiographs

The steps that can be taken to reduce the chance of occupational exposures include:

- Dental operatories should be designed and constructed to meet the minimum shielding requirements of NCRP
  - Walls must be of sufficient density or thickness so that exposure to non-occupational exposed individuals should not be greater than 100% µGy per week
  - Wall of the X-ray rooms on which primary X-ray beam falls is not less than 35 cm thick brick or equivalent
  - Walls of the X-ray room on which scattered X-rays fall is not less than 23 cm thick brick or equivalent
  - There is a shielding equivalent to at least 23 cm thick brick or 1.7 mm lead in front of the doors and windows of the X-ray room to protect the adjacent areas, either used by general public or not under possession of the owner of the X-ray room
  - Walls may be coated with lead and even with gypsum wallboard (dry wall or sheet rock).
- Position and rate distance rule.

The operator should stand at least 6 feet from the patient at an angle of 90 to 135 to the central ray of X-ray beam (in this position, most of the scattered radiations are absorbed by the patients head).

- Operator should never hold the films in place. Film-holding instruments must be used
  - If, correct film placement and retention are still not possible, a parent or any attendant with the patient should be asked to hold the film (lead apron must be given to him).
- While making exposures, the radiographic tube should not be holded
- Film badges to be used
  - These badges contain a piece of sensitive film or a radiosensitive crystal (thermoluminated dosimeter) and a printed report of accumulated exposure at regular intervals
  - Film badges are inexpensive, easy to use and easy to process. Although they are useful for detecting radiation at or above 0.1 mSv, they are not sensitive enough to capture lower levels of radiation.

SHORT ESSAYS

Question 1

What are the factors that influence the effects of radiation?

Answer

The following factors or the factors that influence the effects of radiation:

Dose

- Severity of deterministic damage depends on amount of radiation received
- All individuals receiving doses above threshold level show damage in proportion to dose.

Dose Rate

- Dose rate indicates the rate of exposure
- Exposure of biologic systems to a given dose at high dose rate causes more damage.

Oxygen

The greater cell damage sustained in the presence of O_2 is related to the increased amounts of H_2O_2 and hydroperoxyl free radicals are formed.

Linear Energy Transfer

- Dose required to produce a certain biologic effect is reduced as the linear energy transfer of the radiation is increased
- Thus, higher linear energy transfer radiations are more efficient in damaging biologic system
- Low linear energy transfer radiations, such as X-rays deposit their energy uniformly in the absorber and thus are more likely to cause single strand breakage and less biologic damage

Question 2

Explain radiation caries.

Answer

Radiation caries is a rampant form of dental decay. Occur due to irradiation of salivary gland.

Causes

- Decreased salivary secretions
- Decreased salivary flow
- Decreased pH of saliva 5.5 (Normal 6.5)
- Reduced buffering capacity

- Increased viscosity of saliva
- Acidogenicity of micro-oral flora
- Increased count of acidogenic microflora
- Reduced or absent self-cleansing action of normal saliva
- Radiation of teeth by itself does not initiate the course of radiation caries but is mainly due to change in physical and chemical properties of saliva and microflora.

Types of Radiation Caries

- Widespread superficial lesions involving buccal, occlusal, incisal and palatal surfaces
- Involvement of dentine and cementum primarily in cervical areas
- Progresses circumferentially around the teeth and results in loss of crown
- Dark pigmentation of entire crown is seen. Incisal edges are markedly worn. Some patients develop combination of all these lesions.

Treatment and Prevention

(a) Viscous topical 1% neutral sodium fluoride gel in custom made applicator trays, daily for 5 minutes

(b) Avoidance of dietary sucrose

Both (a) and (b) causes a delay in the irradiation induced elevation of *S. mutans* as well as it decreases the concentration of both *S. mutan* and Lactobacillus.

(c) Dental restorative procedures

(d) Excellent oral hygiene maintenance.

Teeth, which are grossly decayed or periodontally involved, are often extracted before irradiation.

Question 3

Explain radiolysis of water.

Answer

Water is predominant molecule in biologic system.

It frequently participates in interactions between X-ray photon and biological molecule of an organism.

First step: Ionization of water due to absorption of photon or interaction with photoelectron or Compton electron.

Displacement of electron from water result in positively charged water molecule and displace electron.

$$\text{Photon} + H_2O \longrightarrow e^- + H_2O^+$$
$$\text{Photoelectron } e^- + H_2O \longrightarrow 2e^- + H_2O^+$$

Displace electron captured by water and form negatively charged water molecule.

$$e^- + H_2O \longrightarrow H_2O^-$$

not stable ↓ and dissociate

$$H_2O^- \longrightarrow OH^- + H^\cdot$$

Positively charged water molecule react with another molecule and form hydroxyl free radical—

$$H_2O^+ + H_2O \longrightarrow H_2O^+ + OH^\cdot$$

Water may also be excited and dissociate directly into hydrogen and hydroxyl free radical—

$$\text{photon} + H_2O \longrightarrow H_2O^* \longrightarrow OH^\cdot + H^\cdot$$

When dissolved with molecular oxygen (O_2) present in irradia-ted water, hydroperoxyl free radicals may also form—

$$H^\cdot + O_2 \longrightarrow HO_2^\cdot$$

Hydroperoxyl (HO_2) free radical also may contribute to formation of hydrogen peroxide in tissues—

$$HO_2^\cdot + H^\cdot \longrightarrow H_2O_2$$
$$HO_2^\cdot + HO_2^\cdot \longrightarrow O_2 + H_2O_2$$

HO_2 and H_2O_2 are oxidizing agent, can alter biological molecules and cause cell destruction.

CHAPTER 18 X-Ray Films

LONG ESSAYS

Question 1

What is the composition of X-ray film?

Answer

X-ray film is a photographic film consisting of a photographically active, or radiation-sensitive, emulsion that is usually coated on both sides of a transparent sheet of plastic, called base.

Emulsion

- Two important ingredients are *silver halide grains* and *vehicle matrix* in which crystals are suspended
- It is coated on both the sides of the base
- Thickness is not more than 0.5 mm
- Silver halide grains are sensitive to X-radiations
- Mainly composed of silver bromide (AgBr) (90–99%).

Photosensitivity of Films is Increased by Adding

- *Silver Iodide (AgI)*: 1–10% increases sensitivity of film as it disrupts regularity of AgBr crystal structure
- Trace amounts of gold
- In *InSight films*, silver halide grains are flat, tabular structures with mean diameter of 1.8 µm
- *Ultra Speed films* are made up of globular-shaped crystals of 1 µm diameter
- The vehicle, composed of gelatinous and non-gelatinous materials, keeps the silver halide grains evenly dispersed.

Protective Layer

An additional layer of clear gelatin is applied to emulsion as super coat (acts as barrier) which protects film from damage by scratching, contamination or pressure from rollers when an automatic processor is used.

Film Base

- The function of the base is to support the emulsion
- Transparent supporting material composed of polyester polyethylene terephthalate—0.02 mm (0.007 in)
- The base has a slight bluish tint, which makes viewing the films easier on the eye
- The film base must also withstand exposure to processing solutions without becoming distorted.

Adhesive Layer

It is a thin adhesive material on both sides of the base, which ensures good adhesion between emulsion and base.

Sizes of Intraoral Films

- 0: Used in children for both periapical and bitewing radiographs; used for small mouths (22 × 35 mm)
- 1: Used for adult anterior periapicals radiographs (24 × 40 mm)
- 2: Used for adult periapicals and bitewings radiographs (31 × 41 mm)
- 3: Used for extra-long bitewing films; one film covers all teeth on one side of the mouth (27 × 54 mm)
- 4: Used for occlusal films (primarily adults) (57 × 76 mm).

Question 2

Describe the packaging of the intraoral periapical films.

Answer

- The X-ray film packet is made of plastic or paper
- The film is encased in a black paper wrapper followed by an outer white paper or plastic cover
- Between the two wrappers is a thin embossed lead foil
- The foil is positioned in the film packet behind the film, away from the tube

- The lead foil acts as a shield against the back scatter radiations, which reduce the image quality by reducing contrast by fogging of the film
- Lead foil also reduces patient exposure to radiation by absorbing the residual radiations
- A small raised dot is made on one corner of the film
- This dot is use to orient the film in patient's mouth by keeping the dotted side facing the X-ray tube with the depression towards the patient's tongue
- This dot helps in identifying right and left side after the image has been processed.

Question 3

Explain intensifying screens.

Answer

- One of the properties of X-rays is that it causes certain materials to fluoresce (emit light); the phosphor crystals found in intensifying screens are one of these materials
- It creates an image receptor system that is 10–60 times more sensitive to X-rays than the film alone thus substantial reduction in the dose of X-radiation
- The resolving power of screens is related to their speed; the slower the speed of a screen, the greater its resolving power and vice-versa.

Action

- Two intensifying screens are used—one in front of the film and the other at the back
- The front screen absorbs the low-energy X-ray photons and the back screen absorbs the high-energy photons
- The two screens are therefore efficient at stopping the transmitted X-ray beam, which they convert into visible light by the photoelectric effect
- One X-ray photon will produce many light photons, which will affect a relatively large area of film emulsion
- Thus, the amount of radiation needed to expose the film is reduced.

Composition

Base

- Made of polyester plastic that is about 0.25 mm thick
- The base provides mechanical support for the other layers.

Reflecting Layer

- Thin layer of white material—magnesium oxide or titanium dioxide between base and phosphor layer

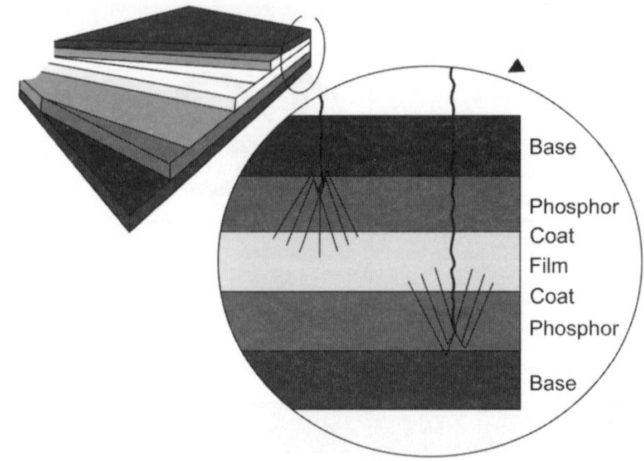

Fig. 18.1: ***

- It reflects light emitted from the phosphor layer back toward the X-ray film
- This has the effect of increasing the light emission of the intensifying screen.

Phosphor Layer

The phosphor layer is composed of phosphorescent crystals suspended in a polymeric binder. When the crystals absorb X-ray photons, they fluoresce.

Three main phosphor materials are used in intensifying screens:

1. Calcium tungstate ($CaWO_4$)—emits blue light and must be used with blue-light sensitive monochromatic radiographic film
2. Rare earth phosphors including gadolinium and lanthanum
3. Yttrium (a non-rare earth phosphor).

Typical Screens Include

- Terbium-activated gadolinium oxysulphide—emit *green* light
- Thulium-activated lanthanum oxybromide—emit *blue* light
- Yttrium (Z = 39), the rare earth-related phosphor, in the form of pure yttrium tantalate emits *ultraviolet* light.

Protective Layer

- A protective polymer coat (up to 15 μ thick) is placed over the phosphor layer
- Function: Helps to prevent static electricity, protect the phosphor, provide a surface that can be cleaned
- The intensifying screens should be kept clean because any debris, spots, or scratches may cause light spots on the resultant radiograph.

Question 4

What are grids?

Answer

- Invented by Dr Gustave Bucky in 1913
- These consist of a series of lead foil strips separated by transparent spacers
- Prevents scatter radiation from reaching film.

Composition

- Composed of a series of a long parallel strips of opaque material (usually lead) held and parallel to each other by an X-ray
- Interspaces of grids are filled either with aluminium or organic compounds
- Lead strip thickness—0.05 mm
- Interspaces are much thicker than Pb strips
- The main purpose of interspace material is to support the thin lead foil.

An X-ray grid absorbs scattered X-ray photons from the primary beam and prevents them from fogging the film. In a focused grid, the absorber plates are angled towards the anode; in a parallel grid, the absorber plates are parallel.

Types

- Focused grids and non-focused grids
- Stationary and moving grids.

Stationary Grids

- Grids are stationary and does not move
- Presence of grid between object and film causes the image of radiopaque absorbing material to be projected on film.

Moving Grids

Synonym—Potter Bucky grid, Bucky grid

- Invented by Dr Hollis E Potter in 1920
- Grid is moved perpendicular to the direction of the grid lines during exposure
- This has the effect of blurring out the radiolucent lines and allowing a more uniform exposure
- Most moving grids are reciprocating, that is, they continuously move 1–3 cm back and forth throughout exposure
- They start moving when X-ray tube head begins to rotate.

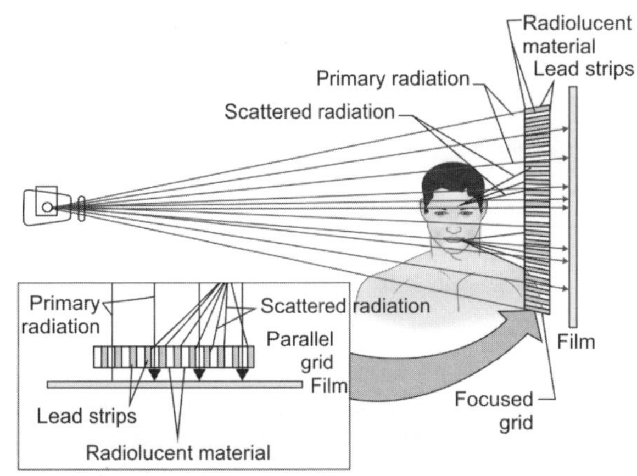

Fig. 18.2: ***

Grid Ratio

- Ratio between height of lead strips and distance between them
- Expressed as two numbers, such as 10:1 with the first number the actual ratio and second number always 1
- It is used to describe grids ability to remove scatter radiation
- Ratio ranges from 4:1 to 16:1
- Higher the ratio, the better is grid function
- Indicated at the top of grid by manufacturers.

Advantages

- Prevents scatter radiation from reaching film
- Scattered radiation causes fog and reduces contrast of film
- This is because the scattered photons have lower energy than primary photons and therefore less penetrating and thus causes fogging of film
- Fine-wired grid when superimposed upon exposing radiographs aid in measurement of relative bone height
- Grid forms 1 mm square, which appear as fine radiopaque lines on resultant radiograph
- This allows quantitative measurement of the position of alveolar bone with respect to dentition.

Disadvantages

- Exposure required is higher when grid is used as compared to absence of grid. This is to compensate for the presence of Pb strips, thus exposure time must be increased
- Bucky grids are costly and may vibrate the X-ray table.

CHAPTER 19 Processing of X-Ray Films

LONG ESSAYS

Question 1

Discuss the processing of X-ray films?

Answer

Processing of an X-ray film describes the process of converting invisible latent image into visible radiographic image from the emulsion in a series of sequential steps.

Processing is Done

- For formation of visible image
- To preserve the image for later correspondence permanently.

Processing Types

There are two types of processing methods:

1. Manual: It consists of
   a. Visual method
   b. Time-temperature method.
2. Automatic processing.

Manual Processing

Visual Method

This kind of processing is performed in a dark room under safe lighting conditions.

- In this method, the exposed X-ray film is immersed in the developing solution and then viewed periodically under the safe light
- Upon the emergence of a clear image, the film is washed followed by immersion into the fixing solution.

Time–temperature Method

- It is a manual processing method in which effective standardization can be achieved
- In this technique, the film is immersed in the developer and is kept at a constant temperature for a fixed amount of time
- Operator has a direct control over the action of development
- This technique requires a dark room, is time consuming and wet film have to be handled.

Time-temperature Chart

Temperature	*Development time*
76°F	3 min
70-72°F	4 min
68°F	5 min
65°F	6 min

Automatic Processing

This technique is performed in automatic processing machines.

- In this method, the exposed film is placed at one end and is then passed automatically in a sequential manner through developer, fixer, water and drier
- The automatic processing machines have a roller system for the transportation of film
- This roller system has a squeezing action too
- The film is transported from the developer to the fixer, the developing solution absorbed by the gelatine of the emulsion will be less
- The film, then comes out from the other end for the processors, which is fully processed, dried and ready for viewing.

Method of Manual Processing

Following are the steps in manual processing of X-ray films:

1. Developing the film
2. Rinsing in water
3. Fixing the film
4. Again rinsing the film in water
5. Drying and maintaining of the film.

Developing the Film

- Exposed film is immersed in developing solution until a clear image emerges
- Developing time ranges from few seconds to few minutes, depending upon the exposure time of film and concentration of the developing solution.

Rinsing in Water

- Film is then rinsed in water for 15–20 seconds
- This helps in removing an alkali of the developing solution before placing in acidic fixer and also slows down process of development.

Fixing of Film

- For about 8–10 minutes, the film is placed in the fixer
- Fixing solution removes the unprocessed silver halide crystals and harden the emulsions
- Film fog and proper contrast can be lost if fixing is done for too long.

Rinsing the Film in Water

- After fixing, the film should be washed properly in running water for sufficient length of time so as to remove any residual fixing solution
- Staining on the film can occur, if the film is not washed properly and if silver compounds are not removed
- Image can also be discoloured because of the presence of thiosulphate and its products.

Drying and Mounting of Film

- It is the final step
- It includes drying of film and mounting it for viewing
- The film should be dried in a relatively dust-free environment
- Driers are also available commercially for drying the film
- Watermarks can lead to artefacts, thus, it becomes very important to dry the films
- The processed films should be properly identified, mounted and then viewed.

Question 2

Discuss about the darkroom.

Answer

The darkroom provides with a completely darkened environment where the X-ray films are handled and processed for the production of radiographs.

Equipment for Darkroom

Darkroom consists of following equipment:

- Safelights
- Visible light source (tube light)
- Working area for loading extraoral cassettes
- Processing tanks
- Thermometer and stop clock
- Dryer
- Storage facility for unexposed films
- Proper ventilation and exhaust.

Requirements of a Darkroom

- Process of processing becomes easier, if a dark room is well planned and well equipped
- An ideal darkroom should have following characteristics:
    - Location should be convenient
    - Size should be adequate with sufficient working space
    - Ample amount of storage space
    - Correct lighting equipment
    - Controlled temperature and humidity
    - A waste basket for disposal of all film wrapping
    - X-ray view box.

Location should be Convenient

A darkroom should be located near a area where X-ray units are installed.

Size should be Adequate with Sufficient Working Space

- The size of the darkroom is determined by following factors:
    - Volume of radiographs processed
    - Number of persons using the room
    - Type of processing equipment used
    - Space required for duplicatin of film and storage.
- Average size should be 6 ft × 8 ft
- The ceiling should not be less than 2.7 m high
- The floor should remain non-slippery and resistant to staining
- The walls should have 2.0 mm equivalency of lead for protection from the ionizing radiation
- A 25-mm thick barium plaster can also be used
- The area where the film are stored should be well covered.

Correct Lighting Equipment

- Darkroom should be light proof and it should have a proper lock system to avoid accidental opening
- There are two types of essential lighting in a darkroom:
    1. Room lighting
    2. Safe lighting.

Room Lighting

- Incandescent room lighting is required for procedures not associated with the act of processing films
- To perform tasks like cleaning, fixing chemicals and stocking materials, and over head white light should be provided, which provides adequate illumination.

Safe Lighting

- Safe lighting is a special type of lighting that provides illumination in the darkroom
- Safe lighting consists of a low wattage (15 watt) bulb and a safe light filter
- A safe light filter removes the short wavelength in the blue-green portion of the visible light spectrum which are responsible for exposing and damaging the X-ray film
- It is important to maintain an adequate safe light illumination distance minimum of 4 ft (12 m) and to keep film handling times to minimum, otherwise they appear fogged, and unwrapped film should be processed immediately under safe light conditions
- A good universal safe light filter should be used in a dark room in which both intraoral screen films and intraoral films can be processed in the GB X-2 safe light filter by Kodak.

Ample Amount of Storage

- There should be ample room space for chemical processing solution, film cassettes and other miscellaneous radiographic supplies
- Opened extraoral film boxes should be shown in the darkroom
- A light tight storage drawer is necessary to protect opened boxes of unexposed extraoral film
- Unopened box of film should not be stored in the darkroom.

A reaction between the fumes from chemical processing solutions in the film emulsion can occur, which would result in film fogging.

Controlled Temperature and Humidity

- To prevent film damage, the temperature and humidity level of the dark room should be controlled
- Recommended room temperature is of 70°F
- Film fog would result, if the room temperature exceeds 90°F
- Humidity level of between 50% and 70% should be maintained
- Film emulsion would not dry, if the humidity levels were too high
- If the humidity levels are too low, static electricity becomes a problem and causes film artefacts
- Darkroom should have provision of both hot and cold water along with mixing valves to adjust the water temperature in the processing tanks.

Question 3

What is the composition and action of developing and fixing solution in the dental radiography?

Answer

Developing Solution

It consists of following:

- Developing agents
- Preservatives
- Activator
- Restrainer
- Hardener
- Fungicide
- Buffer
- Solvent.

Developing Agents

- It is also referred to as reducing agents
- It consists of following chemicals
  - Hydroquinone (para-dihydroxybenzene)
  - Elon or Metol (monomethyl-para-aminophenyl sulphates)
  - Metol/phenidone(1-phenyl 1-3 pyrazolidinone).
- Developing agent reduces the imposed silver halide crystals chemically to black metallic silver
- Hydroquinone acts slowly and produces the black tones and the sharp contrast of the radiographic image
- Hydroquinone is temperature sensitive and is active above 80°F and inactive below 60°F
- Films are best developed at 70°F for 5 min
- Elon is a product of aniline dyes and acts quickly to produce a visible radiographic image
- It helps to develop shadow areas or shades of grey on the film
- It is less sensitive to temperature changes and generates grey tones in the image
- Metol phenidone: It is a byproduct of aniline dyes, works at a faster rate and gives a low contrast
- It is an efficient activator for hydroquinone at a very less concentration and works at a lower alkalinity
- If only Elon is used, image will have shades of grey
- If only hydroquinone is used, image would be black and white

- If a combination of both Elon and hydroquinone is used, image would be black, white and grey shades.

Preservative

- Sodium sulphite is the preservative used
- Since it has a great affinity for oxygen, it prevents oxidation of developer solution and forms sulphonates, when combined with oxygen.

Activator

- Sodium carbonate is used as an activator
- Sodium hydroxide, sodium metaborate and sodium tetraborate can also be used
- Activator provides alkaline medium usually above a pH of 11, which is required for hydroquinone to act and it also soften the gelatin of the emulsion.

Restrainers

- Potassium bromide or benzothiazole is used as a restrainer
- It prevents chemical fogging.

Hardeners

Glutaraldehyde is used as a hardener to prevent emulsion from softening and sticking.

Fungicide

Added to prevent bacterial growth.

Buffers

Added to maintain the pH of developer.

Solvent

Distilled water acts as solvent and as a medium in which the chemicals can react with the silver bromide of the emulsion.

Fixing Solution

Composition:

- Fixing agents
- Preservative
- Hardening agent
- Acidifier.

Fixing Agents

- It is also known as clearing agent and is made up of sodium thiosulphate (hypo) or ammonium thiosulphate
- Its action is to clear all unexposed and undeveloped silver halide crystals from the film emulsion, which allows light to pass through the film image and permits viewing of the radiographic image on a view box.

Preservative

- Sodium sulphite is the preservative
- It prevent the chemical deterioration of the fixing agent
- It also helps to clear the film by binding with any oxidized developer, which is carried to the fixing solution.

Hardening Agents

- Potassium alum, aluminium chloride act as the hardening agent
- It hardens and shrinks the gelatin in the film emulsion to prevent its oxidation and protects it against the scratches
- It also shorten the drying time
- Also neutralizes any contaminating alkali from the developer.

Acidifier

- Acetic acid or sulphuric acid is used as acidifier
- It neutralizes the alkaline developer
- It provides acidic sodium for diffusion of the thiosulphate into the emulsion.

CHAPTER 20 Intraoral Radiographic Techniques

LONG ESSAYS

Question 1

Explain paralleling and bisecting angle technique.

Answer

Paralleling Technique

- Also called as right angle or long-cone technique
- In this technique, the X-ray beam is passed in perpendicular direction to the long axis of teeth and film, which is placed parallel to long axis of the tooth **(Fig. 20.1)**
- This kind of orientation of the tooth, X-ray beam and the film leads to minimum amount of geometric distortion of the image
- To reduce further distortion, the distance between the X-ray source and the object is increased
- Film holders are used to place and stabilize the film in patient's mouth while recording the image
- For maxillary projections, the superior border of the film generally rests at the height of the palatal vault in the midline
- Similarly, for mandibular projections, use the film to displace the tongue toward the midline to allow the inferior border of the film to rest on the floor of the mouth away from the mucosa on the lingual surface of the mandible.

Procedure

Step 1: Film Position

- Vertical dimension:
  - Film is kept parallel to the long axis of the tooth on the lingual/palatal side of the tooth
  - Keep the film far away from the lingual surface of the tooth **(Fig. 20.2)**.

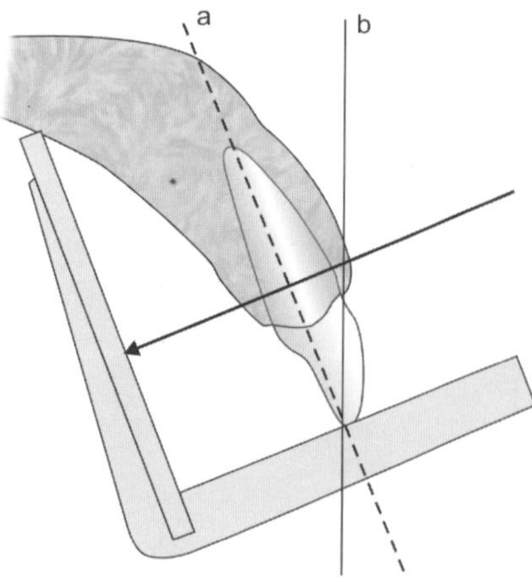

Fig. 20.1: Positions of the film, tooth and the central ray of the X-ray beam in the paralleling technique.

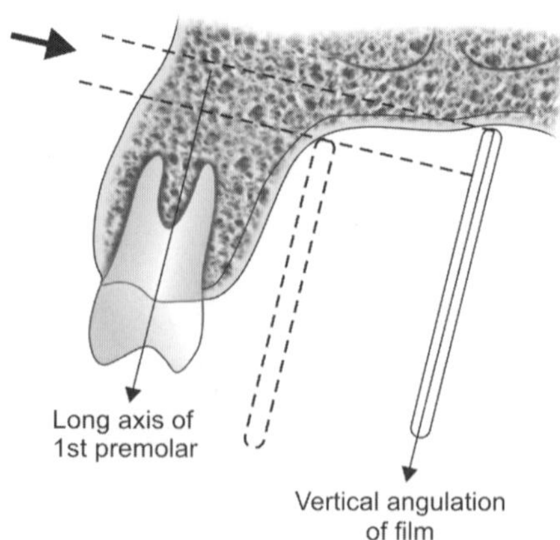

Fig. 20.2: Diagram illustrating the vertical dimension film position

- Two-point contact:
  - A two-point contact is maintained by the film by touching the top edge with the palate and bite portion of the film holder with the occlusal surface **(Fig. 20.3)**.
- Horizontal dimension:
  - The horizontal plane of the film should be placed parallel to the facial surface of the teeth being radiographed **(Fig. 20.4)**.

Step 2: Beam Alignment

- Vertical: Direct the X-ray beam perpendicular to the long axis of the tooth and the film
- Horizontal: Direct the X-ray beam through the contact areas of the tooth.

Bisecting Angle Technique

Based on the geometric theorem, Cieszynski's rule of isometry: This theorem states, "two triangles are equal when they share one complete side and have two equal angles."

Application of the theorem **(Fig. 20.5)**:

- The film is positioned as close to the lingual surface of the tooth as much as possible, resting on the palate or floor of the mouth
- Long axis of the tooth and the plane of the film form an angle with its apex at the point where the film is in contact with the tooth
- Construct an imaginary line that bisects this angle and direct the central ray of the beam at right angles to this bisector
- This forms two triangles with two equal angles and a common side (the imaginary bisector)
- Once these requirements are satisfied, the image cast of the film will be of same size as the object
- To reproduce the length of each root of a multirooted tooth accurately, the central beam must be angled differently for each root
- Another limitation of this technique is that the alveolar ridge often projects more coronally than its true position.

Positioning of the Patient

- Maxillary teeth radiograph: Position the patient's head in upright direction with the sagittal plane vertical and the occlusal plane horizontal **(Figs. 20.6 and 20.7)**
- Mandibular teeth radiograph: The head is tilted back slightly to compensate for the changed occlusal plane when the mouth is opened.

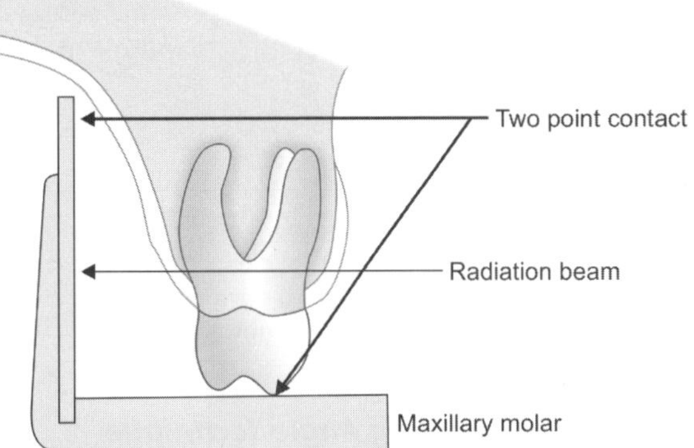

Fig. 20.3: Diagram illustrating the two-point contact film position

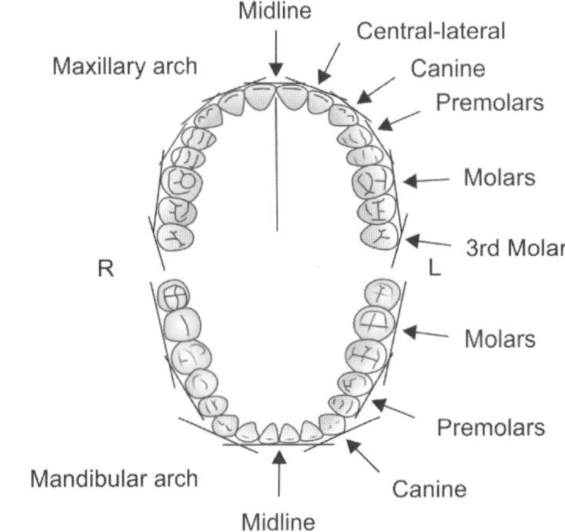

Fig. 20.4: Diagram illustrating position of film and X-ray beam in relation to various teeth in maxillary and mandibular arches

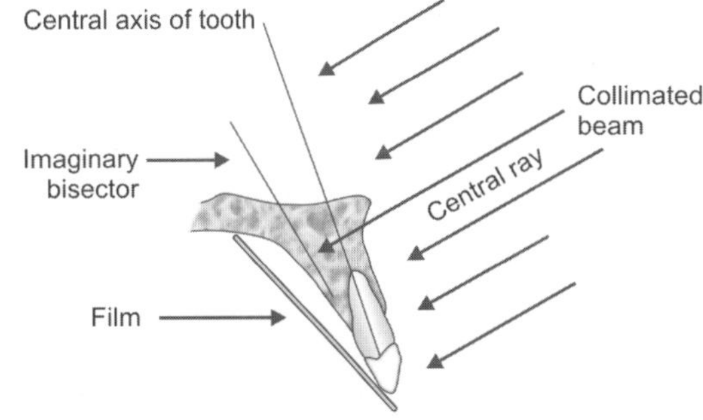

Fig. 20.5: Bisecting angle technique: Position of film, X-ray beam and tooth

Angulation Guidelines of the Tube Head

With occlusal plane being parallel to the floor, the following angles are used for the recording images of different teeth in bisecting angle technique **(Table 20.1)**.

Table 20.1: Angulation guidelines of the tube head		
Projection	**Maxilla (degrees)**	**Mandible (degrees)**
Incisors	+40	–15
Canines	+45	–20
Premolars	+30	–10
Molars	+20	–5

Notes: "+" denotes tube being aimed downwards.
"–" denotes tube being aimed upwards.

Advantages of Bisecting Angle Technique

- Positioning is easy, quick and simple
- Film packet positioning is more comfortable for the patient
- The film packet can be positioned by patient without the need of film holder
- Shorter exposure time.

Disadvantages of Bisecting Angle Technique

- The film packet may deform or move out of place if film holder is not used
- If vertical angulation is increased, it results in foreshortening of the image

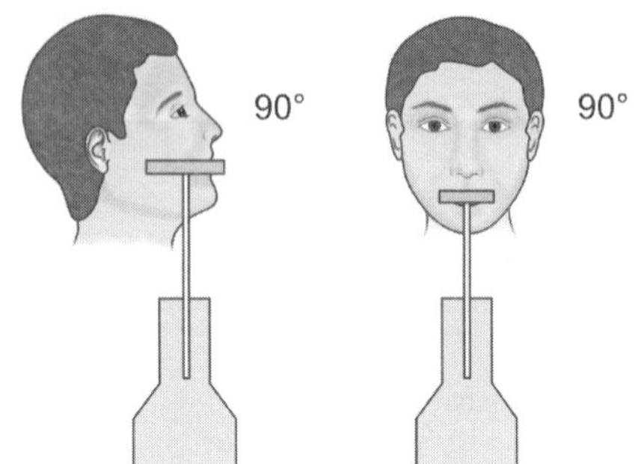

Fig. 20.6: Diagram illustrating position head in occlusal radiography.

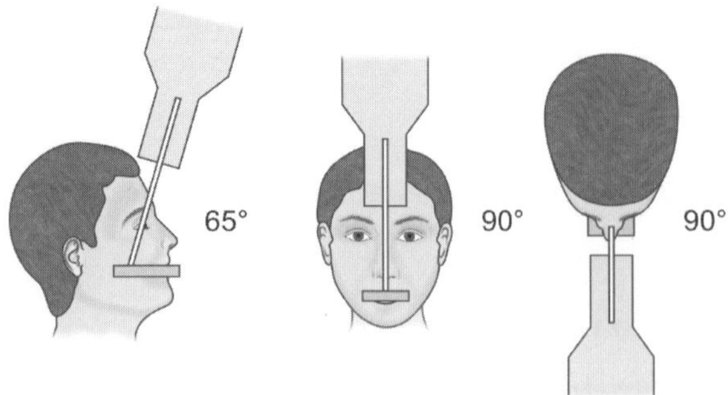

Fig. 20.7: Diagram for positioning of head in occlusal radiography

- In case of reduced vertical angulation, elongation of image occurs.

Question 2

Explain occlusal radiography.

Answer

Occlusal radiographs are used to record the occlusal areas of maxilla and mandible.

Indications

- To locate supernumerary, unerupted or impacted (canine/ third molar) teeth
- To locate salivary stones in Wharton's duct at the floor of mouth
- To locate retained roots of extracted teeth
- To locate and evaluate the extent of lesions (e.g., cyst, tumour, tori, etc.) in the maxilla and mandible
- To locate foreign bodies in either jaws
- To aid in the examination of patient who is unable to open mouth fully or in adults and children who are unable to tolerate periapical films
- As a middle view, when using the parallax method for determining the buccal/palatal position of unerupted/ impacted canines
- To evaluate boundaries of the maxillary sinus
- To examine area of cleft palate
- To evaluate fractures of maxilla and mandible (location, extent and displacement)
- To measure changes in the size and shape of the maxilla and mandible.

Basic Principles

Film Position

- Film is positioned with white side facing the arch, i.e., being exposed
- Film is placed between the occlusal surfaces of the maxillary and mandibular teeth
- Film is stabilized by the patient bite on surface of film.

Patient's Head Position

- For maxilla, the patient's head must be positioned so that the upper arch is parallel to the floor and mid-sagittal plane is perpendicular to the floor
- For mandible, the patient's head must be reclined and positioned so that the occlusal plane is perpendicular to the floor.

Angulation of Tube Head

Table 20.2: Angulation of tube head of occlusal radiography

Projection	Maxilla (degrees)	Mandible (degrees)
Cross sectional	+65	90
Topographic	+45	10
Lateral	+60	–55

Notes: "+" denotes tube being aimed downwards.
"–" denotes tube being aimed upwards.

Maxilla Occlusal Views

Cross-sectional View

Image Field

This view shows the palate, zygomatic process of maxilla, anteroinferior aspects of each antrum, nasolacrimal canals, nasal septum and teeth from right 2nd molar to left 2nd molar.

Film Placement

The film is placed crosswise into the mouth and gently pushed back until it contacts the anterior border of rami.

Projections of the Central Ray

- The central ray is directed at a vertical angulation of +65 and a horizontal angulation of 0 towards the middle of the film
- Generally, central ray enters the patient's face through the bridge of the nose.

Topographic View/anterior

Image Field

- This projection shows the anterior maxilla and its dentition
- It also includes anterior floor of nasal fossa and the teeth from canine to canine.

Film Placement

The film is placed with the exposure side towards the maxilla and long dimension crosswise in the mouth.

Projections of the Central Ray

- The central ray is directed towards the middle of the film
- The vertical angulation is +65 and horizontal angulation is 0
- Generally, central ray enters the patient's face through the tip of nose.

Lateral View

Image Field

This projection shows half of the alveolar ridge of the maxilla, inferolateral aspect of antrum, the tuberosity and the teeth from the lateral incisor to the third molar, zygomatic process of maxilla superimposed with the roots of molars.

Film Placement

- The film is placed with its long axis parallel to the sagittal plane and on the side of interest with the pebbled side towards the maxilla in question
- The lateral border should be positioned parallel to the buccal surface of the posterior teeth and extending lateral approximately 1/4th inch posterior to the buccal cusp.

Projections of the Central Ray

The central ray is projected to a point below the lateral canthus of the eye and directed towards the centre of the film with a vertical angulation of +60.

Mandible Occlusal Views

Cross-sectional View

Image Field

It includes soft tissues of the floor of mouth and lingual and buccal plates of mandible and teeth from 2nd m to 2nd m.

Film Placement

- The film is placed with its long axis perpendicular to the sagittal plane and the pebbled surface towards mandible
- The anterior border of the film should be approximately 1/2 inch approximately anterior to the mandibular central incisor.

Projection of the Central Ray

It is directed at right angles to the centre of the film. The point of entry is in the middle through the floor of the mouth approximately 3 cm below the chin.

Topographic/anterior View

Image Field

It shows anterior portion of mandible.

Film Placement

The film is placed with long axis parallel with the sagittal plane and as far posteriorly as possible with the pebbled side down.

Projection of the Central Ray

Directed towards the middle of the film with –55 angulation in respect to the plane of the film. The point of entry of the central ray in the midline and is through the tip of chin.

Lateral View

Image Field

It includes soft tissues of half of the mandible and teeth from lateral incisor to the 3rd molar.

Film Placement

- The film is placed lengthwise in the mouth with its long axis directed dorsoventrally and the pebbled
- The film is placed as far back as possible, so that the lateral border is parallel to the buccal surfaces of the posterior teeth and extending laterally approximately 1 cm.

Projection of the Central Ray

Directed perpendicular to the centre of the film. The point of entry of central ray is beneath the chin and approximately 3 cm lateral to the midline.

Question 3

Explain tube shift cone technique/Clark's rule/buccal object rule/SLOB.

Answer

The basic principle of this technique is that the relative position of the radiographic images of two separate objects changes when the projection mode is changed.

Method

- Two radiographs of the object are taken **(Fig. 20.8)**
- First using the proper technique and angulations as prescribed
- Second radiograph is taken keeping all other parameters constant and equivalent of those of the central ray either with different horizontal or vertical angulation is used.

Interpretation

- When the dental structure or object seen in the second radiograph appears to have moved in the same direction as the shift of the position-indicating device (PID), the structures or object in question is said to be positioned lingually
- If object appears to have in a direction opposite to the shift of the PID, then the object is positioned buccally
- SLOB rule: Same side lingual opposite side buccal.

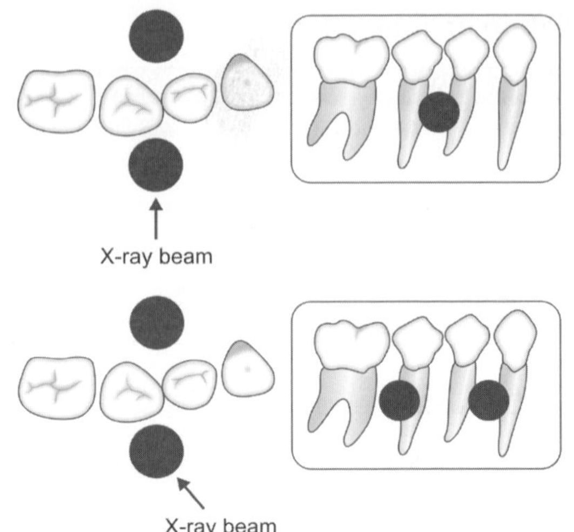

Fig. 20.8: Diagram illustrating the position of tooth and X-ray beem in tube shift cone technique

Indications

- Foreign bodies
- Impacted teeth
- Salivary stones
- Jaw fractures
- Unerupted teeth
- Root positions
- Filling materials
- Broken needles and instruments.

Question 4

Explain bitewing/interproximal radiographs.

Answer

Bitewing radiographs include the crowns of the upper and lower teeth and the alveolar crest on the same film.

Indications

- Detection of interproximal caries
- Detection of secondary caries below restorations
- To detect interproximal calculus
- Monitoring progression of dental caries
- Useful for evaluating alveolar bone crest and changes in bone height can be assessed by comparison with the adjacent teeth
- Evaluating periodontal conditions.

Principle

- The film is placed in mouth parallel to the crowns of both the upper and lower teeth

- The film is stabilized by the patient biting on the bitewing tab of bitewing holder
- The central ray of the X-ray beam is directed through the contacts of the teeth, using a +10 vertical angulation.

Size of Films

- Size 0: Used to study posterior teeth of children, always placed horizontally
- Size 1: Used to examine posterior teeth in mixed dentitions or anterior teeth of adults. It is placed horizontally for the former and vertically to the latter
- Size 2: Used to examine posterior teeth of adults and is always kept horizontally
- Size 3: It is a longer and narrower film used only for bitewing radiographs and spares horizontally from premolar to molar areas results in overlapping of the contacts.

Position Indicating Device and Angulations

- Horizontal angulations: The central ray is perpendicular to the curvature of the arch and through the contact areas of teeth
- Vertical angulations: The central ray is perpendicular to the long axis of tooth, a +10 vertical angulation is recommended for the bitewing radiograph, to compensate for the slight bend of the upper portion of the film and the slight tilt of the maxillary teeth.

Patient Position

- Seated upright and the chair adjusted to a comfortable working position **(Fig. 20.9)**
- Headrest is adjusted to support and position the patient's head so that the upper arch is parallel to the floor and mid-sagittal plane is perpendicular to the floor.

Film Position

The film must be positioned parallel to the crowns of both the upper and lower teeth and stabilized by biting on the film holder or tab.

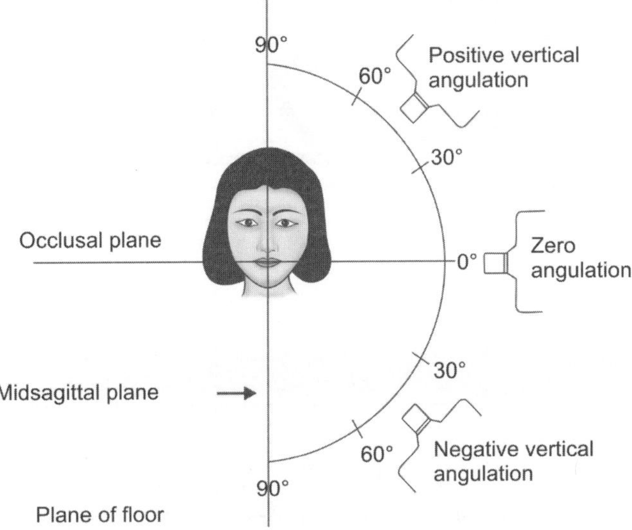

Fig. 20.9: Diagram illustrating the position and negative Vertical angulations

Vertical Angulation

The central ray must be directed at +10.

Horizontal Angulation

The central ray must be directed through the contact areas between the teeth.

Film Exposure

The X-ray beam must be centred on the film to ensure that all the areas of the film are exposed and thus partial image or cone cut is avoided.

Modifications in Technique

- Edentulous spaces: A cotton roll is placed in the area of missing teeth to support the film holder or tab
- Bony outgrowths: In case of mandibular tori, film should be placed in between tori and tongue
- In case of large tori, bitewing film holder is used to place film far away from teeth.

CHAPTER 21 Extraoral Radiography

LONG ESSAYS

Question 1

Describe the methods of extraoral radiographs for mandible.

Answer

The extraoral radiographs techniques used for mandible are:

- PA mandible
- Rotated PA mandible
- Lateral oblique:
  - Anterior body of mandible
  - Posterior body of mandible
  - Ramus of mandible.

PA Mandible

- It shows the posterio-anterior projection of the mandibular body and the ramus
- It is not suitable for showing the facial skeleton, because of superimposition of the base of the skull and the nasal bones.

Indications

- Fractures of the mandible involving the:
  - Posterior 3rd of the body
  - Angles
  - Rami.
- Low condylar neck lesions, such as cysts or tumours in the posterior 3rd of the body or rami to note mediolateral expansion
- Mandibular hypoplasia or hyperplasia
- Maxillofacial deformities.

Film Placement

Film placement is centred so that the lips are centred to the film.

Position of the Patient

- The sagittal plane should be vertical and 90 to the film
- The head is tipped forward so that radiographic baseline is horizontal and perpendicular to the film in the forehead–nose position **(Fig. 21.1)**.

Central Ray

- Centred through the cervical spine at the level of the rami of the mandible **(Fig. 21.2)**.

Exposure parameters: kVp–65, mA: 10 and Sec–2–3.

Rotated PA Mandible

This projection shows the tissues of one side of the face and is used to investigate the parotid gland and the ramus of the mandible.

Indications

- Stones/calculi in the parotid glands
- Lesions, such as cysts or tumours in the ramus to note any medio-lateral expansion
- Submasseteric infection to note new bone formation.

Position of the Patient

- The patient is positioned facing the film, with the occlusal plane horizontal and the tip of the nose touching the film in the so-called normal head position **(Fig. 21.3)**
- The head is then rotated 10° to the side of interest
- This positioning rotates the bones of the back of the skull away from the side of the face under investigation.

Central Ray

- Central ray is directed at 90° to the film, aimed down the side of the face, which is of interest

Exposure parameters: kVp–65, mA–10 and Sec.–2–3.

Mandibular Oblique Lateral Projections

- Two oblique lateral projections commonly used to examine the mandible, one for the body and one for the ramus
- A dental X-ray machine with an open-ended aiming cylinder is best for these projections
- The film: 13 cm × 18 cm (5″ × 7″) or larger
- The patient should hold the cassette.

Indications

- Assessment of the presence and/or position of unerupted tooth
- Detection of fractures of the mandible
- Evaluation of lesions or conditions affecting the jaws including cysts, tumours, giant cell lesions and osteodystrophies
- As an alternative when intraoral views are unobtainable, because of severe gagging/if the patient is unable to open the mouth
- As specific views of the temporomandibular joint (TMJ)
- Oblique laterals are categorized into:
    - Anterior body of mandible
    - Posterior body of mandible
    - Ramus of mandible.

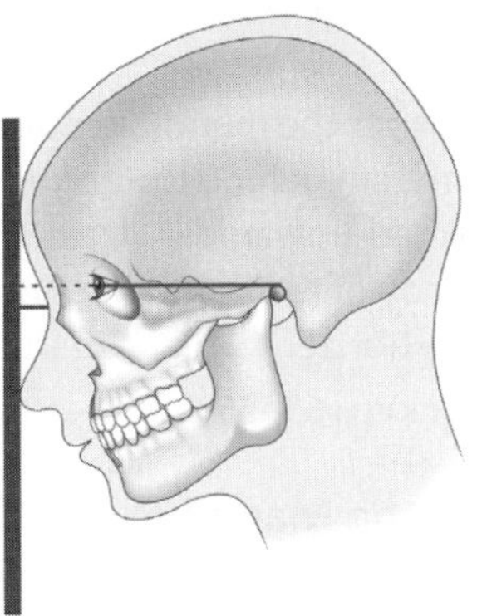

Fig. 21.1: Diagram for positioning of posteroanterior mandible projection

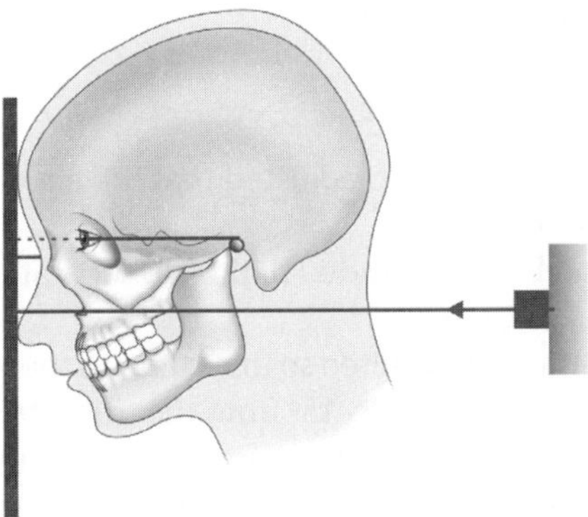

Fig. 21.2: Diagram illustrating PA mandible projection

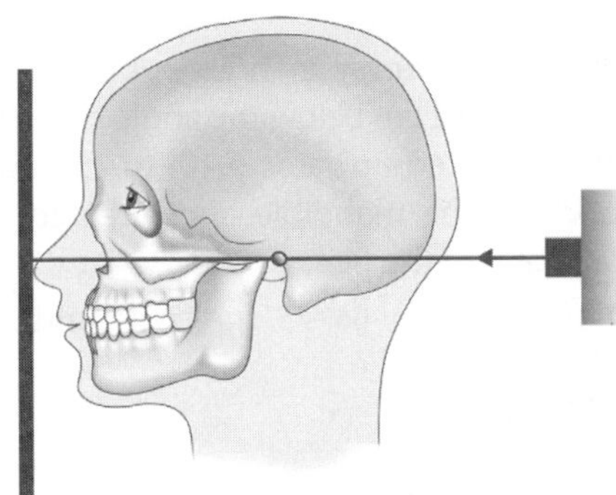

Fig. 21.3: Diagram for positioning of rotated PA mandible

Anterior Body of Mandible

Structures

- Anterior body of the mandible
- Position of teeth in the same area
- Helps to evaluate impacted teeth, fractures and lesions located in the inferior border of the mandible.

Film Placement

- The cassette is placed flat against the patient's cheek and is centred over the body of the mandible overlying the canine teeth
- Should be positioned parallel to the body of the mandible and inferior border of the cassette should be parallel to the lower border and below it.

Position of the Patient

The patient is normally seated upright in the dental chair and is then instructed to:

- Rotate the head to the side of interest to bring the contralateral ramus forwards avoiding its superimposition and to increase the space available between the neck and shoulder
- Raise the chin to increase the triangular space between the back of the ramus and the cervical spine through which the X-ray beam will pass
- The sagittal plane is tilted so that it is 5 to the vertical and rotated 30 from the true lateral position
- The patient must hold the cassette in position with the thumb placed under the edge of the cassette and the palm against the outer surface of the cassette.

Central Ray

- Is directed from under the mandible opposite the side of examination from 2 cm behind the angle of the mandible
- The beam is directed upwards (–10° to 15°) and centred on the anterior body of the mandible. The beam must be directed 90° to the horizontal plane of the film **(Fig. 21.4)**.

Exposure parameters: kVp–65–75, mA–7–10 and Sec.–0.8.

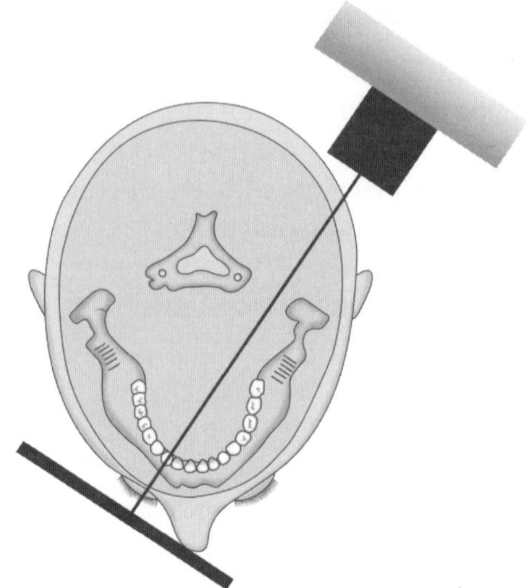

Fig. 21.4: Diagram illustrating positioning of Anterior Body of Mandible

Posterior Body of the Mandible

Structures

- Posterior body of the mandible
- Position of teeth in the same area
- Ramus of the mandible
- Angle of the mandible.

Position of the Patient

- The patient head is so adjusted that the ala tragus line is parallel to the floor
- The mandible is protruded slightly to separate it from the vertebral column
- The sagittal plane is tilted so that it is 5° to the vertical and the head is rotated 10°–15° from the true lateral position
- The patient must hold the cassette in position with the thumb placed under the edge of the cassette and the palm against the outer surface of the cassette **(Fig. 21.5)**.

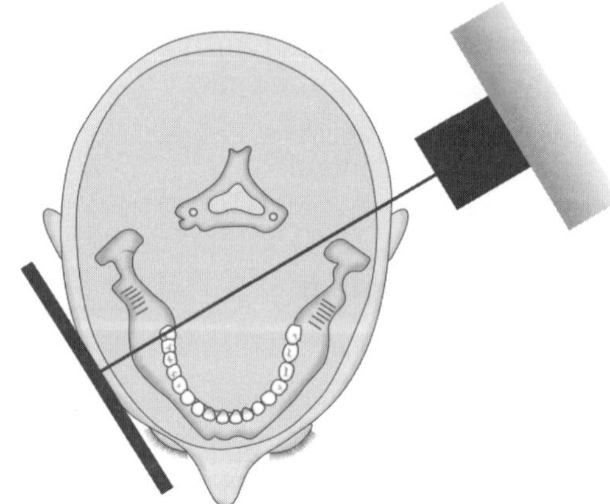

Fig. 21.5: Diagram for the positioning of lateral oblique projection for posterior body of mandible

Central Ray

- Is directed from under the mandible opposite the side of examination, from 2 cm below the angle of the mandible
- The beam is directed upwards (–10° to 15°) and centred on the body of the mandible and directed 90° to the horizontal plane of the film.

Exposure parameters: kVp–65–75, mA–7–10 and Sec.–0.8.

Ramus of Mandible

Structures

Ramus from angle of the mandible to condyles

Position of the Patient

- Ala tragus line
- The mandible is protruded slightly
- The sagittal plane is tilted to 10° to vertical
- Head tilted 5°.

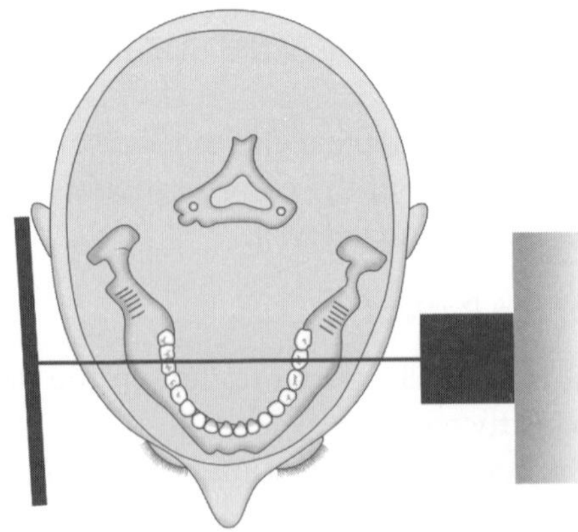

Fig. 21.6: Diagram for the positioning of lateral oblique projection for ramus of the mandible

Central Ray

- Is directed from under the mandible opposite the side of examination, from behind the angle of the mandible to a point posterior to the 3rd molar region on the side opposite to the cassette

- The beam is directed upwards (–10° to 15°) and centred on the ramus of the mandible and directed 90° to the horizontal plane of the film **(Fig. 21.6)**.

Exposure parameters: kVp–65–75, mA–7–10 and Sec.–0.8.

Question 2

What are the imaging techniques of the TMJ?

Answer

Hard Tissue Imaging

- Trans-cranial projection
- Trans-pharyngeal projection
- Trans-orbital projection
- Reverse Towne.

Trans-cranial Projection

- Sagittal view of the lateral aspects of the condyle and temporal component
- Gross osseous changes on the lateral aspect of the joint
- Displaced condylar fractures
- Range of motion.

Film Placement

The cassette is placed flat against the patient's ear and centred over the TMJ of interest, against the facial skin parallel to the sagittal plane.

Head Position

- The patient is placed with the head rotated through 90º so that TMJ under investigation is touching the film and the sagittal plane of the head is parallel to the film **(Fig. 21.7)**
- In open view, the patient's mouth is opened as far as comfortable and even a bite block can also be used for stability.

Central Ray

The X-ray beam is directed downward from the opposite side, through the cranium and above the petrous ridge of the temporal bone, at a +25º angulation through the joint **(Fig. 21.8)**.

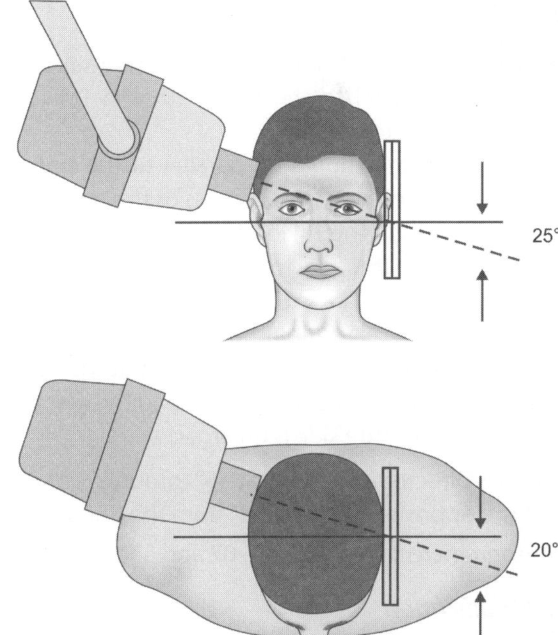

Fig. 21.7: Diagram of illustrating the position of head in trans-cranial pojection

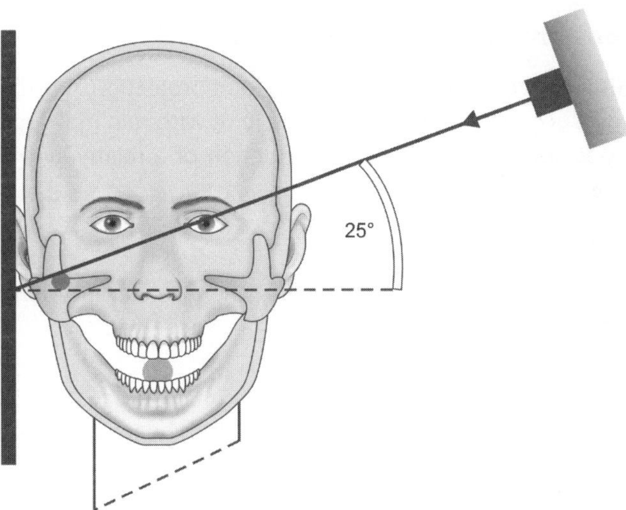

Fig. 21.8: Trans-cranial projection

Trans-pharyngeal (Infra-cranial or McQueen Dell technique or Parma)

Lateral projection of the sagittal view of the medial pole of the condylar head and neck, usually taken in the mouth open position, so that the joint is projected into the shadow of air containing spaces of the nasopharynx, which helps to increase the contrast of the various parts of the joint.

Film Placement

The cassette is placed flat against the patient's ear and is centred to a point ½ inches anterior to the external auditory meatus, over the TM joint of interest, against the facial skin parallel to the sagittal plane.

Position of the Patient

- The patient is positioned so that the sagittal plane is vertical and parallel to the film, with the TM joint of interest adjacent to the film
- The occlusal plane should be parallel to the transverse axis of the film so that the soft parts of the nasopharynx are in one line with the TM joint **(Fig. 21.9)**
- The patient is instructed to slowly inhale through the nose during exposure, so as to ensure filling of the nasopharynx with air during the exposure
- The patient should open his mouth so that the condyles move away from the base of the skull and the mandibular notch of the opposite side is enlarged.

Central ray is directed superiorly at –5° through the sigmoid notch of the opposite side and 7-8° from the anterior.

Exposure parameters: kVp–70, mA–07 and Sec.–0.8.

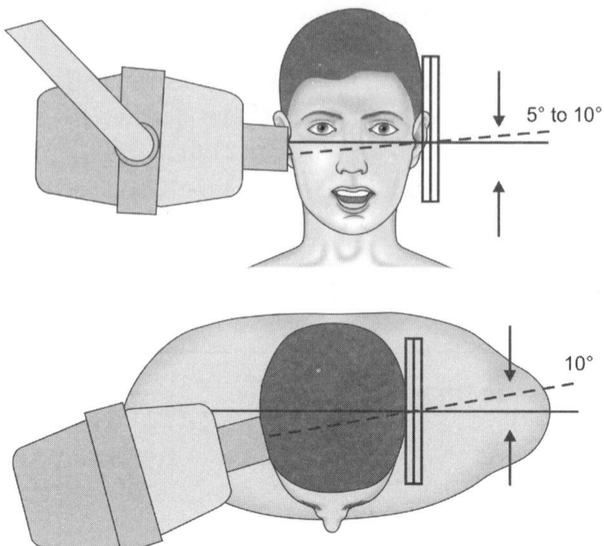

Fig. 21.9: Film placement in trans-pharyngeal projection

Parma Modification

The lead lined open-ended cone is removed and the tube head is brought close to the skin surface, producing magnification of the tube side structures and thereby reducing super imposition.

Trans-orbital (Zimmer Projection)

This is the conventional frontal TM joint projection, which is most successful in delineating the joint with minimal super impositions, leading to the production of a relatively true 'enface' projection.

Structures

The articular surface (convex) and the articular eminence (flat or convex).

Film Placement

The film is positioned behind the patient's head at an angle of 45° to the sagittal plane and perpendicular to the X-ray beam.

Position of Patient

- The patient is positioned so that the sagittal plane is vertical
- The canthomeatal line should be 10° to the horizontal, with the head tipped downwards **(Fig. 21.10)**
- The mouth should be wide open or as an alternative the mandible should be protruded, thereby positioning the condyle at the summit of the articular eminence and avoiding superimposition of the articular eminence or skull base on the condyle.

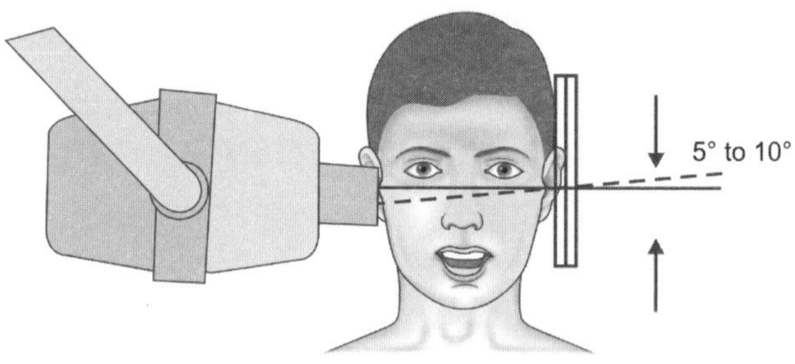

Fig. 21.10: Diagram illustration for trans-orbital projection

Central Ray

The X-ray is directed from the front of the patient through the ipsilateral orbit and TMJ of interest.

The point of entry may be taken at:

- Pupil of the same eye, asking the patient to look straight ahead
- Medial canthus of the same eye.

Exposure parameters: kVp–70, mA–07 and Sec–0.8.

Reverse Towne's Method

Indications

- High fractures of the condylar necks
- Medially displaced condyle
- Intracapsular fractures of the TMJ
- Investigation of the quality of the articular surfaces of the condylar heads in TMJ disorders
- Condylar hypoplasia or hypertrophy.

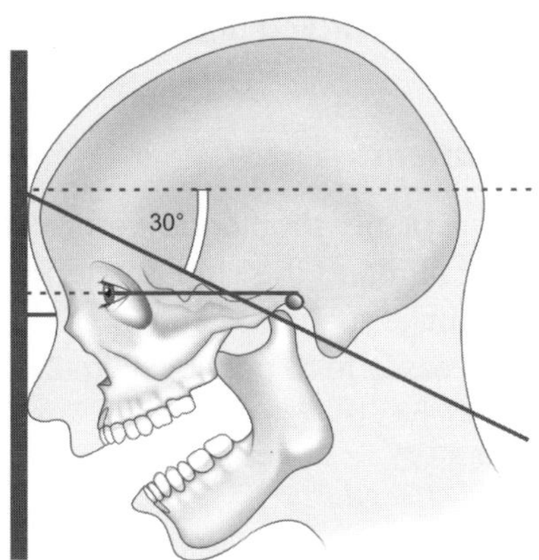

Fig. 21.11: Diagram for positioning of reverse towne's method

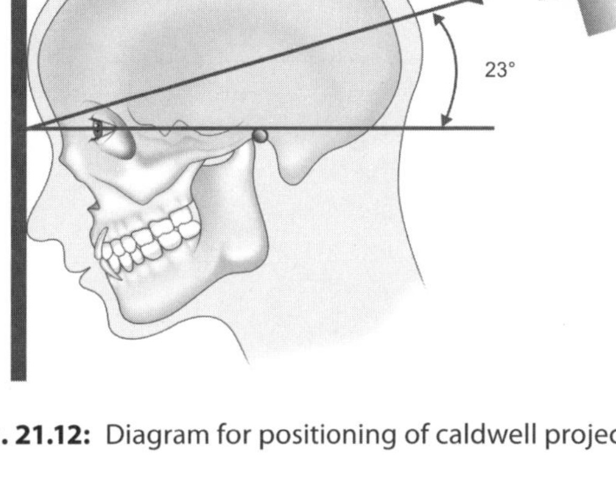

Fig. 21.12: Diagram for positioning of caldwell projection.

Position of the Patient

- The patient is in the PA position, i.e., the head tipped forwards in the forehead-nose position, but in addition, the mouth is open
- The radiographic baseline is horizontal and at right angles to the film
- Opening the mouth takes the condylar heads out of the glenoid fossae so they can be seen.

Central Ray

Is aimed upwards from below the occiput, with the central ray at 30° to the horizontal, centred through the condyles **(Fig. 21.11)**.

Exposure parameters: kVp–50, mA–20–30 and Sec.–0.4 .

Question 3

What are the imaging techniques for maxillary sinus?

Answer

Extraoral radiographic imaging techniques for maxillary sinus are:

- Modified method/Caldwell method
- PA Water's view
- Bregma Menton method.

Modified Method, Inclined Posterior Anterior (Caldwell Projection)

This angulation will cause the petrous ridges to be superimposed on the maxillary sinuses, thus allowing the accurate examination of the orbits and ethmoidal air cells.

- Position of the patient: The mid-sagittal plane is vertical and perpendicular to the cassette
- Canthomeatal line is perpendicular to the cassette

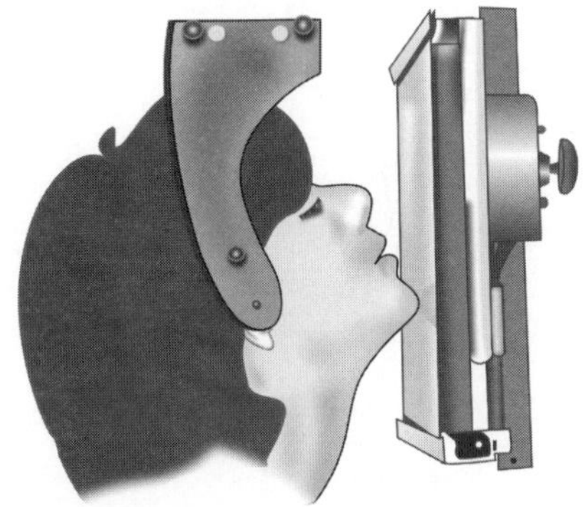

Fig. 21.13: Diagram illustrating film placement for water's view

- Central ray is directed to the 23° to the canthomeatal line, entering the skull about 3 cm above the external occipital protuberance and exiting at glabella **(Fig. 21.12)**.

Exposure parameters: Speed–250, kvp–70, mA–30–50.

Water's View

- Occipitomental view
- It is particularly useful for evaluating maxillary sinuses
- In addition, frontal and ethmoidal sinuses, the orbit, the zygomaticofrontal suture, nasal cavity
- Demonstrates the position of the coronoid process of the mandible between the maxilla and the zygomatic arch.

Film Placement

The long axis of the cassette is positioned vertically **(Fig. 21.13)**.

Head Position

The mid-sagittal plane should be vertical and 90 to the plane of the film. The canthomeatal line should be 37 above the horizontal **(Fig. 21.14)**.

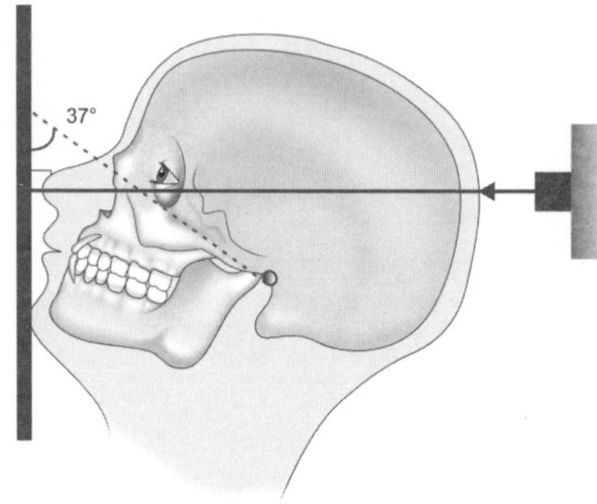

Fig. 21.14: Diagram for positioning of water's projection

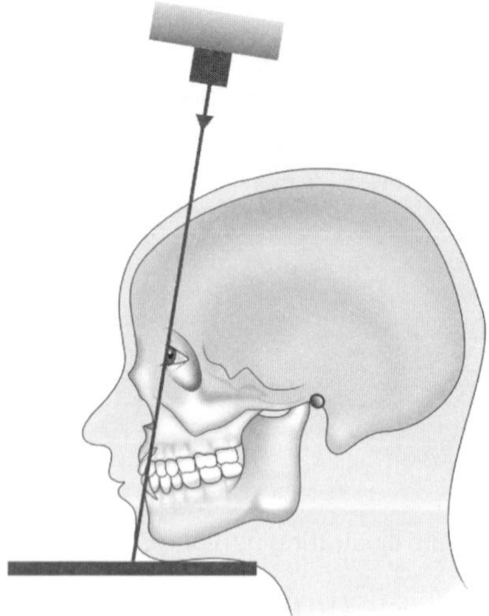

Fig. 21.15: Diagram for positioning of bregma menton projection

Central Ray

The central ray should be perpendicular to the film, through the mid-sagittal plane, and at the level of the maxillary sinus.

Exposure parameters: kVp–65, mA–10 and Sec–2–3.

Bregma Menton

- This projection is primarily used to demonstrate the walls of the maxillary sinus (especially in the posterior areas), the orbits, the zygomatic arches and the nasal septum
- Also demonstrates medial or lateral deviations of any part of the mandible.

Film Placement

- The cassette is placed in a horizontal position on top of a metal table
- The image receptor is tucked under the chin as far back as possible.

Position of the Patient

- The mid-sagittal plane should be vertical and 90 to the plane of the film and the chin is extended as far as comfortable to make the lower border of the mandible as parallel to the cassette as possible **(Fig. 21.15)**
- Only the chin touches the cassette.

Central Ray

Enters at the bregma and exits at the menton.

Exposure parameters: kVp–65, and mA: 10 and Sec.–2–3.

Question 4

What are the extraoral radiographic methods for skull imaging?

Answer

Radiographic techniques for skull are:

- Lateral cephalogram
- True lateral
- PA cephalogram
- PA skull
- Towne's projection
- Submentovertex projection (base of skull view).

Lateral Cephalometric Projection

- To survey the skull and facial bones for evidence of trauma, disease or developmental abnormality
- Nasopharyngeal soft tissues, paranasal sinuses, hard palate
- In orthodontics, to assess facial growth, pre-treatment and post-treatment records
- Conditions affecting the sella turcica, such as tumour of the pituitary gland in acromegaly
- The lateral cephalometric projection reveals the facial soft tissue profile.

Head Position

- Left side of the face near the cassette and mid-sagittal plane parallel to the plane of the film **(Fig. 21.16)**
- For cephalometric projection, patient is positioned within the cephalostat with the sagittal plane of the head vertical and parallel to the film
- Frankfort horizontal plane is kept horizontal to the floor.

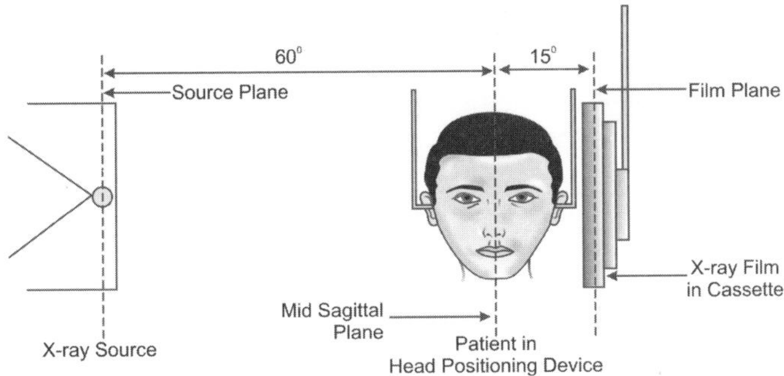

Fig. 21.16: Position of head, X-ray beam and film in lateral cephalometric projection

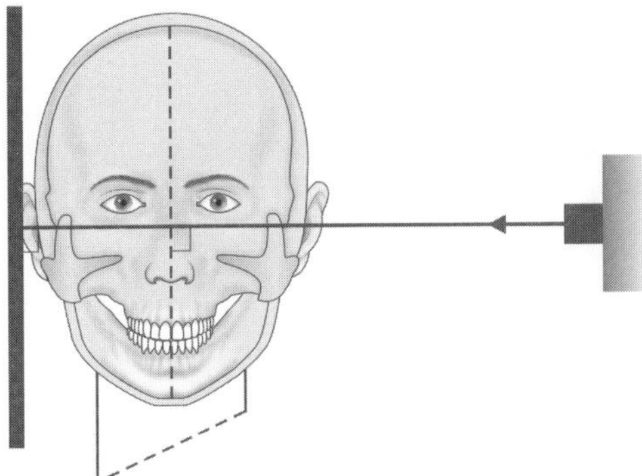

Fig. 21.17: Diagram for the positioning of lateral cephalometric projection

Projection of Central Ray

- Distance between the X-ray source and mid-sagittal plane is 152.4 cm (60 inch)
- Central ray is directed toward the external auditory meatus
- Perpendicular of the film and the mid-sagittal plane **(Fig. 21.17)**.

Exposure parameter: Speed–250, kvp–70, mAs–15–25.

True Lateral Skull

- The image receptor is positioned parallel to the patient's mid-sagittal plane
- The site of interest is placed toward the image receptor to minimize distortion
- The film is adjusted so that the upper circumference of the skull is half inch below the upper border of the cassette
- The central ray is directed perpendicular to the cassette and the mid-sagittal plane and towards the external auditory meatus.

Indications

- Fractures of the cranium and the cranial base
- Middle third facial fractures, to show possible downward and backward displacement of the maxilla
- Investigation of the frontal, sphenoidal and maxillary sinuses
- Conditions affecting the skull vault
  - Paget's disease
  - Multiple myeloma
  - Hyperparathyroidism.
- Conditions affecting the sella turcica.
  - Tumour of pituitary gland in acromegaly.

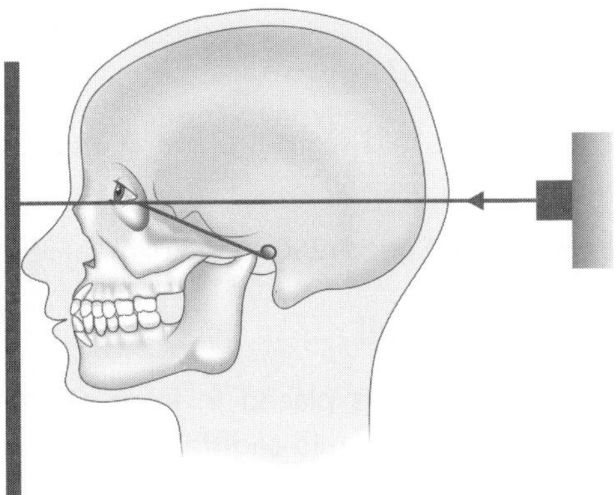

Fig. 21.18: Diagram for the positioning of posterioanterior (PA) cephalogram

Posterioanterior (PA) Cephalogram

Indications

- Examine the skull for disease in trauma or developmental abnormalities in frontal, temporal and parietal bone
- Good record to detect progressive changes in the medi-olateral dimensions of skull, including asymmetric growth
- Visualization of facial structures including the frontal and ethmoidal sinuses, nasal fossae and orbits.

Film Placement

The cassette is positioned vertically in a holding device.

Head Position

- Canthomeatal line parallel to the floor
- For cephalometric applications, the nose should be a little higher so that the anterior projection of the canthomeatal line is 10 above the horizontal plane and Frankfort plane is perpendicular to the film **(Fig. 21.18)**.

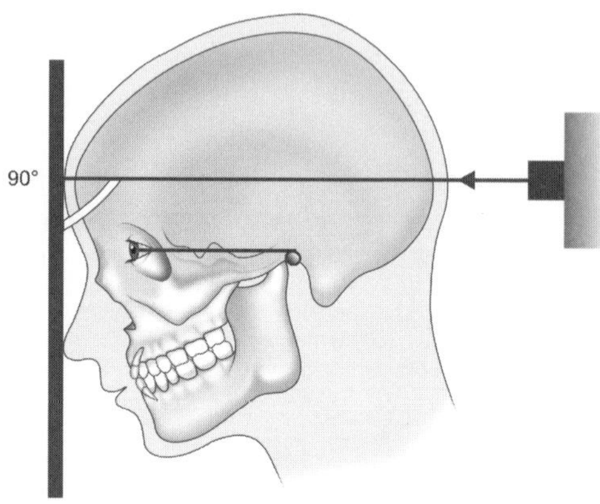

Fig. 21.19: Diagram illustrating posterioanterior skull.

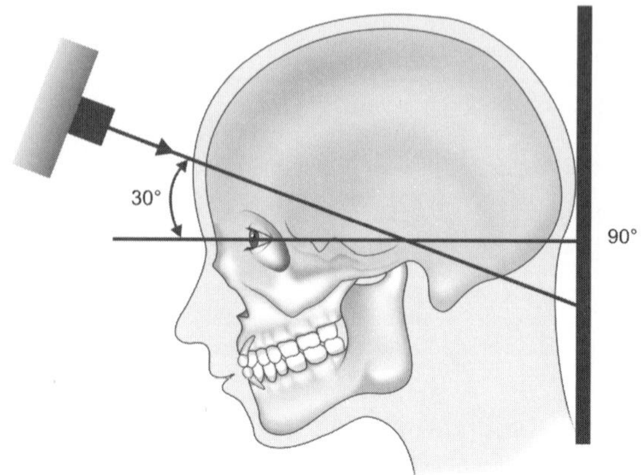

Fig. 21.20: Diagram for positioning of towne's projection

Projection of Central Ray

Coincident with the mid-sagittal plane at the level of the bridge of the nose.

Exposure parameter: Speed–250, kvp–70, mAs–30–50.

Posterioanterior Skull

- The image receptor is placed in front of the patient, perpendicular to the mid-sagittal plane and parallel to coronal plane, so that the canthomeatal line is perpendicular to the image receptor **(Fig. 21.19)**
- Central ray is directed at right angles to the film through the mid-sagittal plane through the occiput.

Indications

- Fractures of the skull vault
- Investigation of the frontal sinuses
- Conditions affecting the cranium
  - Paget's disease
  - Multiple myeloma
  - Hyperparathyroidism.
- Intracranial calcifications.

Towne's Projection

Structures

- Primarily used to observe the occipital area of the skull
- The necks of the condyloid process can also be viewed.

Film Position

- The cassette is placed perpendicular to the floor in a cassette-holding device
- The long-axis of the cassette is positioned vertically.

Position of Patient

- This is an anteroposterior (AP) view, with the back of the patient's head touching the film
- The canthomeatal line is perpendicular to the film.

Central Ray

Is directed at 30° to the canthomeatal line and passes through it at a point between the external auditory canals **(Fig. 21.20)**.

Exposure Parameters: kVp–65, mA–10 and Sec–2–3.

Submentovertex Projection

Structures

- Symmetrical projection of the petrosa
- Mastoid process
- Spinosum canals
- Foramen ovale
- Carotid canals
- Sphenoidal sinuses
- Curvature of mandible
- Lateral wall of maxillary sinuses
- Nasal septum
- Odontoid process of the atlas
- Axial inclination of the mandibular condyles.

Indications

- Destructive expansive lesions affecting the palate, pterygoid region or base of skull
- Any displacement of a fractured zygomatic arch (Jughandle view)
- Investigation of the sphenoidal sinus
- Assessment of the thickness (medio-lateral) of the posterior part of the mandible before osteotomy.

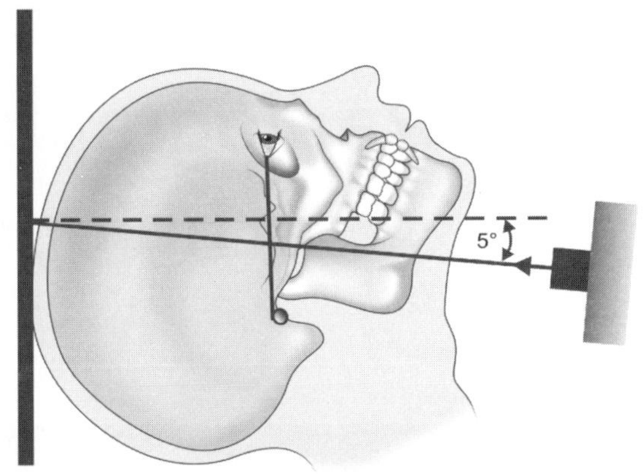

Fig. 21.21: Diagram for positioning of submentovertex projection

Position of the Patient

- The patient is positioned facing away the film
- The head is tipped backwards as far as possible, so the vertex of the skull touches film
- In this position, the radiographic baseline is vertical and parallel to the film.

Central Ray

Is aimed upwards from below the chin, with the central ray at 5 to the horizontal, centred on an imaginary line joining the lower first molars **(Fig. 21.21)**.

Exposure parameters: kVp–50, mA–20–30 and Sec.–0.4.

CHAPTER 22 Specialized Radiographic Techniques

LONG ESSAYS

Question 1

Describe in detail computed tomography (CT).

Answer

Computed tomography was developed for clinical use in 1972 and 1973 by Godfrey Hounsfield. The information presented in a CT image is different from that in a conventional radiographic image.

The most conspicuous difference is that CT shows cross-sectional views of patient anatomy.

Computed tomography is a type of cross-sectional tomographic imaging in which all unwanted planes or layers of a body are completely eliminated using mathematical techniques.

Computed Tomography is Synonymous With:

- Computerized transverse axial tomography (CTAT)
- Computer-assisted tomography or computerized axial tomography (CAT)
- Computerized tomography (CT)
- Reconstructive tomography (RT)
- Computerized transaxial transmission reconstructive tomography (CTT)
- The term computed tomography has been established by Radiology and The American Journal of Roentgenology.

Basic Physical Principles

- CT is essentially a tomographic technique giving images of slices of the patient's anatomy (as a loaf of bread may be sliced) **(Fig. 22.1)**
- Each slice may then be examined separately
- In the CT scanner, the slice location is determined by moving the patient in or out of the gantry housing
- At a given slice location, the gantry rotates around the patient with the transmitted radiation that passes through the patient measured by an array of many hundreds of detectors
- The result is some 3 million measurements of transmitted radiation taken at multiple angles
- From these measurements, the computer makes calculations to fill in each square in a matrix 512 × 512 in size

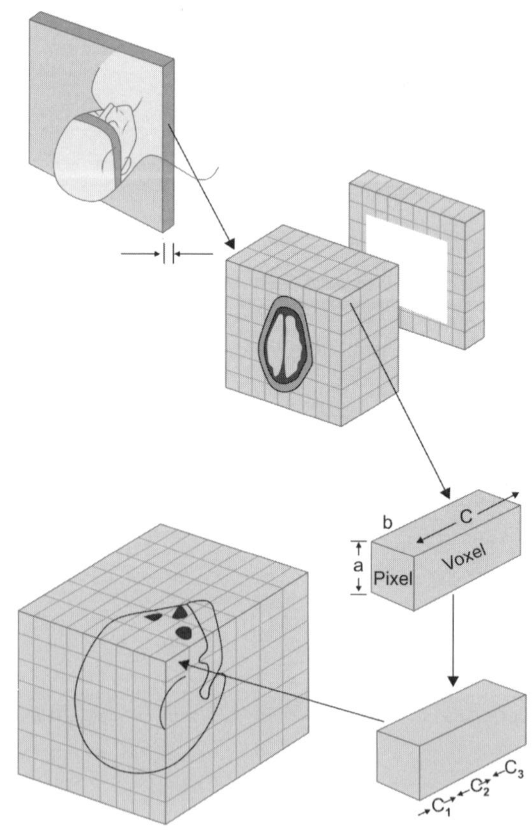

Fig. 22.1: Schematic sequence for computed tomography image acquisition

- Each square in this matrix is called a pixel or picture element
- After necessary calculations, each pixel is assigned a digital value
- This represents the X-ray absorption coefficient of all the tissue present within 1 voxel in the patient
- A *VOXEL* is defined as the "*volume of tissue bounded by the dimensions of a pixel and the width of the X-ray beam*"
- Each pixel is approximately 0.5 mm × 0.5 mm in dimensions
- Pixel size is the limiting factor in spatial resolution in CT
- For a standard head scan, the best CT resolution currently obtainable is of the order of 0.3–0.5 mm
- The width of the X-ray beam is usually 10 mm and hence each pixel value corresponds to the absorption coefficient of a volume or voxel of tissue measuring approximately 0.5 × 0.5 × 10 mm
- The width of the X-ray beam and thus the slice thickness is easily adjusted and most scanners give options of between 1 and 10 mm slice thickness.

Hounsfield Unit (HU)

- The digital value ascribed to each pixel is called the Hounsfield value, which lies on a scale where pure water has a value 0 and air has a value of –1,000
- Bone has a value of the order of +1,000 **(Fig. 22.2)**
- CT numbers based on a magnification constant of 1,000 are also called *Hounsfield units*
- The CT scan calculates from the collected data, the linear attenuation coefficient (μ) of each pixel

Positive ↑ White		
	+1000	Bone/Calcification
	+70	Congealed blood
	+45	Grey matter
	+35	
	+30	White matter
Displayed on spectrum of shades of grey (grey scale)	+20	
	+8	CSF
	0	Reference point (pure water)
	—70	Fat
	—1000	Air
Black ↓ Negative	Hounsfield values, in units (Hu) Not to scale	

Fig. 22.2: Hounsfield unit

- Now, the value is converted to a new number called CT number
- This allows the computer to present the information as a picture with a large gray scale
- The Hounsfield value reflects directly the X-ray attenuation coefficient or electron density and thus the physical composition of the voxel of tissue that the pixel represents
- The values for different tissue types are measurable and reproducible
- Present scanners have a measurement range of –1,000 HU to +3,095 HU
- For easy visual interpretation, each pixel is then ascribed a shade of grey, depending on its Hounsfield value and the windowing technique chosen
- Displayed in this form the electronic image is transferred to hard copy film using a matrix or laser camera.

Axial Plane

- The axial plane is the one most readily available on CT and can easily be obtained in most supine patients
- The axial plane offers the advantage of direct left-right comparison, which is useful in a symmetrical structure like the head.

Coronal Plane

It also allows left-right comparisons and has the geometric advantage of offering scans at right angles to major bony structures, such as the floors of the anterior and middle cranial fossae, the orbital roof and floor and the hard palate.

Sagittal Plane

- Sagittal images are splendid for midline unpaired structures, such as the corpus callosum, pineal, pituitary, aqueduct and spinal cord
- Due to anatomic constraints, direct sagittal scans are almost impossible in cranial CT, and one has to rely on reformations
- Contiguous slices (with no inter-slice gaps) are required and a slight degree of overlap helps smooth the reformatted image.

Cone Beam CT (CBCT)

- CBCT is an apparatus designed by Arai et al. in 1997 for the specific usage in dentistry
- CBCT uses a round or rectangular cone-shaped X-ray beam centred on a two-dimensional X-ray sensor to scan a 360° rotation about the patient's head

- During the scan, a series of 360° exposure or projections, one for each degree of rotation, is acquired, which provides the raw digital data for reconstruction of the exposed volume by computer algorithm
- Depending on the equipment, scan time ranges from 17 seconds to approximately more than one minute
- Visual resolving power of these systems varies up to about 2 lp/mm, four times that of CT
- The final image may be printed on a 1:1 scale with geometric accuracy to about 2% or less.

Advantages

- Low radiation dose
- Less exposure time
- High resolution images
- Reduction of artefacts
- Seated patient position
- Useful in assessment of thickness of glenoid fossa
- Pressure-sensitive floor activates "fast stop" for the patient safety during scanning
- Excellent contrast resolution (for bone and soft tissues)
- Presence of implant mode helps in implant placement
- Useful in assessment of range and type of condyle movement.

Indications of CT in Head and Neck Region

- Investigations of intracranial diseases including tumours, haemorrhage and infarcts
- Investigations of suspected intracranial and spinal cord damage following trauma
- Assessment of fractures
  - The orbit and naso-ethmoidal complex
  - Cranial base
  - Cervical spine.
- Tumour staging—assessment of the site, size and extent of tumours, both benign and malignant, affecting:
  - Maxillary antrum
  - Base of skull
  - Pterygoid region
  - Pharynx
  - Larynx.
- Investigation of tumours, intrinsic and extrinsic to the salivary gland
- Investigation of osteomyelitis
- Investigation of TMJ
- Preoperative assessment of alveolar bone level and thickness before inserting implants.

Advantages Over Conventional Film-Based Tomography

- Detailed imaging of intracranial lesions
- Imaging of hard and soft tissues
- Excellent differentiation between different types of tissues
- Images can be manipulated
- Axial tomographic sections are obtainable
- Reconstructed images can be obtained
- Images can be enhanced by the use of contrast media.

Disadvantages

- Very thin slice imaging may result in high-dose investigation
- Metallic restorations may produce artefacts
- Inherent risks associated with contrast media.

Question 2

What are the uses of ultrasound in dentistry?

Answer

- Medical ultrasound, also called sonography, is a mode of medical imaging that has a wide array of clinical applications, both as a primary modality and as an adjunct to other diagnostic procedures
- The basis of its operation is the transmission of high frequency sound into the body followed by the reception, processing, and parametric display of echoes returning from structures and tissues within the body
- Ultrasound is primarily a tomographic modality, meaning that it presents an image that is typically a cross-section of the tissue volume under investigation
- It is also a soft-tissue modality, given that current ultrasound methodology does not provide useful images of or through bone or bodies of gas, such as found in the lung and bowel.

Indications in the Head and Neck Region

- Evaluation of swellings of the neck, particularly those involving the thyroid, cervical lymph nodes or the major salivary glands
- Detection of salivary gland and duct calculi
- Determination of the relationship of vascular structures and vascularity of masses with the addition of colour flow Doppler imaging
- Assessment of blood flow in the carotids and carotid body tumours
- Assessment of ventricular system in babies by imaging through the open fontanelles

- Therapeutically, in conjunction with the newly developed sialolithotripter, to break up salivary calculi
- Ultrasound-guided fine-needle aspiration biopsy
- In temporomandibular disorders.

Advantages

- Sound waves are NOT ionizing radiation
- There is no known harmful effects on any tissues at the energies and doses currently used in diagnostic ultrasound
- Images show good differentiation between different soft tissues and are very sensitive for detecting focal disease in the salivary glands
- Technique is widely available and inexpensive
- Ultrasound scanning is non-invasive (no needles or injections in most cases) and is usually painless
- It renders "live" images, where the operator can dynamically select the most useful section for diagnosing and documenting changes, often enabling rapid diagnoses
- It shows the structure of organs
- It has no known long-term side effects and rarely causes any discomfort to the patient.

Disadvantages

- Ultrasound has limited use in the head and neck region because sound waves are absorbed by bone
- It is therefore restricted to superficial structures
- Technique is operator-dependent
- Image can be difficult to interpret for inexperienced operators because image resolution is often poor
- Real-time imaging means that the operator should be present during the investigation
- Ultrasound performs very poorly when there is a gas between the scan head and the organ of interest, due to the extreme differences in acoustical impedance.

Question 3

Explain magnetic resonance imaging.

Answer

Magnetic resonance imaging or scanning (MRI) is a method of looking inside the body without using surgery, harmful dyes or X-rays. The MRI scanner uses magnetism and radiowaves to produce clear pictures of the human anatomy.

Imaging Principles

- In contrast to other imaging techniques, magnetic resonance imaging uses non-ionizing radiation from the radio-frequency (RF) band of the electromagnetic spectrum
- To produce an MR image, the patient is placed inside a large magnet, which induces a relatively strong external magnetic field
- This causes the nuclei of many atoms in the body, including hydrogen, to align themselves with the magnetic field
- After application of an RF signal, energy is released from the body, detected, and used to construct the MR image by computer
- The high-contrast sensitivity of MRI to tissue differences and the absence of radiation exposure are the main advantages of MRI over CT.

T1-weighted Images

- A short repetition time (TR) of 500 msec between pulses and a short echo or signal recovery time (TE) of 20 msec produces a T1-weighted image
- T1-weighted images are fat images because fat has the shortest T1 relaxation time and the highest signal relative to the other tissues and thus appears bright in the image
- High anatomic detail is possible in this type of image because of good image contrast
- T1-weighted images are useful for depicting small anatomic regions (e.g., TMJ) where high spatial resolution is required.

T2-weighted Image

- A long repetition time of 2,000 msec and a long echo or signal recovery time of 80 msec produces a T2-weighted image
- T2 weighted images are called *water images* because water has the longest T2 relaxation time and thus appear bright in the image
- T2 weighting are most commonly used when the practitioner is looking for inflammatory or other pathologic changes.

Indications of MRI

- Assessment of intracranial lesions involving particularly the posterior cranial fossa, the pituitary and the spinal cord
- Tumour staging—evaluation of site, size and extent of all soft tissue tumours including nodal involvement, involving all areas in particular:
  - The salivary glands
  - Tongue and floor of mouth
  - Pharynx

- Larynx
- Sinuses
- Orbits.

- Implant assessment
- Investigation of TMJ to show both the bony and soft tissue components of the joint including the disc position.
  - When diagnosis of internal derangement is in doubt
  - As a preoperative assessment before disc surgery.

Advantages of MRI

- Improved soft tissue contrast—MRI shows a rather excellent soft tissue contrast as compared to CT
- It can differentiate between soft tissue structures like muscle, fat, neurovascular or lymphoid structures
- It does not use any form of ionizing radiation; hence, all the risks associated with it are avoided like altered cellular function, somatic and genetic changes, desquamation of skin and erythema
- It is capable of performing multiplanar imaging, i.e., Images are obtained in axial, coronal and sagittal plane for imaging, without moving the patient
- MRI is non-invasive
- No known biological hazard
- Normal control volunteers can be imaged
- Possibility of tissue characterization and blood flow imaging measurements possible
- Imaging of tissues in their function
- Vascular imaging can be done non-invasively to image the morphology of the vascular system (MRangiography).

Disadvantages of MRI

- Lack of signal from the cortical bone as normal cortical bone produces no signal and appears black on MRI
- Limitations of its use in patients with cardiac pacemakers, spinal implants, aneurismal clips or metallic foreign body as these metallic objects interfere with the imaging procedure
- It is very expensive and the services are not easily available
- Long imaging time
- Reduced patient co-operation as MRI is a lengthy time consuming procedure due to which patient may exhibit motion and result in artefacts
- The patient co-operation is reduced because of the claustrophobia due to the closed chamber and the constant noise associated with it
- Many protocol options
- Correct choice of machine parameters essential
- Difficult to image and monitor patients who are critical
- Bone, teeth, air and metallic objects all appear black, making differentiation difficult.

Question 4

Explain sialography.

Answer

Sialography can be defined as the radiographic demonstration of the major salivary glands by introducing a radiopaque contrast medium into their ductal system.

Indications

- To determine the presence and/or position of calculi or other blockages, whatever their radiodensity
- To assess the extent of ductal and glandular destruction secondary to an obstruction
- To determine the extent of glandular breakdown and as a crude assessment of function in cases of dry mouth
- To determine the location, size, nature and origin of a swelling or mass
- This indication is somewhat controversial as other investigations often prove more useful.

Contraindications

- Allergy to compounds containing iodine
- Periods of acute infection/inflammation, when there is discharge of pus from the duct opening
- When clinical examination or routine radiographs have shown a calculus close to the duct opening, as injection of the contrast medium may push the calculus back down the main duct where it may be inaccessible.

Phases

- The preoperative phase
- The filling phase
- The emptying phase.

Preoperative Phase

- Take preoperative (scout) radiographs, before the introduction of the contrast medium, for the following reasons:
  - To note the position and/or presence of any radio-paque obstruction
  - To assess the position of shadows cast by normal anatomical structures that may overlie the gland, such as the hyoid bone
  - To assess the exposure factors.

Parotid: Radiographs taken

- Dental panoramic tomograph
- Oblique lateral
- Rotated PA or AP
- Intraoral view of the cheek.

Submandibular gland: Radiographs taken
- Dental panoramic tomograph
- Oblique lateral
- Lower 90° occlusal (to show the duct)
- Lower oblique occlusal (to show the gland)
- True lateral skull with the tongue depressed.

Filling Phase

- Orifice of duct is found probed and dilated and then cannulated
- Contrast medium can then be introduced
- When this is complete, the filling phase radiographs are taken, ideally at least two different views at right angles to one another.

Emptying Phase

- The cannula is removed
- Patient allowed to rinse out
- Lemon juice is used as an aid excretion of the contrast medium
- After 1 and 5 minutes, the emptying phase radiographs are taken, usually oblique laterals
- These films can be used as a crude assessment of function.

Sialographic Techniques

There are three main techniques available:
1. Simple injection technique
2. Hydrostatic technique
3. Continuous infusion pressure—monitored technique.

Simple Injection Technique

Oil-based or aqueous contrast medium is introduced using gentle hand pressure until the patient experiences tightness or discomfort in the gland *(about 0.7 mL for parotid gland, 0.5 mL for the submandibular gland)*.

Advantages

- Simple
- Inexpensive.

Disadvantages

- The arbitrary pressure which is applied may cause damage to the gland
- Reliance on patient's response may lead to underfilling or overfilling of the gland.

Hydrostatic Pressure

Aqueous contrast media is allowed to flow freely into the gland under the force of gravity until the patient experiences discomfort.

Advantages

- The controlled introduction of contrast medium is less likely to cause damage or give artefactual picture
- Simple
- Inexpensive.

Disadvantages

- Reliant on the patient's responses
- Patient has to lie down during the procedure, so they need to be positioned in advance for the filling phase.

Continuous Infusion Pressure— Monitored Technique

Using aqueous contrast medium, a constant flow rate is adopted and the ductal pressure monitored throughout the procedure.

Advantages

- The controlled introduction of contrast media at known pressures is not likely to cause damage
- Does not cause overfilling of the gland
- Does not rely on the patient's responses.

Disadvantages

- Complex equipment is required
- Time consuming.

Contrast Media Used

- Ionic aqueous solutions
  - Diatrizoate (Urografin®)
  - Metrizoate (Triosil®)
- Non-ionic aqueous solutions, including:
  - Iohexol (Omnipaque®)
- Oil-based solutions, including:
  - Iodized oil, e.g., Lipiodol® (iodized poppy seed oil).

Oil-Based Contrast Media

Advantages

- Densely radiopaque, thus, show good contrast
- High viscosity, thus slow excretion from the gland.

Disadvantages

- Extravasated contrast may remain in the soft tissues for many months, and may produce a foreign body reaction
- High viscosity means considerable pressure needed to introduce the contrast, calculi may be forced down the main duct.

Aqueous-Based Contrast Media

Advantages

- Low viscosity, thus easily introduced
- Easily and rapidly removed from the gland
- Easily absorbed and excreted if extravasated.

Disadvantages

- Less radiopaque, thus show reduced contrast
- Excretion from the gland is very rapid unless used in a closed system.

Sialographic Interpretation

- Normal parotid gland: Tree in winter appearance
- Normal submanibular gland: Bush in winter
- Sialodochitis: Sausage-like appearance
- Sialadenitis: Dots or blobs seen in parotid gland called sialectasis
- Sjogren's syndrome: The main duct is normal and there are widespread dots or blobs of contrast medium throughout the gland, the snowstorm appearance of punctate sialectasis
- Tumour: Ball-in-hand appearance in tumour.

CHAPTER 23 Image Principles and Characteristics

LONG ESSAYS

Question 1

Explain in detail about artefact, blemishes and faults in dental radiography.

Answer

Artefacts

Artefact is an abnormal radiographic appearance, which is seen in a radiograph due to some artificial means and is normally not present.

Blank Radiograph

- Unexposed film
- Exposed film immersed into the fixer before it was placed into the developer.

Partial Image

When only a part of the film has been immersed into the developer.

Blurred Image

When movement of tube head or patient takes place or there is twice exposure on the same film.

Spot on the Radiograph

It can be seen due to:

- Finger prints
- Bending of the film excessively
- Due to contamination of the film with the developer solution before the processing
- When film comes in contact with another film or tank walls during the fixing procedure.

Blisters on the Film

- Air bubbles present on the film surface while developing
- Increased acidity of the developer solution
- Films have not been agitated when first immersed in fixer.

Light Spots on the Radiograph

- Film exposed to the fixer solution before the process of development
- Film in contact with another film or tank wall in the developing procedure.

Black Lines and Mark

Moisture contamination.

Yellow or Brown Stain

It can be due to:

- Less amount of fixer
- Oxidized or exhausted developer
- Contaminated solutions
- Insufficient washing/rinsing.

Blemishes

They are the errors or faults or defects on the radiograph.

They can be:

- Errors in film storage and handling
- Errors in film placement and projection technique
- Errors in exposure parameters and processing technique.

Errors in Film Storage and Handling

- Film fog
  - Out-dated films
  - When films have been stored at high temperature or exposed to radiation.
- Emulsion peel
  - Wet film comes in contact with finger nails.
- Dark spots or line.
  - Occurs due to contamination with finger prints.

Errors in Film Placement and Projection Technique

- Type mark pattern
  - Occurs when wrong side or opposite side of the film has been exposed to radiation.
- Cone cut
  - Due to improper placement of the film or position-indicating device (PID).
- Shortened image
  - Occurs due to increased vertical angulation used in bisecting angle technique
  - When film has not been placed parallel to the long axis of the tooth in the paralleling technique.
- Elongated image
  - Occurs due to decreased vertical angulation in bisecting angle technique
  - Film has not been placed parallel to the long axis of the tooth in paralleling technique.
- Overlapping of the teeth
  - Incorrect horizontal angulation.
- Blurred image
  - Because of movement of the film or patient during the exposure
  - Excessive bending of the film.
- Crown portion of the teeth or apical ends of the teeth not imaged
  - Improper placement of the film
  - Vertical angulation is less.
- Tyre track effect (Herring bone effect)
  - Opposite side of film placed towards tube.
- Double images.
  - When film is exposed two times to a radiation.

Errors in Exposure Parameters and Processing Technique

- Film fog
  - Improper wattage of the safelight
  - Prolonged exposure of the film to safelight
  - Safelight not at a proper distance from the working place
  - Light leaks from cracked safelight filters or ventilators.
- Dark Radiographs
  - Exposure Errors
    - Excessive mA, kVp and exposure time
    - Insufficient film and X-ray source distance.
  - Processing Errors.
    - Improper safe lighting and accidental exposure to light
    - high developer temperature and concentration
    - Film developed for a longer period
    - Longer developing time
    - Inadequate fixation.
- Light Radiograph
  - Exposure Errors
    - Insufficient mA, kVp and exposure time
    - Film packet placed with the wrong side facing the X-ray source.
  - Processing Error.
    - Excessive fixation
    - Depleted and diluted or contaminated developer solution
    - Too low temperature of the developer solution.
- Low Contrast Radiographs.
  - kVp too high
  - Under exposure or under development.

Question 2

Define ideal radiograph. What are the characteristics of an ideal radiograph?

Answer

According to HM Worth, an ideal radiograph is one which has desired density and overall blackness and which shows the part completely without distortion with maximum details and has the right amount of contrast to make the details fully apparent.

Following are the characteristics of an ideal radiograph:

- Visual characteristics
- Geometric characteristics
- Anatomic accuracy of radiographic image
- Adequate coverage of the anatomic region of interest.

Visual Characteristics

- Density
- Contrast.

Density

Factors effecting the density of a radiograph are:

First-degree Factors

- Milliamperage (mA)
- Exposure time
- Operating kilo-voltage peak (kVp)
- Source–film distance.

Milliamperage (mA):

- Increased mA produces more X-ray that exposes the film and result in increased film density
- Increase in mA leads to increase in film density.

Exposure time:

- An increase in the exposure time increases the film density
- If exposure time is increased, then film density is increased and if exposure time is decreased, then film density is decreased.

Operating kilo-voltage peaks (kVp):

- Increased kVp increases the penetrating power of X-rays, thereby increasing the density
- If kVp increases, then film density increases
- If kVp decreases, then film density decreases.

Source–film distance:

The intensity of an X-ray beam varies inversely as the square of the source film (S-F) distance, density also varies inversely as the square of the (S-F) distance

$$\text{Hence, Density} = \frac{(\text{kVp})^2 \times \text{mA} \times \text{S}}{[(\text{S}-\text{F})\ \text{distance}]^2}.$$

Second-degree Factors

- Subject thickness
- Development conditions
- Type of film
- Screens
- Grids
- Amount of filtration used
- Fog.

Subject thickness:

- In a patient with an increased amount of soft tissue or thick dense bones, fewer X-ray would reach the film and the radiograph would appear light and have less density
- If the subject thickness increases, then density decreases, if subject thickness decreases, then density increases.

Development conditions:

Under or over development of the radiograph results in a light or dark radiograph.

Type of film:

- Film speed: High-speed films require less mA/s in order to obtain a density change
- Film latitude: It is measured as a range of exposures that can be recorded as distinguishable densities on a film
- Radiographic noise: It is appearance of uneven density of a uniformly exposed radiographic film.

Screens:

Use of screens requires less mA in order to obtain a density change.

Grids:

The use of grids requires more mAs in order to obtain a density change.

Amount of filtration used:

Reduction in the amount of added filtration used will increase the density.

Fog:

Film fog may result in an undesirable form of darkening of the film.

Characteristic Curve

- Relationship between film density and exposure has been described by Hurter and Driffield in 1890
- A graphical relationship between film density and exposure is known as characteristic curve or Hand D curve
- This curve is a screen-film combination, and reveals information about film contrast, speed and latitude.

Contrast

- The difference in the degree of blackness or densities between adjacent areas on a dental radiograph is known as contrast
- A radiograph has a high contrast when there are areas, which are very dark and very light, because the dark and the light areas are very different
- A radiograph has a low contrast when it does not have very dark and very light areas, instead has many shades of grey
- Final visual difference between the various shades of black, white and grey shadows depends upon:
    - Subject contrast
    - Film contrast
    - Fog and scatter.

Geometric Characteristics

Sharpness/Details

It is referred to as the ability of the X-ray film to define an edge.

Resolution or Definition

- It is the measure of films ability to differentiates between different structure and record separate images of small objects placed very close together
- It is measured in lines pair per mm.

Magnification

It means the radiographic image, which appears larger than the actual size of the object it represents.

The image magnification on a dental radiograph is influenced by:

- Target film distance
- Object film distance.

Distortion

Dimensional distortion of a radiographic image is a variation in the true size and shape of the object being radiographed.

The factors that influence dimensional distortion are:

- Object–film alignment
- X-ray beam angulation.

Anatomic Accuracy of Radiographic Images

- It means when the anatomical structures are reproduced on the film in exact relationship as they normally appear
- A radiograph with anatomical accuracy will have a minimum superimposition of images of adjacent tissues.

Adequate Coverage of the Anatomic Region

- It is essential that the area of interest is well covered in the radiograph
- Adequate coverage of the area of interest depends upon:
  - Proper alignment of the film and the radiation beam to the area of interest
  - Proper selection of the film types and projection techniques.

CHAPTER 24 Radiolucencies of Jaws

LONG ESSAYS

Question 1

What are the normal radiolucent structures seen in maxilla, mandible and common to both jaws?

Answer

Structures Peculiar to Maxilla

- Intermaxillary suture
- Incisive foramen, incisive canal and superior foramina of incisive canal
- Nasal cavity
- Nasolacrimal duct/canal
- Maxillary sinus
- Lateral fossa.

Structures Peculiar to Mandible

- Mandibular foramen
- Mandibular canal
- Mental foramen
- Lingual foramen
- Submandibular fossa
- Mental fossa
- Midline symphysis
- Medial sigmoid depression
- Pseudocyst of mandible.

Structures Common to Both Jaws

- Periodontal ligament space
- Marrow space
- Nutrient canal
- Follicular space.

Structures Peculiar to Maxilla

Airway Shadow

- Bilateral, relatively radiolucent
- Seen on panoramic, lateral oblique and cephalometric radiographs
- Results from lack of soft tissue between the posterolateral surface of tongue and region of soft palate and posterior pharynx.

Intermaxillary Suture

- Intermaxillary/median suture between right and left maxillary bones, can be identified as thin vertical radiolucency in midline between central incisors
- Usually delineated by two thin, vertical radiopaque lines (cortical bone)
- Generally fuses later in life and then no longer seen on radiograph.

Incisive Foramen

- Incisive foramen (anterior palatine foramen) frequently shows as a round, oval, diamond-shaped or heart-shaped radiolucency that is well defined on occlusal and periapical radiographs
- The position of foramen on radiograph ranges from between the roots of central incisors, close to alveolar ridge to the level of apices
- Variability in position of foramen on radiograph is due to the angulation of the rays and position of foramen.

Superior Foramina of Incisive Canals

- The nasopalatine canal originates at two foramina at the floor of nasal cavity
- Openings are at each side of nasal septum, and each branch passes downward anteriorly and medially to unite with canal from other side in incisive (nasopalatine) foramina
- Superior foramina of canal sometimes appear in projections of maxillary incisors, especially if vertical angle is increased sharply

- On radiograph, they are seen as two round or oval radiolucent areas above the apices of central incisors in the floor of nasal cavity near its anterior border and both sides of nasal septum
- In IOPA, their image can be superimposed over apices of incisors, which may be misinterpreted as periapical pathosis.

Nasal Cavity/fossa

- Inferior aspect of nasal cavity is seen on periapical radiographs of incisors and canine regions, especially, if vertical angulation is increased
- Seen as bilateral radiolucencies separated by the radiopaque septum and are delimited by radiopaque cortical bone
- Inferior border is often projected over the apices of incisors and canines.

Nasolacrimal Duct/canal

- Nasal and maxillary bones form the nasolacrimal canal
- Seen on maxillary occlusal radiograph, projected onto the posterior hard palate near the 1st or 2nd molar as well-defined radiolucency bilaterally well-defined by sharp radiopaque borders
- On periapical radiographs, it may be seen in the region above the apex of canine, especially if steep angulation is used.

Lateral Fossa

- Lateral/incisive fossa is a gentle depression in the maxilla near the apex of lateral incisor
- On intraoral periapical (IOPA), it is seen as diffuse radiolucency
- It can be differentiated from periapical pathosis by presence of intact lamina dura of lateral incisor.

Maxillary Sinus

- Appear as well defined radiolucency with thin, sharp radiopaque borders
- It shows considerable variation in size
- They enlarge in childhood, achieving mature size by age of 15–18 years
- Floors of maxillary sinus and nasal cavity are seen at approximately same level at age of puberty in radiograph
- In adults, sinuses are usually seen to extend from the distal aspect of canine to the posterior wall of maxilla above tuberosity.

Structures Peculiar to Mandible

Mandibular Foramen

- Usually situated just above the mid-point in the medial surface of the ramus and just posterior to the mid-point between the anterior and posterior borders
- Seen on panographic and lateral oblique films
- Outline of foramen varies from triangular to oval to funnel shaped
- Radiographic image is usually up to 1 cm in diameter
- It is associated with relatively radiolucent mandibular canal that passes from it in an anteroinferior direction
- Lingula may be detected as a triangular radiopacity of variable density at the foramen's anterior border
- These associated structures with mandibular canal and lingula can be mistaken for pathology.

Mandibular Canal/inferior Dental Canal

- Largest of the nutrient canals
- Seen on panoramic or periapical radiographs of molar region
- Appears as relatively radiolucent channel bounded by definite, thin radiopaque lines (cortical bones) throughout its length
- Its course can be followed anteroinferiorly to a point where it frequently appears to sweep upward to meet the mental foramen (now called mental foramen).

Mental Foramen

- Anterior limit of mandibular canal
- Mandibular canal send off the mental canal in the premolar region
- This smaller, short canal runs in superior buccal direction, terminating with the mental foramen
- It is usually located on the radiograph in the vicinity of premolar apices
- It may be mistaken for periapical pathosis when it occurs at the apex of premolars.

Lingual Foramen

- Seen in relation to lower central incisors often on periapical views
- Located well below the apices of these teeth in the midline
- Seen as radiolucency measuring usually 1–2 mm in diameter surrounded by prominent radiopaque ring of cortical bone
- Occasionally two or more foramina are seen.

Submandibular Gland Fossa

- Submandibular fossa is concave area on the lingual side of the mandible below the molar area, which accommodates the submandibular salivary gland
- Lies between inferior alveolar canal and lower cortical margin of mandible
- This is seen as relatively radiolucent area with sparse trabecular pattern, which is sharply limited superiorly by the lower border of mylohyoid ridge and inferiorly by lower border of mandible
- Shape is round, ovoid or triangular (rarely)
- Rarely occurs bilaterally.

Mental Fossa

- Depression on the labial aspect of midline of mandible just above the mental tubercle
- Due to relative thinness of bone over in this area, it may be seen as radiolucency over the incisor roots, which may be mistaken for periapical pathology.

Midline Symphysis

- Seen on the midline of the mandible of infants
- Seen as radiolucent line which may be misinterpreted for fracture line
- Symphysis usually ossifies by age of 1 year and then is no longer apparent.

Medial Sigmoid Depression

- It is a radiolucency that appears below and just anterior to greatest depth of sigmoid notch of ramus
- Seen on approximately 10% of panoramic radiographs
- It is defined by temporal crest and crest of mandibular neck
- Its degree of expression is variable depending upon prominence of these two crests.

Sublingual Gland Depression

- First reported by Richard and Ziskind (1957)
- It may develop to accommodate sublingual salivary gland tissue that lies in close proximity to the lingual cortex of mandible in canine region
- Most often associated with canines, followed by incisors and 2nd premolars (rare), in apical 1/3rd of root
- Average size 1.2 cm
- Trabeculation may be present within radiolucency
- Have punched out appearance or corticated margin.

Pseudocyst of the Condyle

- Friedlander, Monson, Friedlander and Esquerra identified and reported the pseudocyst of condyle
- Appears as well-defined radiolucency in the anterior aspect of condyle on panoramic radiographs
- Seen in 1 out of 100 patients
- More common in older people
- Measure approximately 0.4–0.5 cm and are surrounded partially or completely by discrete sclerotic rim
- Image represents marked cupping of anterior surface of condyle
- Cupping is produced by pterygoid fovea and dense medial and lateral ridges.

Structures Common to Both Jaws

Marrow Space

- Marrow spaces between trabeculae of bone appear as radiolucent region
- Varies greatly in shape, size and distribution
- Radiographically, in maxilla, they are generally relatively uniform in size
- In mandible, marrow spaces are smaller and more numerous in the anterior portion and larger in the posterior portion
- In some persons trabecular spaces just above and below the roots of molars are so large and trabeculae so sparse that the combined appearance may resemble and be misinterpreted as cysts and other pathosis
- These are referred as *focal osteoporotic bone marrow defects*.

Nutrient Canal

- Appear as ribbon-like radiolucencies of fairly uniform width
- Carry neurovascular bundles
- Seen more often on periapical mandibular radiographs
- Canals become more marked when teeth are missing
- If the beam of radiograph is directed parallel to a canal and through its foramen in the cortical bone, the canal appears as small, round radiolucency, which may be confused with pathology.

Pericoronal/follicular Space

- The crowns of unerupted teeth are surrounded by dental follicle—remnant of reduced enamel epithelium
- It is composed of soft myxomatous to dense collagenous fibrous connective tissue or cords of odontogenic epithelium

- On radiograph, it appears as homogeneous radiolucent halo
- Surrounded by thin outer radiopaque border representing compact bone continuous with lamina dura
- Radiolucent halo merges with periodontal ligament space
- Width of halo varies because of varying thickness of the follicles and accumulation of fluid between the capsule of reduced enamel epithelium and tooth crown.

Developing Tooth Crypt

- Seen in radiographs of developing dentitions so seldom present in patients over the age of 15 years
- If developing tooth is uncalcified, the crypt appears as roundish homogeneous radiolucency
- If just tips are calcified, radiographically a well-defined radiolucency containing radiopaque foci is seen.

Question 2

Describe periapical radiolucencies.

Answer

Pulpoperiapical radiolucencies

- Periapical granuloma
- Radicular cyst
- Scar
- Dentoalveolar abscess
- Surgical defect
- Osteomyelitis
- Periapical cemento-osseous dysplasia
- Non-radicular disease.

Periapical Abscess

- The primary abscess develops in a periapical region that is normal on radiographic examination
- The infection is usually acute and exudative, involving the periodontal tissues at the apex of the tooth with necrotic pulp
- The infection and inflammation in the apical area forces the tooth slightly from its socket, creating an increased periodontal ligament space around the entire root that is usually apparent on the radiograph
- The secondary abscess may be of the chronic or the acute type
- Related tooth shows features, such as deep restorations, caries, narrowed pulp chamber, or canals, which suggest that the pulp is non-vital
- The roots of these teeth may show resorption at the apex
- The tooth is painful on percussion and the patient complains that it seems 'high' to bite on
- Tooth does not respond to electric pulp test
- The tooth may demonstrate increased mobility
- In untreated cases, the abscess may penetrate the cortical plate at the thinnest and closest point to the apex and form a space infection in the adjacent soft tissue.

Radiographic Features

- Periapical radiolucency is a feature of the secondary abscess
- The radiolucency may vary from small to quite large to involve much of the jaw
- The initial periapical lesion may cause expansion of cortical plate
- In case of acute lesion, the margins of the radiolucency may be well defined with possibly a hyperostotic border
- The borders are poorly defined in case of chronic conditions
- Sometimes the radiolucency is represented as a blurred area of somewhat lessened density than that of surrounding bone.

Periapical Granuloma

- Represents between 69.7% and 94% of allpulpoperiapical lesions
- It is a result of successful attempt by the periapical tissue to neutralize and confine the irritating toxic products that are escaping from the root canal
- Continual discharge of chronic irritating products from the canal into the periapical tissue is sufficient to maintain a low-grade inflammation in the tissues, which results in formation of periapical granuloma.

Radiographic Features

- Well-circumscribed radiolucency somewhat rounded and surrounding apex of tooth
- May be surrounded by thin radiopaque (hyperostoic) border
- Cannot be differentiated from radicular cyst radiographically alone
- Cysts tend to be larger than granulomas but differentiation on basis of size is not possible as some cysts are small and granulomas large
- Granulomas are rarely larger than 2.5 cm in diameter
- Involved tooth is non-vital and asymptomatic.

Radicular Cyst

- Synonyms—
  - Periapical cyst
  - Apical periodontal cyst
  - Dental cyst.

- Most common type of cyst in jaw
- It results when cell rests of Malassez in the periodontal ligament (PDL) are stimulated to proliferate and undergo cystic degeneration by inflammatory products by non-vital tooth
- Usually asymptomatic unless secondary infection occurs
- Incidence is greater in 3rd to 6th decade with slight male predilection
- Most radicular cysts involve apices of permanent teeth
- 58% involve lateral incisors
- History and clinical features are similar to those of periapical granuloma
- Studies by Lalonde show that such a lesion is more likely to be a radicular cyst if the periapical radiolucency tends to be at least 1.6 cm in diameter
- An untreated cyst may enlarge slowly and cause expansion of cortical plates
- In these cases, a dome-like swelling is seen on the alveolus over the periapical region of alveolus of involved tooth
- Swelling is initially bony hard on palpation but later it may demonstrate crackling sound (crepitus) as cortical plate is thinned
- In these cases swelling is rubbery and fluctuant because of cystic fluid.

Radiographic Features

- Location
  - Most common site—maxilla (60%) especially incisors (58%) and canines
  - In deciduous teeth, most commonly molars are involved
  - Epicentre is located at the apex of non-vital tooth
  - Occasionally, it appears on the mesial or distal surface of root, at the opening of accessory canal, or infrequently in a deep periodontal pocket.
- Periphery and shape
  - Usually has well-defined cortical border
  - When cyst becomes secondarily infected due to inflammatory reaction of surrounding bone, cortex may be lost or become more sclerotic
  - Outline is usually curved or circular.
- Effect on surrounding structures.
  - If cyst is large, displacement and resorption of roots of adjacent teeth may occur
  - Outer cortical plate of maxilla or mandible may expand in curved or circular shape
  - Cyst may displace the inferior alveolar canal in an inferior direction.

Differential Diagnosis

- Periapical granuloma and radicular cyst cannot be distinguished radiographically alone, although radiolucency with well-defined corticated border, more than 2 cm diameter, is more likely to be cyst
- Periapical scars associated with teeth that have received non-surgical endodontic treatment and are well-sealed
- A persistent non-enlarging radiolucency is most likely scar
- Surgical defect: Asymptomatic radiolucency that persist after root resection is likely surgical defect
- Periapical cemento-osseous dysplasia: Difficult to distinguish radiographically from periapical granuloma and radicular cyst in its early lytic stage. Tooth is vital in PCOD. Lower teeth especially incisors more commonly involved
- Traumatic bone cyst: Teeth associated with lesion are vital. Most commonly seen in mandibular region in molar, premolar and incisor regionPeriapical granuloma does not have predilection for lower jaw and more common in anterior region. Lamina dura is intact in traumatic bone cyst
- Mandibular infected buccal cyst: Located on buccal aspect of mandibular molar tooth. Pulp of involved tooth is usually vital. Lamina dura of involved tooth is intact. Occlusal surface of involved tooth is tipped towards mandible.

Periapical Scar

- Composed of dense fibrous tissue
- Situated at the periapex of a pulpless tooth which has been treated endodontically
- It represents a previous periapical granuloma, cyst, or abscess whose healing has terminated in formation of dense scar instead of bone
- Accounts for 2–5% of periapical radiolucent lesions
- Frequently occurs in cases initially by periapical curettage or root resection.

Radiographic Features

- Seen as well-circumscribed round radiolucency resembling periapical granuloma or cyst
- Usually smaller than periapical granuloma or cyst
- Remains constant in size or may shrink slightly
- Tooth is asymptomatic
- Most often in anterior region of maxilla.

Surgical Defect

- It is area in bone that fails to fill in with osseous tissue after surgery
- Accounts for approximately 3% of all periapical radiolucencies
- Seen periapically after root resection procedures especially when both labial and lingual plates are destroyed

- 25% of the surgical defects resulting from root resection procedures do not heal completely
- Tooth and periapical area is asymptomatic
- Defect may be detected on palpation if it is large enough.

Radiographic Features

- Radiolucency is rounded in appearance, smoothly contoured with well-defined borders
- Usually does not measure more than 1 cm in diameter
- Frequently, it resolves to certain size and then remains constant.

Osteomyelitis

- Osteomyelitis is inflammation of bone
- The inflammatory process may spread through the bone to involve the marrow spaces, cortex, cancellous portion and periodontium
- In the jaws, osteomyelitis may be caused by pyogenic organisms that reach the bone marrow from abscessed teeth or post-surgical infection. In some cases, haematogenous spread may be the source of infection
- The bacteria and their products stimulate an inflammatory reaction in bone, causing destruction of the endosteal surface of the cortical bone
- This destruction may progress through the cortical bone to the outer periosteum
- The hallmark of osteomyelitis is the development of sequestra
- A sequestrum is a segment of bone that has become necrotic because of ischemic injury caused by the inflammatory process
- Phases of osteomyelitis: Acute and chronic.

Acute Phase

- Synonyms
  - Acute suppurative osteomyelitis
  - Pyogenic osteomyelitis
  - Subacute suppurative osteomyelitis
  - Garre's osteomyelitis
  - Proliferative periostitis
  - Periostitis ossificans.
- The acute phase of osteomyelitis is caused by infection that has spread to the bone marrow
- The medullary spaces of the bone contain an inflammatory infiltrate consisting predominantly of neutrophils and mononuclear cells
- In the younger patients, it is believed that the inflammatory exudate spreads subperiosteally, elevating the periosteum and stimulating formation of new bone as the periosteum is loosely attached to the bone surface and has greater osteogenic potential.

Clinical Features

- Affects people of all ages
- Has strong male predilection
- Common in mandible than in the maxilla.

Signs of Acute Osteomyelitis

- Rapid onset
- Pain
- Swelling of the adjacent soft tissues
- Fever
- Lymphadenopathy
- Leucocytosis
- Associated teeth may be mobile and sensitive to percussion
- Purulent drainage may also be present
- Paraesthesia of the lower lip may be present.

Radiographic Features

- Very early in the disease, no radiographic changes may be identifiable
- The bone may be filled with inflammatory exudate and inflammatory cells and may show no radiographic changes.

Chronic Phase

Synonyms

- Chronic diffuse sclerosing osteomyelitis
- Chronic non-suppurative osteomyelitis
- Chronic osteomyelitis with proliferative periostitis
- Garre's chronic non-suppurative sclerosing osteitis.

The chronic phase of osteomyelitis may be sequelae of inadequately treated acute osteomyelitis, or it may arise de novo.

Diffuse sclerosing osteomyelitis refers to chronic osteomyelitis in which the balance in bone metabolism is tipped towards increased bone formation, producing a subsequent sclerotic radiographic appearance.

Clinical Features

- Intermittent, recurrent episodes of swelling
- Pain
- Fever
- Lymphadenopathy
- Paraesthesia and drainage with sinus formation may also occur.

Radiographic Features

Location:

- Most common site is posterior mandible Periphery
- Better defined than seen in the acute phase
- Usually a gradual transition is seen between the normal surrounding trabecular pattern and the dense granular pattern characteristic of the disease
- When the disease is active and spreading through bone, the periphery may be more radiolucent and have poorly defined.
- Internal structure:
  - Comprises regions of greater and lesser radiopacity compared with surrounding normal bone
  - Most of the lesion usually is composed of more radiopaque or sclerotic bone pattern
  - In older lesions, the internal bone density can be exceedingly increased to cortical bone. In these cases, no region of radiolucency may be seen
  - In other cases, small regions of radiolucency may be scattered throughout the radiopaque bone
  - The radiolucent regions may show islands of bone or sequestrum within the centre.
- Chronic osteomyelitis may demonstrate four distinct radiographic pictures:
  - Completely radiolucent
  - Mixed radiolucent and radiopaque
  - Completely radiopaque
  - Proliferative periosteitis.
- Effect on surrounding structure.
  - The outer contour of the mandible is altered, assuming an abnormal shape and girth may be larger than on the unaffected side
  - The roots of teeth may undergo external resorption, and the lamina dura may become less apparent as it blends with the surrounding granular sclerotic bone
  - If a tooth is non-vital, the periodontal ligament space usually is enlarged in the apical region
  - Chronic lesions may develop a draining fistula, which may appear as a well-defined break in the outer cortex or in the periosteal new bone.

Periapical Cemanto-osseous Dysplasia

- Synonyms
  - Periapical cemento-osseous dysplasia
  - Cementoma
  - Fibrocemento-osseous lesion
  - Periapical osteofibrosis
  - Periapical fibrous dysplasia
  - Periapical fibro-osteoma
  - Most common fibrocemento-osseous lesion.
- Periapical cemental dysplasia is the localized lesion of cemento-osseous dysplasia often confined predominantly to the anterior mandible
- There is striking predilection for both females and black patients
- Seen in patients beyond 30 years of age
- It predominantly involves apical areas of mandibular incisor teeth
- Lesion is asymptomatic and mild expansion of bone may be seen
- Associated with vital teeth.

Radiographic Features

- Three radiographic stages of periapical cemental dysplasias
  - Osteolytic: Appear as well-circumscribed radiolucent
  - Cementoblastic: Appears as mixed radiolucent/radiopaque
  - Mature stage: Radiopaque lesions.
- Location.

Epicentre lies at the apex of tooth.

In most cases, lesion is multiple and bilateral.

- Periphery and shape
  - In most cases, the periphery of a periapical cemento-osseous dysplasia lesion is well-defined
  - Often a radiolucent border of varying width is present, surrounded by a band of sclerotic bone that also can vary in width
  - The sclerotic bone represents a reaction of the immediate surrounding bone
  - The lesion may be irregularly shaped or may have an overall round or oval shape.
- Internal structure
  - Internal structure varies, depending on the maturity of the lesion
  - In the early stage, normal bone is resorbed and replaced with fibrous tissue that usually is continuous with the periodontal ligament (causing loss of lamina dura)
  - Radiographically, this appears as radiolucency at the apex of the involved tooth
  - In cementoblastic and mature stage, lesion appears as mixed radiolucent/radiopaque and radiopaque lesions, respectively.
- Effects on surrounding structures
- The lamina dura of the teeth involved with the lesion is lost, making the periodontal ligament space either less apparent or giving it a wider appearance
  - Tooth structure usually is not affected, although in rare cases some root resorption may occur resulting in spiking or widened apices

- Occasionally hypercementosis occurs on the root of a tooth positioned within the lesion.
- Effects on surrounding structures.

Small lesions do not cause expansion of the involved jaw. However, larger lesions may cause expansion of the jaw, an area, which is always bordered by a thin, intact outer cortex similar to that seen in fibrous dysplasia.

Question 3

Describe inter-radicular radiolucencies.

Answer

Various inter-radicular radiolucencies are:

- Traumatic bone cyst
- Incisive canal cyst
- Median mandibular cyst
- Globulomaxillary cyst
- Lateral periodontal cyst
- Lateral radicular cyst
- Furcation involvement
- Rarities.
  - Adenomatoid odontogenic tumours
  - Buccal cyst
  - Histiocytosis X
  - Osteoradionecrosis
  - Paradental cyst.

Traumatic Bone Cyst

Synonyms

- Simple bone cyst
- Haemorrhagic bone cyst
- Extravasations cyst
- Progressive bone cavity
- Solitary bone cyst
- Unicameral bone cyst.

Radiographic Features

Location

Found in mandible, most often in ramus and posterior region.

Periphery and Shape

- Margins vary from well-defined delicate cortex to ill-defined border that blends into the surrounding bone
- Shape is most often smooth and curved with an oval and scalloped border
- Lesion often scallops between roots.

Internal Structure

- Totally radiolucent
- Occasionally may appear multilocular due to pronounced scalloping of endosteal surface of either buccal or lingual plate.

Effects on Surrounding Structure

- Usually no effect on surrounding structures
- Rarely root displacement and resorption seen
- Lamina dura is either intact or partly destroyed
- Grows along the long axis of the bone causing minimal expansion.

Incisive Canal Cyst

Synonyms

- Median anterior maxillary cyst
- Nasopalatine duct cyst
- Median palatal cyst.

Radiographic Features

Location

- Found in nasopalatine foramen or canal
- If it extends posteriorly to involve hard palate it is referred as *median palatal cyst*
- It may expand anteriorly between the central incisors, destroying or expanding the labial plate and causes teeth to diverge (*median anterior maxillary cyst*)
- May be asymmetrical.

Periphery

- Well defined
- Usually corticated
- Circular or oval in shape
- Shadow of nasal spine may be superimposed on the cyst, giving it a heart-shape.

Effect on Surrounding Structures

- Causes divergence of roots of central incisors
- Root resorption occurs occasionally
- It may expand labial as well as palatal cortex
- Floor of nasal fossa may be displaced in superior direction.

Median Mandibular Cyst

Radiographic Features

- Most commonly associated with mandibular symphyseal region

- Seen as unilocular expansile radiolucency underlying vital mandibular central incisor
- Sharply defined and corticated margin
- Lamina dura around mandibular central incisors is intact.

Globulomaxillary Cyst

Radiographic Features

- Located between maxillary lateral incisors and canines
- Appears as inverted pear-shaped radiolucency
- Inferior margin is situated at or near the alveolar crest, while the upper border may invaginate the floor of nasal fossa or antrum
- Size is variable and may reach a maximal lateral diameter of 3–4 mm
- Causes root divergence.

Lateral Periodontal Cyst

Radiographic Features

Location

- More commonly seen in mandible (50–75%), in region of lateral incisor to second premolar
- Occasionally, seen in maxilla, especially between lateral incisor and canine.

Periphery and Shape

- Well-defined radiolucency with prominent cortical boundary
- Round or oval in shape.

Effects on Surrounding Structures

Small cyst may efface the lamina dura of adjacent teeth. Large cyst can displace the adjacent teeth and cause expansion.

SHORT ESSAYS

Question 1

Explain radiographic features and differential diagnosis of dentigerous cyst.

Answer

Radiographic features of dentigerous cyst are:

Location

- Mandibular 3rd molar or maxillary canines are most commonly involved
- Epicentre is found just above the crown of involved tooth
- Cyst is attached to the cemento-enamel junction (CEJ)
- Some cysts are eccentric developing from the lateral aspect of crown so that they occupy an area besides the crown instead of above the crown.

Periphery and Shape

- It has well-defined cortex with a curved or circular outline
- Cortex may be missing if infection is present.

Internal Structure

Completely radiolucent except the crown of involved tooth.

Effects on Surrounding Structure

- Displaces tooth involved usually in apical direction
- It may also resorb the adjacent teeth
- The floor of maxillary antrum may be displaced as the cyst invaginates the antrum and displace inferior alveolar canal in inferior direction
- It tends to expand outer cortex of involved jaw.

Differential Diagnosis

Hyperplastic Follicle

- Size of normal follicular space is 2–3 mm
- If follicular space exceeds 5 mm, it is more likely to be dentigerous cyst
- Tooth displacement and expansion is associated with dentigerous cyst.

Odontogenic Cyst

- Sometimes associated with unerupted tooth with lesion present at pericoronal position
- Does not cause expansion of bone
- Less likely to resorb teeth
- May attach further apically on root than at CEJ.

Ameloblastic Fibroma

- May be present around the crown of an unerupted tooth
- Difficult to differentiate radiographically.

Unicystic Ameloblastoma

- Unilocular ameloblastoma located around the crown of an unerupted tooth is difficult to differentiate
- Causes apical displacement of teeth.

Calcifying Epithelial Odontogenic Tumour

- 52% associated with impacted tooth
- Molar and premolar region most often involved
- Seen in older age group (40 years).

Adenomatoid Odontogenic Tumour

- When completely radiolucent and associated with impacted tooth difficult to differentiate
- Attached apical to CEJ.

Radicular Cyst Associated with Primary Tooth

- Radicular cyst at the apex of primary tooth surrounds the crown of permanent tooth positioned apical to it may resemble dentigerous cyst
- Seen in deciduous molars and developing premolars
- Presence of deep caries indicate radicular cyst.

Question 2

Explain radiographic features and differential diagnosis of adenomatoid odontogenic tumour.

Answer

Radiographic features of adenomatoid odontogenic tumour are:

Location

- 75% occur in maxilla especially in incisor-canine-premolar region
- Has follicular relationship with impacted tooth but does not attach at CEJ, most often canine is involved or sclerotic border.

Periphery

Lesion is well defined with corticated or sclerotic border.

Internal Structure

- One-third of cases show completely radiolucent lesions
- In rest, radiopacities are present within the lesion.

Effect on Surrounding Structures

- Causes displacement of teeth
- Root resorption rare
- May inhibit eruption of tooth
- Expansion of jaw may occur.

Differential Diagnosis

- Dentigerous cyst: Associated with impacted teeth but radiolucent lesion is more apical than CEJ
- Odontogenic keratocyst: Difficult to differentiate pericoronal odontogenic keratocyst from adenomatoid odontogenic tumour, radiographically.

Question 3

Explain radiographic features of ameloblastic fibroma.

Answer

Synonym

- Soft odontoma
- Soft mixed odontoma
- Mixed odontogenic tumour
- Fibroadmantoblastoma
- Granular cell ameloblastic fibroma.

Radiographic Features

Location

- Mandibular premolar–molar region is most common site
- Tumour may involve ramus in some cases
- Common location is crest of alveolar process or in follicular relationship with an unerupted tooth
- It can also arise in an area where tooth failed to develop.

Periphery

Borders are well defined and corticated.

Internal Structure

More commonly present as unilocular radiolucency but may be multilocular with indistinct curved septa.

Effects on Surrounding Structure

- Large lesion can cause expansion of cortical plates without bone destruction
- Associated tooth may fail to erupt or is displaced apically.

Question 4

Describe radiographic features of ameloblastoma.

Answer

Synonyms

- Adamantinoma
- Adamtoblastoma

- Odontomas embryolastiques
- Epithelial odontomas.

Radiographic Features

Location

- About 80% develop in mandibular molar—ramus region and may extend into the symphyseal region
- In maxilla, 3rd molar area is involved and extends in the maxillary sinus and nasal floor.

Periphery

- Well defined and delineated with a cortical border
- Border is often curved and in small lesions it may be indistinguishable from a cyst
- Maxillary lesions are more ill-defined.

Internal Structure

- Varies from totally radiolucent to mixed with bony septae creating internal compartments
- These septae are usually coarse and curved and originate from the normal bone that has been trapped within the tumour
- Since ameloblastoma frequently has internal cystic components, these septae are often remodelled into curved shape giving a honeycomb or soap bubble appearance
- Generally, loculations are larger in posterior mandible than in anterior part.

Effects on Surrounding Structures

- Causes extensive root resorption and tooth displacement
- Common point of origin is occlusal to tooth; teeth may be displaced apically
- Occlusal radiograph may show cyst-like expansion and thinning of adjacent cortical plate, leaving a thin eggshell of bone
- In late stages, perforation of bone into surrounding soft tissues or anatomic spaces occurs
- Unicystic types may cause extreme expansion of mandibular ramus.

Question 5

Describe radiographic features of cherubism.

Answer

Location

- Lesion is bilateral
- Often both the jaws are affected
- When present in only one jaw, mandible is more commonly affected
- Epicentre is always in posterior part of jaws, in ramus of mandible, or tuberosity of maxilla
- Lesion grows in anterior direction
- In severe cases may extend up to midline.

Periphery

Well defined and in some instances corticated.

Internal Structure

Fine granular bony and wispy trabeculae present giving a soap-bubble appearance.

Effects on Surrounding Structure

- Expansion of maxillary and mandibular cortex occurs resulting in severe enlargement of jaws
- Maxillary lesion enlarges into maxillary sinus
- Teeth are displaced in anterior direction as epicentre is placed in posterior part of jaw
- Degree of expansion can be severe resulting in destruction of tooth buds and incipient follicles.

Question 6

Describe radiographic features of odontogenic myxoma.

Answer

Location

- Most commonly affects mandible (3:1)
- Occurs in premolar and molar areas and rarely in ramus and condylar area
- In maxilla, alveolar process in premolar and molar regions and zygomatic process is involved.

Periphery

- May be well defined and corticated or poorly defined (in maxilla)

Internal Structure

- It may produce several pattern
  - Unicystic
  - Multilocular
  - Pericoronal
  - Radiolucent—radiopaque
- Residual bone trapped within the bone remodels into curved or straight, coarse or fine septae giving multilocular appearance

- Characteristically septae are straight and thin (tennis racket or step ladder appearance), but this pattern is rarely seen
- Majority of septae are curved and coarse, but finding one or two of these straight septa help in identification.

Effects on Surrounding Structure

- Causes displacement and loosening of teeth but rarely resorption
- Lesion frequently scallops between the roots of adjacent structure
- Tendency to grow along the bone without causing much expansion.

Question 7

Describe radiographic features of central haemangioma.

Answer

Location

- Mandible twice more affected than maxilla
- Posterior body and ramus and within the inferior alveolar canal.

Periphery

- Periphery is well-defined and corticated or ill-defined
- Variation is related to the amount of residual bone around the blood vessels
- Formation of linear spicules of bone emanating from the surface of the bone in sunray-like appearance can occur when haemangioma breaks through the outer cortex and displace the periosteum.

Internal Structure

- Multilocular appearance is due to entrapment of residual bone trapped around the blood vessels
- Small radiolucent locules may resemble marrow spaces surrounded by coarse, dense and well-defined trabeculae
- These trabeculae produce honeycomb pattern composed of small circular radiolucent spaces that represent blood vessels oriented in the same direction as X-ray beams
- Width of inferior alveolar canal, if involved, is increased and shape becomes serpiginous path
- Phleboliths are formed when soft tissue is involved
- They develop from thrombi that become organized and mineralized and consist of calcium phosphate and calcium carbonate.

Effects on Surrounding Structures

- Roots of teeth are resorbed or displaced
- Width of inferior alveolar canal, if involved, is increased and shape changes to serpiginous path
- Mandibular and mental foramen may be enlarged
- Involved bone may be enlarged and have coarse internal trabeculae
- Developing teeth in contact with haemangioma may be larger and erupt earlier.

Question 8

Describe radiographic features of aneurysmal bone cyst.

Answer

Location

Mandible is more commonly involved than maxilla (3:2) in molar and ramus region.

Periphery and Shape

Periphery is usually well-defined and shape is circular and hydraulic.

Internal Structure

- Small initial lesion may show no evidence of an internal structure
- Often internal structure is multilocular
- Septa is wispy and ill-defined and perpendicular to outer expanded border.

Effects on Surrounding Structures

- Causes expansion of outer cortical plates
- Displaces and resorbs teeth.

Question 9

Describe radiographic features of central giant cell granuloma.

Answer

Location

- More common in mandible (2:1)
- Epicentre of lesion is usually anterior to 1st molar, although large lesion can extend posterior to 1st molar
- Most maxillary lesion arise anterior to canines
- Lesions can cross midline.

Periphery

- Well-defined margin in mandible
- Lesions in maxilla have ill-defined borders.

Internal Structure

- Small lesions are completely radiolucent
- Larger lesion show subtle granular pattern of calcification
- Occasionally, these calcifications are organized into ill-defined wispy septa which are at right angles to the periphery of the lesion
- Sometimes, these septa are well defined and divide the internal aspect into compartments, creating a multilocular appearance.

Effects on Surrounding Structures

- Often displace and resorb teeth
- Resorption of roots not common but when it occurs, it may be profound and irregular in outline
- Lamina dura of involved teeth is absent
- Inferior alveolar canal may be displaced in an inferior direction
- Causes of cortical boundaries of jaw
- Expansion is uneven or undulating in nature, which may give appearance of a double boundary when seen in occlusal radiograph
- Outer cortical plate is destroyed in some cases and is seen more often in maxilla.

Question 10

Describe radiographic features of odontogenic keratocyst.

Answer

Location

- Site—posterior body of mandible (90% occur posterior to canine) and ramus (> 50%)
- Epicentre is located superior to inferior alveolar canal.

Periphery and Shape

- Cortical border is intact unless they have become second-arily affected
- Has smooth round or oval shape.

Internal Structure

- Most commonly radiolucent
- In some cases, curved internal septa may be present, giving lesion a multilocular appearance.

Effects on Surrounding Structures

- Grows along the internal aspect of jaws, causing minimal expansion
- Can displace and resorb teeth
- This occurs throughout the mandible except for the upper ramus and coronoid process, where considerable expansion may occur
- Inferior alveolar canal may be displaced inferiorly
- In maxilla, it may invaginate and occupy maxillary antrum.

Question 11

Describe radiographic features of multiple myeloma.

Answer

Location

- Incidence of jaw involvement varies from 2–78%
- More frequently seen in mandible
- In mandible, posterior body and ramus are favoured site
- Maxillary lesions usually occur in posterior sites.

Periphery and Shape

- Well defined and non-corticated
- Lesions appear "punched out"
- Many appear as ragged or even infiltrative
- Some lesions have oval or cystic shape
- Untreated or aggressive areas may become confluent, giving multilocular appearance.

Internal Structure

- Completely radiolucent
- Occasionally, islands of residual bone, yet unaffected by tumour, give appearance of presence of new trabecular bone within the mass
- Very rarely lesion appears radiopaque internally.

Effects on Surrounding Structure

- Lamina dura is lost
- Follicles of impacted teeth and mandibular canal may lose its corticated border completely or partly
- Mandibular lesions cause thinning of lower border of mandible or endosteal scalloping
- Periosteal reaction is uncommon, but if present, it takes form of single radiopaque line or rarely sunray appearance.

Question 12

Describe radiographic features of fibrous dysplasia.

Answer

Location

- Maxilla twice more commonly affected than mandible
- Occurs frequently in posterior aspect
- Lesions are unilateral.

Periphery

- Periphery of lesion is commonly ill-defined, with gradual blending of normal trabecular bone into abnormal trabecular pattern.
  - Occasionally boundary between bone and lesion may appear sharp and even corticated, especially in young lesions.

Internal Structure

- Density and trabecular pattern vary considerably
- Variation is more pronounced in mandible than in maxilla
- Three distinct patterns are seen depending on stage of maturation
- The ill-defined radiolucent pattern represents the early lesion of fibrous dysplasia, which shows a radiolucent area with poorly defined borders in which a few faint granular trabeculae may be visible giving multilocular appearance
- Abnormal trabeculae are thinner, irregularly shaped and more numerous than normal trabeculae giving ground glass, peau d'orange or cotton wool appearance.

Effects on Surrounding Structures

- If the lesion is small, it may have no effect on surrounding structures (subclinical variety)
- The effects on the involved bone may include expansion with maintenance of a thinned outer cortex
- May expand into the antrum by displacing its cortical boundary and subsequently occupying part or most of the maxillary sinus
- Occasionally trabeculae may arrange into swirling pattern similar to fingerprint
- Extension into the maxillary antrum usually occurs from the lateral wall, and the last section of the sinus to be involved usually is the most posterosuperior portion
- Cortical boundaries such as the floor of the antrum may be changed into the abnormal bone pattern
- Often the bone surrounding the teeth is altered without affecting the dentition
- Lamina dura is lost
- If the fibrous dysplasia increases the bone density, the periodontal ligament space may appear to be very narrow
- Fibrous dysplasia can displace teeth or interfere with normal eruption, complicating orthodontic therapy
- In rare cases, some root resorption may occur
- Displaces the inferior alveolar nerve canal in a superior direction.

Question 13

Describe radiographic features of chondrosarcoma.

Answer

- Involvement of facial bone not common (10%)
- Occur in equal frequency in maxilla and mandible
- In maxilla, lesions are present in anterior region
- In mandible, coronoid process, condylar head and neck and occasionally symphyseal region is involved
- Generally, it has well-defined corticated borders
- Occasionally, peripheral periosteal new bone may present perpendicular to original cortex, giving sunray or hair-on-end appearance
- Aggressive lesions have non-corticated ill-defined borders
- Early lesions are radiolucent because neoplastic cartilage is yet not calcified
- Later lesions have mixed radiolucent–radiopaque appearance
- Causes expansion of cortex
- Inferior alveolar canal is expanded
- Maxillary lesions may push the walls of maxillary sinus or nasal fossa and impinge on infratemporal fossa
- Lesions of condyle causes its expansion and perhaps remodelling of corresponding articular fossa and eminence
- If lesion occurs in articular disk region, a widened joint space may be present with remodelling of condylar neck
- Erosion of articular fossa may also occur
- If lesions occur near the teeth, root resorption and tooth displacement may occur
- Causes band-like widening of periodontal membrane space.

Question 14

Describe radiographic features of osteogenic sarcoma.

Answer

Location

- Mandible more commonly affected than maxilla
- Posterior part of mandible, including tooth bearing region, angle and vertical ramus most commonly involved
- In maxilla, posterior alveolar ridge, antrum, palate is affected commonly
- Lesions may cross midline.

Periphery and Shape

- Ill-defined borders
- Lesion is usually radiolucent with no peripheral sclerosis or encapsulation

- Sunray spicules or hair-on end trabeculae is seen if periosteum is involved
- If periosteum is elevated and maintains its osteogenic potential but it is breached in centre, a Codman's triangle is formed.

Internal Structure

- May be entirely radiolucent, mixed or completely radiopaque
- Internal osseous structure may take the appearance of granular or sclerotic appearing bone, cotton balls, wisps or honeycomb internal structure.

Effects on Surrounding Structure

- Widening of PDL space
- Antral or nasal wall cortices may be lost
- Mandibular lesions may destroy the cortex of neurovascular canals or cause its widening
- Adjacent lamina dura is lost.

SHORT NOTES

Question 1

Explain radiographic features of unicystic ameloblastoma.

Answer

Radiographic features of unicystic ameloblastoma are:

- Mandible is more commonly involved
- 77% were in molar ramus region, 10% in premolar area, 13% in symphysis
- There is pericoronal radiolucency associated with an unerupted mandibular 3rd molar
- Associated teeth is displaced
- Adjacent erupted 2nd or 3rd molar may show knife-edge pattern of root resorption
- Expansion is often present, which tends to be greatest on buccal aspect
- There may be perforation of anterior margins of ramus or at retromolar pad area.

Question 2

What are different multilocular radiolucencies?

Answer

Commonly occurring multilocular radiolucencies are:

- Ameloblastoma
- Cherubism
- Odontogenic myxoma
- Central haemangioma
- Aneurysmal bone cyst
- Central giant cell granuloma
- Odontogenic keratocyst.

SECTION 3

RECENTLY ASKED QUESTIONS

CHAPTER 25 Recently Asked Questions

ULCERATIVE, VESICULAR AND BULLOUS LESIONS

Long Essays

1. Classify oral ulceration with a suitable example of each condition. Describe the clinical features and management of recurrent aphthous ulcers. [RGUHS; TN]
2. What are the oral causes of halitosis? How are you going to treat a case of ANUG. [RGUHS]
3. Classify vesiculobullous lesions. Write in detail about the aetiology, clinical features and management of pemphigus vulgaris. [OS]
4. Classify vesiculobullous lesions of oral cavity and site in detail about erythema multiforme. [NTR]
5. Enumerable various vesiculobullous lesions of oral cavity. Describe erythema multiforme in detail. [NTR; RGUHS]
6. Classify the vesiculobullous lesions of oral caving. Add a note on the management of oral mucous mem-brane pemphigoid. [NTR]
7. Classify vesiculobullous lesions. Discuss in detail aetiopathogenesis, clinical features and management of pemphigus vulgaris. [NTR]
8. Classify vesiculobullous lesions of the oral mucosa. Describe in detail the clinical picture and treatment of any one of the mucocutaneous ocular lesions. [BUHS]
9. Classify vesiculobullous lesions. Write briefly about aetiology, clinical features and treatment of erythema multiforme. [BUHS]
10. Define ulcer. Classify the ulcers of the oral cavity. Write the clinical features and management of erythema multiforme. [RGUHS]
11. What are the bullous lesions of oral mucosa? Describe the clinical features, differentia] diagnosis and treatment of pemphigus vulgaris. [BUHS]
12. Define an autoimmune disease and enumerate autoimmune disease that has indirect and direct effects on the oral cavity. Give the clinical features and investigations of pemphigus vulgaris. [RGUHS]
13. Discuss the differential diagnosis of multiple ulcers of oral mucosa. [NTR]
14. Classify ulcers of the oral mucosa. Discuss the differential diagnosis of recurrent multiple ulcer. [NTR]
15. Define an autoimmune disease and enumerate autoimmune diseases that have indirect and direct effects on the oral cavity. Give the clinical features and investigations of pemphigus vulgaris. [RGUHS]
16. Classify ulcerative and vesiculobullous lesions of the oral cavity. Write in detail clinical features, diagnosis, investigations, differential diagnosis and treatment of herpetic gingivostomatitis. [TN]
17. Classify the vesiculobullous lesions. Write in detail about the aetiopathogenesis, clinical features, differen-tial diagnosis, investigations and management of herpes infection. [TN]
18. Classify oral ulcers. Discuss the differential diagnosis of acute multiple ulcers of the oral cavity. [TN]
19. Define vesicle. Write the pathogenesis, clinical features, investigations and management of primary herpetic infection. [NTRUHS]
20. Define ulcer. Classify ulcers of oral cavity. Write the clinical features and management of erythema multiforme. [RGUHS]
21. Classify vesiculobullous lesions. Write briefly about aetiology, clinical features and treatment of erythema multiforme. [RGUHS]
22. Classify the ulcerative and vesiculobullous lesions of oral cavity. Describe in detail recurrent aphthous stomatitis. [RGUHS]
23. List the common viral infections that may involve the oral cavity. Discuss in detail the differential diagnosis of herpes simplex. [RGUHS]

24. Enumerate the various vesiculobullous lesions of oral cavity. Give differential diagnosis of primary acute herpetic stomatitis, erythema multiforme and aphthous stomatitis. [MUHS]
25. Enumerate the various vesiculobullous lesions of oral cavity. Discuss in detail the clinical features, differential diagnosis and treatment plan of primary herpes simplex infection. [MUHS]
26. Enumerate ulcerative regions of oral cavity. Discuss in detail any two of them. [MUHS]
27. Classify ulcerative and vesiculobullous lesions of the oral cavity. Give the differential diagnosis between acute necrotizing ulcerative gingivostomatitis and primary herpes infection and give treatment plan for each. [MUHS]
28. Clinical features and management of erythema multiforme. [MUHS]
29. Classify vesiculobullous lesions and discuss the aetio-pathogenesis, clinical features and management of erythema multiforme. [RGUHS]
30. Classify vesiculobullous and ulcerative lesion of oral cavity. Discuss in detail primary herpes simplex infection. [NTRUHS]
31. Enumerate the conditions which cause multiple ulcers in the oral cavity. Discuss in detail the aetiology, clinical features, investigations and management of erythema multiforme. [NTRUHS]
32. Classify vesiculobullous lesions of oral mucosa. Describe in detail the clinical picture and treatment of any one of the mucocutaneous ocular lesions. [RGUHS]
33. What are the bullous lesions of oral mucosa? Describe the clinical features, differential diagnosis and treatment of pemphigus vulgaris. [RGUHS]
34. Enumerate the various bullous lesions and describe the aetiology, clinical features differential diagnosis and management of pemphigus. [TN]
35. Classify ulcerative lesions of oral mucosa and write the differential diagnosis of recurrent multiple ulcers. [TN]
36. Classify ulcerative and vesiculobullous lesions of oral cavity. Describe the aetiology, clinical features and treatment plan for recurrent aphthous stomatitis. [MUHS; TN]
37. Classify oral ulcerations with a suitable example. Describe clinical features and management of recurrent aphthous ulcer. [TN]
38. Classify ulcerative and vesiculobullous lesions of oral cavity. Discuss in detail the aetiology, clinical features and management of erythema multiforme. [TN]
39. Classify the ulcerative and vesiculobullous lesions of oral cavity. Describe in detail recurrent aphthous ulcers. [RGUHS]
40. Classify oral ulcerations with a suitable example of each condition. Describe clinical features and manage-ment of recurrent aphthous ulcer. [RGUHS; TN]
41. Define ulcer. Classify ulcers of oral cavity. Write the clinical features and management of erythema multi-forme. [RGUHS]
42. Classify ulcerative and vesiculobullous lesion of oral cavity and discuss the differential diagnosis between acute necrotizing ulcerative gingivitis and primary heipes simplex infection. Mention the treatment for both these conditions. [MUHS]
43. Classify ulcerative and vesiculobullous lesion of oral cavity. Describe the aetiology, clinical features and treatment plan for recurrent aphthous stomatitis. [MUHS]
44. Enumerate the various ulcerative and vesiculobullous lesion of oral cavity. Give the clinical features, differential diagnosis and treatment of pemphigus vulgaris. [MUHS]

Short Essays

1. Clinical features of erythema multiforme. [MUHS]
2. Describe the differences of oral ulcer and oral wound. [RGUHS]
3. Investigations and management of primary herpetic gingivostomatitis. [RGUHS]
4. Classify vesiculobullous lesions of oral cavity. [MUHS]
6. Describe clinical features of Stevens-Johnson syndrome. [RGUHS]
5. Discuss in detail the clinical features, differential diagnosis and treatment of erythema multiforme. [MUHS]
7. Give treatment plan for ANUG. [RGUHS; MUHS]
8. Give treatment plan for pemphigus vulgaris. [RGUHS]
9. Examination of ulcer. [RGUHS]
10. Pemphigus. [RGUHS]
11. Recurrent oral ulcers. [MUHS]
12. Erythema multiforme. [MUHS]
13. Aphthous ulceration. [MUHS]
14. Recurrent aphthous stomatitis. [MUHS]
15. Define vesicle and papule. Give two examples of each. [MUHS]
16. Bell's palsy. [RGUHS]
17. Aphthous ulcer. [NTRUHS]
18. Ulceration on the lower lip. [MUHS]
19. Pemphigus vulgaris. [RGUHS; MUHS]

20. Recurrent aphthous stomatitis. [RGUHS]
21. Give the treatment plan for erosive lichen planus. [MUHS]
22. Herpes zoster. [RGUHS]
23. Herpetic gingivostomatitis. [RGUHS]
24. Nikolsky's sign. [RGUHS]
25. Classification and treatment of recurrent aphthous stomatitis. [RGUHS]
26. Describe clinical features of ANUG. [RGUHS]
27. Subepithelial dermatoses. [RGUHS]

Short Notes

1. Pemphigus vulgaris. [RGUHS]
2. Erythema multiforme. [RGUHS]
3. Postherpetic neuralgia. [RGUHS; TN]
4. Gangrenous stomatitis. [RGUHS]
5. Treatment of gangrenous stomatitis. [RGUHS]
6. Treatment of aphthous ulcer major. [RGUHS]
7. Differences between herpes simplex and zoster. [RGUHS]
8. Oral manifestations of Stevens-Johnson syndrome. [RGUHS]
9. How will you manage a case of gangrenous stomatitis? [RGUHS]
10. Classify pemphigus and describe benign mucous membrane pemphigoid. [RGUHS]
11. Outline the clinical features of herpetic gingivitis and Vincent's infection. [RGUHS]
12. ANUG. [RGUHS; NTRUHS]
13. Patch test. [RGUHS]
14. Tzanck test. [RGUHS]
15. Tzanck smear. [RGUHS]
16. Investigations with the result of pemphigus vulgaris. [NTR]
17. How do you manage the pemphigus or pemphigoid? [NTR]
18. Lipschutz bodies. [RGUHS]
19. Herpes zoster. [RGUHS]
20. Nikolsky's sign. [RGUHS; NTRUHS]
21. Acute pemphigus. [RGUHS]
22. Enumerate four differences between pemphigus vulgaris and benign mucous membrane pemphigoid. [RGUHS]
23. Nikolsky's sign. [NTR]
24. Erythema multiforme. [NTR; RGUHS]
25. Aphthous ulcer. [BUHS; RGUHS; TN]
26. Target lesions. [RGUHS]
27. Stevens-Johnson syndrome. [NTR]
28. Describe the oral manifestations of pemphigus vulgaris. [NTR]
29. Describe briefly the classification and management of vesiculobullous lesions of the mouth. [NTR]
30. Oral manifestations of Stevens-Johnson syndrome. [BUHS]
31. Describe the clinical features of Stevens-Johnson syndrome. [RGUHS]
32. Give treatment plan for pemphigus vulgaris. [RGUHS]
33. Classify pemphigus and describe benign mucous pemphigoid. [BUHS]
34. Recurrent aphthous stomatitis. [NTR]
35. Management of recurrent aphthous ulcers. [NTR]
36. Describe the differences of oral ulcer and oral wound. [BUHS]
37. Classification and treatment of recurrent aphthous stomatitis. [RGUHS]
38. Enumerate the important differences between the herpetic stomatitis and aphthous stomatitis. [BUHS]
39. Aphthous stomatitis. [TN]
40. Sarcoidosis. [RGUHS]
41. Major aphthous ulcers. [RGUHS]
42. Treatment of aphthous ulcer major. [BUHS]
43. Discoid lupus erythematosus. [BUHS]
44. Ectodermal dysplasia. [TN; NTRUHS]
45. Various syndromes associated with erythema multiforme. [TN]
46. Differential diagnosis of vesiculobullous lesions of oral cavity. [TN]
47. Tzanck test. [RGUHS]
48. Tzanck smear. [RGUHS]
49. Target lesions. [RGUHS]
50. Acute pemphigus. [BUHS]
51. Pemphigus vulgaris. [BUHS; TN]
52. Oral manifestations of Stevens-Johnson syndrome. [BUHS]
53. Laboratory findings of pemphigus vulgaris. [RGUHS]
54. Enumerate four differences between pemphigus vulgaris and benign mucous membrane pemphigoid. [RGUHS]
55. Erosive lichen planus. [NTRUHS]
56. Erythema multiforme. [NTRUHS]
57. Psoriatic arthritis. [OS]
58. Smoker's palate. [RGUHS]
59. Paterson-Kelly syndrome. [RGUHS]
60. Keratoacanthoma. [RGUHS]

RED AND WHITE LESIONS

Long Essays

1. Classify oral mucosal candidiasis: Write the aetiopathogenesis, clinical features investigations and management of chronic atrophic candidiasis. [TN]
2. Classify white lesions of the oral cavity. Describe the aetiology, clinical features, differential diagnosis, investigations and treatment of oral lichen planus. [TN]
3. Classify white lesions of the oral mucosa and describe the aetiology, clinical features, diagnosis and management of oral lichen planus. [TN; NTR]
4. Enumerate the various white lesions which can be scrapped. Describe the clinical features, differential diagnosis and treatment of candidiasis. [TN]
5. Classify and write briefly on the clinical features, investigations and treatment of oral candidiasis. [TN]
6. What are the keratinizing lesions of the oral cavity? Write about oral leukoplakia. [TN]
7. Classify red and white lesions of the oral mucosa. Describe in detail aetiology, clinical features and management of oral submucous fibrosis. [TN]
8. Classify white lesions of the oral mucosa and describe the aetiology, clinical features, diagnosis and management of acute atrophic candidiasis. [TN]
9. Classify oral white lesions, write about the clinical features, differential diagnosis and management of oral submucous fibrosis. [RGUHS]
10. Describe clinical features of lichen planus in buccal mucosa. [RGUHS]
11. Describe the clinical features and differential diagnosis of oral lichen planus. [RGUHS]
12. Classify white lesions of the oral cavity. Describe the aetiology, clinical features and management of leukoplakia. [RGUHS]
13. Enumerate oral precancerous lesions and conditions. Describe clinical features and management of oral submucous fibrosis. [RGUHS]
14. Name some of the white lesions of oral mucosa. Describe the clinical features, differential diagnosis and treatment of leukoplakia of hard palate. [RGUHS]
15. What conditions may produce trismus. Describe in detail the predisposing factors, clinical features, treatment of oral submucous fibrosis. [RGUHS]
16. Classify oral white lesions. Write the clinical features, differential diagnosis and management of oral submucous fibrosis. [TN]
17. Write an essay on oral candidiasis. [TN]
18. Classify white lesions. Discuss in detail the aetiopathogenesis, clinical features, diagnosis and management of oral submucous fibrosis. [RGUHS]
19. Enumerate predisposing factors of candidiasis. Mention the various types and discuss in detail the treatment plan. [NTRUHS]
20. Classify candidiasis. Write in detail about the aetiology, clinical features and management of oral thrush. [RGUHS]
21. Give the differential diagnosis of psoriasis. [NTR]
22. Enumerate the white lesions of the oral mucosa. Write about aetiology, clinical features, investigations and management of oral thrush. [NTR]
23. Classify white lesions of the oral cavity. Describe the aetiology, clinical features, diagnosis and management of lichen planus. [RGUHS; TN]
24. Classify white lesions of the oral cavity. Describe the aetiology, clinical features and management of leukoplakia. [RGUHS]
25. Name some of the white lesions of oral mucosa. Describe the clinical features, differential diagnosis and treatment of leukoplakia of hard palate. [BUHS]
26. Classify candidal lesions of the oral mucosa. Write in detail the clinical features, lab diagnosis and management of oral candidiasis. [RGUHS]
27. Classify white lesions and discuss in detail about the clinical features and management of leukoplakia. [RGUHS]
28. Classify white lesions. Describe in detail the aetiology, classification, clinical features and management of leukoplakia [RGUHS]
29. Define premalignant lesions and conditions. Describe oral lichen planus in detail. [RGUHS]
30. Enumerate the 'white lesions' of the oral cavity. Describe leukoplakia in detail, giving differential diagnosis. [MUHS]
31. Classify white lesions and give clinical features, laboratory diagnosis tests and treatment of oral candidal infection. [MUHS]
32. Treatment of acute pseudomembranous moniliasis. [MUHS]
33. Define leukoplakia. Discuss the aetiopathogenesis, clinical features and treatment of oral leukoplakia. [RGUHS]
34. Candidiasis. [MUHS]
35. Treatment option for oral thrush. [MUHS]
36. Moniliasis. [MUHSH]

37. Describe the clinical features and management of:
    a. Oral leukoplakia
    b. Oral submucous fibrosis. [NTR-GR]
38. Classify the red and white lesions of the oral cavity. Describe in detail the aetiology, clinical features, treatment plan and prognosis of submucous fibrosis. [MUHS]
39. Discuss in detail the clinical features, differential diagnosis and treatment of erythema multiforme. [MUHS]
40. Classify oral candidiasis. Describe the aetiology, clinical features, differential diagnosis and management of oral thrush. [MUHS]
41. Classify ulcerative and vesiculobullous lesions of the oral cavity. Give the differential diagnosis between acute necrotizing ulcerative gingivostomatitis and primary herpes infection and give treatment plan for each. [MUHS]
42. Define oral precancerous lesions and conditions. Discuss in detail the clinical features and management of oral submucous fibrosis. [RGUHS]

Short Essays

1. Mention the treatment plan for submucous fibrosis. [MUHS]
2. Classify red and white lesions. Describe in detail oral submucous fibrosis. [MUHS]
3. Define leukoplakia. [MUHS]
4. Treatment of candidiasis. [MUHS]
5. Predisposing factors of moniliasis. [MUHS]
6. Management of oral lichen planus. [MUHS; NTRUHS]
7. Define vesicle and papule. Give two examples of each. [MUHS]
8. Predisposing factors of candidiasis. [RGUHS]
9. Smear examination for Candida albicans. [RGUHS]
10. Pathogenesis and management of oral leukoplakia. [RGUHS]
11. Investigation and management of oral candidiasis. [RGUHS]
12. Aetiology and management of oral submucous fibrosis. [RGUHS]
13. Mention' the predisposing factors of candidiasis. [MUHS]
14. Leukoplakia. [RGUHS; TN; MUHS; NTRUHS]
15. Lichenoid reactions. [MUHS; RGUHS]
16. Discoid lupus erythematosus. [RGUHS]
17. Lupus erythematosus. [RGUHS]
18. Erythroplakia. [RGUHS]
19. Oral thrush. [RGUHS]
20. Oral hairy leukoplakia. [NTRUHS]
21. White spongy naevus. [NTRUHS]
22. Behcet's syndrome. [NTRUHS]

Short Notes

1. Oral manifestations of oral submucous fibrosis. [RGUHS]
2. Outline four differences between leukoplakia and lichen planus. [RGUHS]
3. White sponge naevus. [NTR]
4. Thrush. [NTR]
5. Atrophic candidiasis. [NTR]
6. Describe the clinical features and management of oral moniliasis. [NTR]
7. Enumerate the important differences between the Auspitz's sign and Tzanck test. [NTR]
8. Enumerate the white lesions of oral cavity. [BUHS]
9. Describe the white lesions of the oral cavity. [BUHS]
10. Predisposing factors of candidiasis. [RGUHS]
11. Smear examination for Candida albicans. [RGUHS]
12. Investigation and management of oral candidiasis. [RGUHS]
13. Moniliasis. [RGUHS]
14. Auspitz's sign. [RGUHS]
15. White spongy naevus. [RGUHS]
16. Erosive lichen planus. [RGUHS]
17. Grinspan's syndrome. [RGUHS; TN]
18. Chronic atrophic candidiasis. [RGUHS]
19. Treatment of mondial granuloma. [RGUHS]
20. Lichen planus in buccal mucosa. [RGUHS]
21. Treatment of oral submucous fibrosis. [RGUHS]
22. Clinical features of erosive lichen planus. [RGUHS]
23. Enumerate the white lesions of oral cavity. [RGUHS]
24. Describe clinical features and management of denture sore mouth. [RGUHS]
25. Candidiasis. [NTR; TN; NTRUHS]
26. Auspitz's sign. [NTR]
27. White spongy naevus. [NTR]
28. Id reaction. [RGUHS]
29. Moniliasis. [BUHS; RGUHS]
30. Monilial granuloma. [BUHS]
31. Types of oral candidiasis. [RGUHS]
32. Chronic atrophic candidiasis. [BUHS]
33. Treatment of monilial granuloma. [BUHS]
34. Lichen planus. [OS]
35. Target lesions. [RS]
36. Id reaction. [RS]
37. Sturge-Weber syndrome. [RS]
38. Lichenoid reaction. [RGUHS]
39. Mucous membrane pemphigoid. [RGUHS]
40. Classify oral candidiasis. [NTRUHS]

41. Leukoplakia. [NTRUHS; RGUHS]
42. Stomatitis venenata. [NTRUHS]
43. Mucous patches. [NTRUHS]
44. Cancrum oris. [RGUHS]
45. Erythroplakia. [RGUHS]
46. Oral hairy leukoplakia. [RGUHS; TN]
47. Treatment of oral lichen planus. [TN; RGUHS]
48. Erythema multiforme. [TN]
49. Oral thrush. [TN; RGUHS]
50. Investigations of oral candidiasis. [TN]
51. Ectodermal dysplasia. [TN]
52. Management of lichen planus. [TN]
53. SLE (systemic lupus erythematosus). [TN]
54. Behcet's syndrome. [TN]
55. Lichen rubber planus. [TN]
56. Management of oral candidiasis. [TN]
57. Stevens-Johnson syndrome. [TN]
58. Treatment plan of erosive lichen planus. [TN]
59. Leukodema. [TN]
60. Hairy leukoplakia. [TN; RGUHS]

PIGMENTATION OF THE ORAL TISSUE

Long Essays

1. What are the causes of pigmentation of oral mucosa? [RGUHS]
2. 'Pigmentation in oral structure' diagnostic clue to diagnose systemic diseases. Discuss. [RGUHS]
3. General and oral manifestations of bismuthism. [RGUHS]
4. Discuss the conditions which cause pigmentations of the oral mucosa. [RGUHS]
5. Discuss the differential diagnosis of oral mucosal pigmentation. [NTR]
6. Enumerate the various causes of pigmentation of the oral cavity. Discuss in detail endogenous pigmentation. [MUHS]
7. Enumerate the various factors that cause endogenous pigmentation of the oral tissues. Describe in detail the oral manifestations of bismuth, lead and mercury intoxication. [MUHS]
8. Discuss in detail the diseases causing oral pigmentation. [RGUHS]
9. Classify orofacial pigmentation. Describe various type of endogenous pigmentation. [RGUHS]

Short Essays

1. Enumerate diseases with cafe-au-lait pigmentation. [RGUHS]
2. Classification and clinical significance of endogenous pigmentation. [RGUHS]
3. Different diagnosis of oral pigmentation. [RGUHS]
4. Oral mucosal pigmentations. [NTR]

Short Notes

1. Exogenous pigmentation of oral cavity. [RGUHS]
2. Pigmented lesions of orofacial pain. [NTR]
4. In Addison's disease there is deposition of which pigment. [MUHS]
5. Endocrinopathic pigmentation. [MUHS]
6. Cafe-au-lait spots. [TN; RGUHS]
7. Albright's syndrome. [RGUHS]
8. Endogenous pigmentation. [NTR; MUHS]
9. Oral mucosal pigmentations. [NTR; TN]
10. Intrinsic stains and extrinsic stains. [NTR]
11. Filters. [TN]
12. Discolouration of teeth. [RGUHS]
13. Cafe-au-lait spots. [NTR]

BENIGN TUMOURS OF THE ORAL CAVITY INCLUDING GINGIVAL ENLARGEMENTS

Long Essays

1. Give differential diagnosis of growth in gingiva.[RGUHS]
2. Give differential diagnosis of growth in gingiva. [BUHS]
3. Give differential diagnosis of desquamation of gingiva. [BUHS]
4. What are the oral causes of halitosis? How are you going to treat a case of ANUG? [BUHS]
5. Enumerate the conditions which produce multiple ulcers in the oral cavity. Describe the clinical features, investigations and management of acute herpetic gingivostomatitis. [RGUHS]

6. Give differential diagnosis of desquamation of gingiva. [RGUHS]
7. Describe the aetiology, clinical features, radiological and histological features of ameloblastoma. [RGUHS]
8. What are the premalignant lesions of the oral cavity? What precautions should be taken in the prevention of oral malignancies? [RGUHS]
9. Write briefly histopathology of:
   a. Adenomatoid odontogenic tumour
   b. Pleomorphic adenoma. [RGUHS]
10. Classify the cysts of the jaws. Write in detail about ameloblastoma. [TN]
11. Classify the cysts of the jaws. Write in detail about the aetiopathogenesis, clinical features, investigations, management and prognosis of ameloblastoma. [TN]
12. Classify the cysts of the jaws. Describe the clinical and radiographic features of 'dental cysts'. [TN]
13. Discuss differential diagnosis of the swelling at the angle of mandible along with diagnostic aids. [TN]
14. Give the differences between benign and malignant tumours. Describe the clinical and radiographic features of a squamous cell carcinoma. [RS2]
15. Enumerate the clinical features and radiological features of
   a. Fibrous dysplasia
   b. Radiopaque lesions of the jawbone
   c. Chronic osteomyelitis at the angle of the mandible. [NTR-GR]
16. Enumerate the benign tumours of the jaws and describe in detail ameloblastoma. [RGUHS]
17. Classify cysts of the jaws and describe in detail:
   a. Dentigerous cyst
   b. Primodial cyst [MUHS]
18. Name the nonodontogenic cysts of jaw bones. Discuss any one of them in detail. [MUHS]
19. What are the aetiological factors of osteomyelitis of mandible? [RGUHS]
20. Define osteomyelitis. Describe various types, aetiology, clinical features, diagnosis and management of osteomyelitis of mandible. [BUHS]
21. Classify osteomyelitis. Write in detail about the aetiology, clinical features, radiographic features and management of chronic suppurative osteomyelitis. [RGUHS]
22. Define osteomyelitis. Describe the various types, aetiology, clinical features, diagnosis and management of osteomyelitis of mandible. [BUHS]
23. Describe the aetiological factors of osteomyelitis of mandible. Describe the clinical features and management of actinomycosis of jaws. [BUHS]
24. Describe the aetiology, clinical features, radiological and histological features of ameloblastoma. [BUHS]
25. Classify the cysts of the jaws and discuss in detail the odontogenic keratocyst. [MUHS]

Short Essays

1. Discuss the differential diagnosis of gingival enlargement. [MUHS]
2. Enumerate the various causes of gingival enlargement. Discuss differential diagnosis of inflammatory and noninflammatory gingival enlargement. [MUHS]
3. What are the causes of bleeding from the gums? Discuss in detail 'acute necrotizing ulcerative gingivosto-matitis'. [MUHS]
4. Classify gingival enlargements and discuss in detail the inflammatory gingival enlargement of systemic background. [MUHS]
5. Enumerate the local and systemic causes of gingival enlargement. Describe the clinical features and oral changes seen in leukaemia and scurvy. [MUHS]
6. Acute necrotizing ulcerative gingivostomatitis (ANUG). [MUHS]
7. Primodial cyst. [MUHS]
8. Differential diagnosis between periapical cysts and periapical abscess. [MUHS]
9. Multilocular lesions. [MUHS]
10. Differentiate between radicular cyst and maxillary sinus. [MUHS]
11. Differential diagnosis between periapical cyst with maxillary molar and maxillary sinus. [MUHS]
12. Enumerate various benign tumours affecting the oral cavity. Describe in detail ameloblastoma. [MUHS]
13. Enumerate the benign tumours of the oral cavity; describe the clinical features, radiographic appearance and differential diagnosis of ameloblastoma. [MUHS]
14. Classify vesiculobullous lesions of oral cavity. Describe ANUG in detail. [MUHS]
15. Give the differential diagnosis of conditions that cause gingiva] enlargement. [MUHS]
16. Differential diagnosis between condensing osteitis and diffuse sclerosing osteomyelitis. [MUHS]
17. Differential diagnosis between cementifying dysplasia (Id stage) and condensing osteitis. [MUHS]
18. Enumerate the fibro-osseous lesions that involve the jaws. Discuss the aetiology, pathogenesis and clinical features of Paget's disease. Add a note on its complications. [TN]
19. Gingival bleeding. [MUHS]
20. Treatment plan of ANUG. [MUHS]

21. Differential diagnosis between ANUG and primary herpes simplex lesions. [MUHS]
22. Differential diagnosis between leukaemic and Dilantin gingival enlargement. [MUHS]
23. Leukaemic gingival enlargement. [MUHS]
24. Fibrous dysplasia. [MUHS]
25. Paget's disease. [MUHS]
26. Periapical cementifying dysplasia. [MUHS]
27. Describe the clinical features, differential diagnosis and treatment plan of acute necrotizing ulcerative gingivostomatitis. [NTRUHS]

Short Notes

1. Torus mandibularis. [RGUHS]
2. Ameloblastoma in mandible. [RGUHS]
3. Biochemical investigations of Paget's disease. [RGUHS]
4. ANUG. [NTR-QR; NTRUHS]
5. Acute necrotizing ulcerative gingivitis. [NTR-NR]
6. Pregnancy tumour and gingivitis. [NTR-QR]
7. Treatment of Dilantin gingival enlargement. [RGUHS]
8. Name four drugs causing gingival enlargement. [RGUHS]
9. Cementoma. [RGUHS]
10. Nasopalatine cyst. [RGUHS]
11. Multilocular cyst. [RGUHS]
12. Periapical cemental dysplasia. [RGUHS]
13. Cafe-au-lait spots. [RGUHS]
14. Carcinoma in situ. [RGUHS]
15. Herpetic gingivostomatitis. [NTR-NR]
16. Clinical features of acute herpetic gingivostomatitis. [NTR-NR]
17. Vincent's infection (trench mouth). [BUHS, RGUHS]
18. Describe the clinical features of ANUG. [RGUHS]
19. Describe the treatment plan for ANUG. [RGUHS]
20. Describe the role of osteoradionecrosis in intraoral anaesthesia. [NTR-QR]
21. Osteosarcoma. [RGUHS]
22. Clinical features and radiographic appearance of osteosarcoma. [RGUHS]
23. Types of osteomyelitis and their features. [RGUHS]
24. Describe the radiographic appearance of chronic osteomyelitis. [RGUHS]
25. Describe the radiographic appearance of acute and chronic osteomyelitis. [BUHS]
26. Pathogenesis and management of osteoradionecrosis. [RGUHS]
27. Dentigerous cyst. [NTR-OR; TN]
28. Radiographic appearance of ameloblastoma. [NTR-GR]
29. Odontogenic keratocyst. [NTR-GR]
30. Describe the radiographic features of ameloblastoma. [NTR-OR]
31. Name the drugs causing gingival enlargement. [RGUHS]
32. Treatment of Dilantin gingival hyperplasia. [BUHS]
33. Investigations and management of primary herpetic gingivostomatitis. [RGUHS, RGUHS]
34. Cherubism. [NTR-QR]
35. Fibrous dysplasia. [NTR-QR, NTR-QR; RGUHS]
36. Describe the radiographic features of fibrous dysplasia. [NTR-QR]
37. Garre's osteomyelitis. [NTR-QR]
38. Condensing osteitis. [NTR-QR]
39. Osteoradionecrosis. [NTR-QR, NTR-QR, NTR-QR]
40. Radiographic appearance of odontogenic keratocyst. [NTR-NR]
41. Describe radiographic appearance of dentigerous cyst. [RGUHS]
42. Describe radiographic features of cementoma and hypercementosis. [BUHS]
43. Write briefly histopathology of:
    a. Adenomatoid odontogenic tumour
    b. Pleomorphic adenoma. [BUHS]
44. Name two drugs causing gingival enlargement. [MUHS]
45. Give the treatment plan of ANUG. [MUHS]
46. ANUG. [NTR-NR]
47. Cancrum oris. [NTR-NR]
48. Gingival hyperplasia. [NTR-NR; TN]
49. Desquamative gingivitis. [RGUHS]
50. Gangrenous stomatitis. [BUHS]
51. Myxoma. [NTR-GR]
52. Pleomorphic adenoma of palate. [NTR-GR]
53. Ossifying fibroma—clinical features. [NTR-NR]
54. Describe the radiographic features of myxoma. [NTR-GR]
55. Carcinoma in situ of buccal mucosa. [RGUHS]
56. Enumerate periapical lesions. [MUHS]
57. Mention any four causes of generalized gingival enlargement. [MUHS]
58. Treatment of gangrenous stomatitis. [BUHS]
59. How will you manage a case of gangrenous stomatitis? [BUHS]
60. Why hydrogen peroxide mouthwash is given in ANUG? [RGUHS]
61. How will you investigate herpetic gingivostomatitis? [BUHS]
62. Outline the clinical features of herpetic gingivitis and Vincent's infection. [BUHS]
63. Write briefly the osteomyelitis of mandible. [NTR-NR]
64. Radiographic appearance of Paget's disease. [NTR-NR]
65. Nasopalatine cyst. [BUHS]
66. Ameloblastoma in mandible. [BUHS]

67. Periapical cemental dysplasia. [BUHS; TN]
68. Describe radiographic appearance and clinical features of cementoma. [BUHS]
69. Describe radiographic appearance of periapical cementoma. [RGUHS]
70. Radiographic appearance of fibrous dysplasia. [NTR-NR; TN]
71. Cafe-au-lait spots. [RGUHS]
72. Biochemical investigations of Paget's diseases. [RGUHS]
73. Radiographic appearance of osteogenic sarcoma. [RGUHS]
74. Explain why sequestrum appears more radiopaque than adjacent bone. [RGUHS]
75. Radiographic appearance of periapical cemental dysplasia. [NTR-NR]
76. Cementoma. [BUHS]
77. Multilocular cyst. [RGUHS]
78. Fibroma. [RGUHS; TN]
79. Torus mandibularis. [BUHS]
80. Cherubism. [RGUHS]
81. Ossifying fibroma. [RGUHS; TN]
82. Albright's syndrome. [TN; RGUHS]
83. Giant cell granuloma. [TN]
84. Radiographic appearance of reparative granuloma. [TN]
85. Drug-induced gingival hyperplasia. [RGUHS]
86. Periapical granuloma. [RGUHS]
87. Multiple myeloma. [NTRUHS]
88. Pyogenic granuloma. [NTRUHS]
89. Median mandibular cyst. [NTRUHS]
90. Fibromatosis gingivae. [TN]
91. Adenomatoid odontogenic tumour. [TN]
92. Residual cyst. [RGUHS]
93. Von Recklinghausen's disease. [RGUHS]
94. Paget's disease. [TN]
95. Fibrous inflammatory hyperplasias. [RGUHS]
96. Pregnancy gingivitis and tumour. [NTR-OR]
97. Drug-induced gingival enlargement. [TN]
98. Drug-induced gingival hyperplasia. [RGUHS]
99. Epulis. [TN]
100. Polyostotic fibrous dysplasia. [TN]
101. Amelogenesis imperfecta. [TN]
102. Pyogenic granuloma. [TN]
103. Multiple myeloma. [TN]
104. Infectious mononucleosis. [TN]
105. Fissural cysts. [TN]
106. Nonodontogenic cysts of the jaws. [TN]
107. Giant cell. [RGUHS]
108. Cherubism. [RGUHS]
109. Cleidocranial dysplasia. [RGUHS]
110. Lipoma. [RGUHS]
111. Compound odontome. [RGUHS]
112. Papilloma. [RGUHS]
113. Pierre Robin syndrome. [RGUHS]
114. Pseudocysts. [NTR]
115. Pyogenic granuloma. [MUHS]
116. Paul-Bunnell test. [RGUHS]
117. TNM staging. [RGUHS]
118. Odontomes. [RGUHS]
119. Mural ameloblastoma. [RGUHS]
120. Midline lethal granuloma. [RGUHS]
121. Complex composite odontome. [NTRUHS]
122. Fibroti'c gingival enlargement. [NTRUHS]
123. Gingival enlargement. [RGUHS]

ORAL CANCER

Long Essays

1. Describe the clinical varieties of leukoplakia and mention the treatment of different types of leukoplakia. Add a note on aetiology of leukoplakia. [NTR-NR]
2. Classify white lesions of the oral cavity. Describe the aetiology, clinical features, diagnosis and management of lichen planus. [NTR-NR]
3. Classify the white lesions of the mouth. Describe in detail the clinical features, differential diagnosis and management of oral lichen planus. [NTR-OR]
4. Describe the clinical features and management of oral submucous fibrosis. Discuss the aetiological factors of this condition. [NTR-NR]
5. Enumerate premalignant lesions and premalignant conditions. Describe the aetiology, clinical features and treatment of oral submucous fibrosis. [NTR-NR]
6. Describe the clinical features and management of:
   a. Oral leukoplakia
   b. Oral submucous fibrosis. [NTR-OR]
7. Describe clinical features of lichen planus in buccal mucosa. [BUHS]
8. Describe the medical management of malignant tumours of the mouth. [RGUHS]
9. Describe the aetiology, clinical features and management of oral carcinomas. [RGUHS]
10. Treatment for leukoplakia. [MUHS]

11. Enumerate premalignant lesions and premalignant conditions. Describe the aetiology, clinical features and treatment of oral submucous fibrosis. [NTR-NR; TN]
12. Enumerate malignant tumour of the oral cavity. Describe the clinical and radiographic features of squamous cell carcinoma involving the mandibular alveolus. Briefly mention the modalities of treatment and complications of the treatment modalities. [MUHS]
13. Enumerate premalignant conditions and lesions of oral mucosa. Describe in detail any two of them. [TN]
14. Enumerate premalignant conditions and premaligqant lesions of oral mucosa. Describe in detail any two of them. [NTR-GR]
15. Describe the clinical features and differential diagnosis of oral lichen planus. [BUHS]
16. Classify white lesions of the oral cavity. Describe the aetiology, clinical features and management of leukoplakia. [RGUHS]
17. Name some of the white lesions of oral mucosa. Describe the clinical features, differential diagnosis and treatment of leukoplakia of hard palate. [BUHS]
18. Enumerate oral precancerous lesions and conditions. Describe clinical features and management of oral submucous fibrosis. [RGUHS]
19. What conditions may produce trismus? Describe in detail the predisposing factors, clinical features and treatment of oral submucous fibrosis. [BUHS]
20. Clinical picture and treatment plan of erosive lichen planus. [MUHS]
21. Classify the causes for cervicofacial lymphadenopathy and discuss in detail Hodgkin's disease. [TN]
22. Describe differential diagnosis and mention the necessary investigations for leukoplakia and lichen planus. [MUHS]
23. Differentiate between leukoplakia and leukoedema. [MUHS]
24. Oral manifestation of leukoplakia. [MUHS]
25. Clinical features and management of leukoplakia. [MUHS]
26. Rodent ulcer. [MUHS]
27. Squamous cell carcinoma. [MUHS]
28. Basal cell carcinoma. [MUHS]
29. Describe differential diagnosis and mention the necessary investigations for cancrum oris and carcinoma. [MUHS]
30. Treatment of squamous cell carcinoma. [MUHS]
31. Describe the clinical features and management of oral cancers. [NTR-NR]
32. Describe the medical management of malignant tumours of the mouth. [BUHS]
33. Describe the aetiology, clinical features and management of oral carcinomas. [BUHS]
34. What are the premalignant lesions of the oral cavity? What precautions should be taken in the prevention of oral malignancies? [BUHS]
35. Describe the differential diagnosis of oral precancerous lesions and conditions. [TN]
36. Classify the red and white lesions of the oral cavity. Describe in detail the aetiology, clinical features, treatment plan and prognosis of submucous fibrosis. [MUHS]
37. Describe differential diagnosis and treatment plan of benign mucous membrane pemphigoid. [MUHS]
38. Classify the white lesions of the oral cavity and discuss in detail the aetiology, clinical features, treatment plan and differential diagnosis of lichen planus. [MUHS]
39. Submucous fibrosis. [MUHS]

Short Essays

1. Malignant melanoma. [RGUHS]
2. Kaposi's sarcoma. [NTRUHS]
3. Osteogenic sarcoma. [NTRUHS]
4. Kaposi's sarcoma. [RGUHS]
5. X. Pathogenesis and management of osteoradionecrosis. [RGUHS]
6. Clinical features and radiographic appearance of osteosarcoma. [RGUHS]
7. Clinical features and radiographic appearance of osteoradionecrosis. [RGUHS]
8. Mention various forms of lichen planus. [MUHS]
9. Mention the treatment plan for submucous fibrosis. [MUHS]
10. Give the treatment plan for erosive lichen planus. [MUHS]
11. Define leukoplakia. [MUHS]
12. Name two premalignant conditions. [MUHS]
13. Management of oral submucous fibrosis. [NTRUHS]
14. TNM staging of oral cancer. [NTRUHS]
15. Radiotherapy. [RGUHS]
16. Oral submucous fibrosis. [RGUHS]
17. Treatment plan for oral submucous fibrosis. [MUHS]
18. Define premalignant lesions of oral cavity. [MUHS]
19. Causes of perforation of palate. [MUHS]
20. Precancerous lesions. [RGUHS]
21. Oral precancerous conditions. [NTRUHS]
22. Investigations of oral cancer. [NTRUHS]
23. Toluidine blue test. [NTRUHS]
24. Lugol's iodine test. [NTRUHS]

Short Notes

1. Treatment plan of leukoplakia. [NTR-OR]
2. Write briefly the identification and management of leukoplakia. [NTR-OR]
3. How do you manage the speckled leukoplakia and erosive lichen planus? [NTR-OR]
4. Lichen planus. [NTR-OR]
5. Lichenoid reaction. [NTR-OR]
6. Diagnosis of oral lichen planus. [NTR-OR]
7. Submucous fibrosis. [NTR-OR; NTR-NR]
8. Management of submucous fibrosis. [NTR-OR]
9. Enumerate the important differences between the submucous fibrosis and scleroderma. [NTR-OR]
10. Carcinoma in situ of buccal mucosa. [BUHS]
11. Reticular lichen planus. [RGUHS]
12. Clinical features of erosive lichen planus. [RGUHS]
13. Give the treatment plan for erosive lichen planus. [RGUHS]
14. Brachytherapy. [RGUHS]
15. Verrucous carcinoma. [RGUHS]
16. Aids in diagnosis of oral malignancies. [RGUHS]
17. Oral precancerous lesions. [NTR-OR, NTR-NR]
18. Erythroplakia. [NTR-OR]
19. Speckled leukoplakia. [NTR-OR]
20. Leukoplakia treatment. [NTR-OR]
21. Pathogenesis and management of oral leukoplakia. [RGUHS]
22. Outline the clinical features of leukoplakia and lichen planus. [BUHS]
23. Describe the clinical features of oral submucous fibrosis. [RGUHS]
24. Clinical features of erosive lichen planus. [RGUHS]
25. Treatment of oral submucous fibrosis. [BUHS]
26. Management of oral submucous fibrosis. [RGUHS]
27. Oral manifestations of oral submucous fibrosis. [BUHS; RGUHS]
28. Outline four differences between leukoplakia and lichen planus. [RGUHS]
29. Lichenoid reaction. [RGUHS]
30. Lichen planus in buccal mucosa? [BUHS]
31. Tumour markers. [TN]
32. Infectious mononucleosis. [TN]
33. Prevention and control of oral cancer. [TN]
34. Precancerous oral lesions. [TN]
35. Clinical features of patients suffering from oral submucous fibrosis. [TN]
36. TNM staging. [BUHS]
37. Define a premalignant lesion and a condition. [RGUHS]
38. Oncogenes. [RGUHS]
39. Oral precancerous conditions. [RGUHS]
40. Treatment of leukaemic ulcer. [RGUHS]
41. Chemopreventive agents. [NTRUHS]
42. Brachytherapy. [RGUHS]
43. TNM staging. [RGUHS; TN]
44. Brachytherapy. [RGUHS]
45. Verrucous carcinoma. [RGUHS]
46. Aids in diagnosis of oral malignancies. [BUHS]
47. Periapical osteofibrosis. [TN]
48. Oral submucous fibrosis. [TN]
49. Aetiology and management of oral submucous fibrosis. [RGUHS]
50. Kaposi's sarcoma. [NTR-NR]
51. Oral cancer—predisposing factors. [NTR-NR]
52. Erosive lichen planus. [NTR-NR]
53. Atrophic lichen planus. [NTR-NR]
54. Management of submucous fibrosis. [NTR-NR]
55. Carcinoma in situ. [RGUHS]
56. Oral hairy leukoplakia. [RGUHS; TN]
57. Grin span syndrome. [BUHS]

DISEASES OF THE TONGUE AND LIPS

Long Essays

1. Black hairy tongue. [MUHS]
2. Glossodynia. [MUHS 1987]
3. Benign migratory glossitis. [MUHS]
4. Discuss tongue lesions in various anaemiae. [RGUHS]
5. How will you diagnose carcinoma of tongue? Mention treatment planning of carcinoma of tongue. [RGUHS]
6. Enumerate the papillae that take part in the atrophic changes on the tongue. Name the various conditions causing such changes. [NTR]
7. Describe the appearance of tongue in:
   a. Geographic tongue
   b. Amyloidosis
   c. Hunter's glossitis. [RGUHS]
8. Describe the appearance of tongue in:
   a. Amyloidosis
   b. Hunter's glossitis
   c. Geographic tongue [BUHS]
9. How will you examine the tongue? Describe the various developmental anomalies of the tongue. [MUHS]

10. Describe the papillae of the tongue. Enumerate and describe the conditions in which there are atrophic changes in the papillae (tongue coating). [MUHS]
11. Describe in detail the anatomy of the tongue and the detail examination and tests required in various diseases and conditions affecting the tongue. [MUHS]
12. Discuss the importance of examination of tongue. Give differential diagnosis of loss of papillae on the tongue. [MUHS]
13. Discuss tongue lesions in various anaemiae. [BUHS]
14. How will you diagnose carcinoma of tongue? Mention treatment planning of carcinoma of tongue. [RGUHS]
15. Differential diagnosis of bald tongue. [MUHS]
16. How can the clinical examination of the tongue be carried out? Describe the differential diagnosis of glossodynia. Mention the treatment plan in brief. [RGUHS]

Short Essays

1. Glossodynia. [NTR-NR; TN; RGUHS]
2. Glossopyrosis and glossodynia. [NTR-NR]
3. Fissured tongue. [RGUHS]
4. Migratory glossitis. [BUHS]
5. Depapillation of tongue. [RGUHS]
6. Ankyloglossia. [RGUHS]
7. Black hairy tongue. [NTR]
8. Angioneurotic oedema. [BUHS]
9. Tuberculosis ulcers on the tongue. [RGUHS]
10. Clinical features of carcinoma of tongue. [BUHS]
11. Differential diagnosis of nonscrapable white patch on tongue. [RGUHS]
12. Give four causes of depapillation of tongue. [MUHS]
13. Mention the causes of 'bald tongue'. [MUHS]
14. Angular cheilitis. [BUHS; RGUHS]
15. Causes for angular cheilitis. [RGUHS]
16. Treatment of angular cheilitis. [BUHS]
17. Treatment of atrophic glossitis and angular cheilitis. [BUHS]
18. Treatment planning of carcinoma of tongue. [BUHS]
19. Treatment of atrophic glossitis and angular cheilitis. [BUHS]
20. Four causes of macroglossia. [RGUHS]
21. Recurrent aphthous stomatitis. [TN]
22. Allergic stomatitis. [TN]
23. Actinic cheilitis. [RGUHS]
24. Burning mouth syndrome. [RGUHS]

Short Notes

1. Bald tongue. [NTR-OR]
2. Hairy tongue. [NTR-OR]
3. Glossopyrosis. [NTR-OR]
4. Geographic tongue. [NTR-NR; TN]
5. Benign migratory glossitis. [NTR-NR; TN]
6. Differential diagnosis of smooth tongue. [NTR-NR, RGUHS]
7. How do you manage a case of carcinoma of tongue? [NTR-OR]
8. Carcinoma of tongue. [BUHS]
9. Hairy leukoplakic tongue. [BUHS]
10. Differential diagnosis of nonscrapable white patch on tongue. [RGUHS]
11. Angular cheilitis. [RGUHS]
12. Causes for angular cheilitis. [RGUHS]
13. Treatment of angular cheilitis. [RGUHS]
14. Hairy tongue. [RGUHS]
15. Migratory glossitis. [RGUHS]
16. Angioneurotic oedema. [RGUHS]
17. Tuberculous ulcers on the tongue. [RGUHS]
18. Clinical features of carcinoma of tongue. [RGUHS]
19. Treatment planning of carcinoma of tongue. [RGUHS]
20. Actinic cheilitis. [NTRUHS]
21. Mucocele. [NTRUHS; RGUHS]
22. Pseudocysts. [NTRUHS]
23. Mucocele. [NTRUHS]
24. Actinic cheilitis. [NTRUHS]
25. Differential diagnosis of macroglossia. [RGUHS]
26. Management of glossodynia. [RGUHS]
27. Glossodynia. [RGUHS]
28. Treatment of atrophic glossitis and angular cheilitis. [RGUHS]
29. Angioedema. [NTR]
30. Angioneurotic oedema. [NTR]
31. Angular stomatitis. [RGUHS]
32. Halitosis. [RGUHS]
33. Bald tongue. [RGUHS]
34. Dysgeusia. [TN]
35. Cheilitis granulomatosa. [TN]
36. Management of a patient suffering from glossodynia. [TN]
37. Name the papillae of tongue. [RGUHS]
38. Ankyloglossia. [RGUHS]
39. Differential diagnosis of bald tongue. [RGUHS]
40. Diascopy. [RGUHS]

SALIVARY GLAND DISEASES

Long Essays

1. Mucocele. [MUHS]
2. Xerostomia. [MUHS]
3. Pleomorphic adenoma. [MUHS]
4. Parotitis. [MUHS]
5. Treatment option for xerostomia. [MUHS]
6. Enumerate the cause for xerostomia. Describe the clinical features, investigations and management of Sjogren's syndrome. [TN]
7. Describe in detail sialography and its significance in various diseases of salivary glands. [RGUHS]
8. Clinical features differential diagnosis and management of functional disturbance of salivary glands. [RGUHS]
9. Classify functional disorders of the salivary glands. Describe the aetiology, clinical features, diagnosis and management of Sjogren's syndrome. [TN; NTRUHS]
10. Describe differential diagnosis of inflammation of parotid salivary gland. [TN]
11. What are the functions of saliva? Enumerate the causes of xerostomia and add a note on its management? [NTR-NR]
12. Enumerate the clinical features and radiological features of functional disturbances of salivary glands. [NTR-OR]
13. Describe the procedure for sialography of parotid gland. [NTR-OR]
14. Describe sialography in detail and write briefly on its significance in various salivary gland disorders. [NTR-NR]
15. Describe clinical features, differential diagnosis and management of functional disturbance of salivary glands. [BUHS]
16. Describe the indications and contraindications of sialography. Describe the technique briefly. [RGUHS]
17. Describe in detail sialography and its significance in various diseases of salivary glands. [BUHS, RGUHS]
18. Enumerate the autoimmune disorders of the oral cavity. Discuss the clinical features, diagnosis and management of Sjogren's syndrome. [RGUHS]
19. Name the various diseases of salivary glands. Discuss clinical features, diagnosis, differential diagnosis and treatment of parotitis. [MUHS]
20. Classify salivary gland diseases. Describe the various causes, clinical features and the management of sialadenitis. [TN]

Short Essays

1. Treatment of xerostomia. [MUHS]
2. Clinical features and investigations of submandibular sialolithiasis. [RGUHS]
3. Bacterial sialadenitis [RGUHS]
4. Sialography. [RGUHS]
5. Liths in orofacial region. [RGUHS]
6. Indications of sialography. [RGUHS]
7. Indications and contraindications of sialography. [RGUHS]
8. Sialolithiasis. [MUHS; RGUHS]
9. Sialadenosis. [RGUHS]
10. Sjogren's syndrome. [NTRUHS; RGUHS]
11. Xerostomia. [NTRUHS]

Short Notes

1. Treatment of ptyalism. [RGUHS]
2. Clinical appearance of actinomycosis. [RGUHS]
3. Aetiology and clinical features of sialolithiasis. [RGUHS]
4. Sialography. [NTR-NR]
5. Sialolithiasis. [NTR-QR; TN]
6. Sialometaplasia. [NTR-NR]
7. Necrotizing sialometaplasia. [NTR-OR]
8. Ranula. [TN; RGUHS]
9. Xerostomia—causes and management. [TN]
10. Sialadenosis. [TN; RGUHS]
11. Necrotizing sialometaplasia. [RGUHS]
12. Why sialolithiasis is more common in submandibular gland? [RGUHS]
13. Sialorrhoea. [RGUHS]
14. Causes for reduced salivary flow. [RGUHS]
15. Liths in orofacial region. [RGUHS]
16. Mumps. [RGUHS]
17. Xerostomia. [RGUHS, NTR-OR; BUHS; TN]
18. Mucous cyst. [RGUHS, BUHS]
19. Schirmer's test. [RGUHS]
20. Sjogren's syndrome. [NTR-QR; TN; NTRUHS]
21. Liths in orofacial region. [RGUHS]
22. Indications of sialography. [BUHS]
23. Indications and contraindications of sialography. [RGUHS]
24. Contraindications of sialography. [RGUHS]
25. Ptyalism. [TN]

DISORDERS OF TMJ AND MPDS

Long Essays

1. Describe TMJ disorders in detail. [RGUHS]
2. Classify TMJ disorders. Describe in detail myofacial pain dysfunction syndrome. [RGUHS]
3. Define pain. Enumerate the causes of facial pain. Write clinical features and management of MPDS. [RGUHS]
4. Classify TMJ disorders. Describe in detail myofacial pain dysfunction syndrome. [RGUHS]
5. Classify temporomandibular disorders. Discuss the management of TMJ arthritis. [TN]
6. Describe radiographic techniques to diagnose temporomandibular ioint diseases and disorders. [TN]
7. Enumerate the clinical features, differential diagnosis and management of oral and myofacial pain dysfunction syndrome. [RGUHS]
8. Management of myofacial pain dysfunction syndrome. [RGUHS]
9. What conditions may produce trismus. Describe in detail the predisposing factors, clinical features, treatment of oral submucous fibrosis. [NTR]
10. Describe in detail TMJ disorders. [BUHS]
11. Enumerate the causes of trismus. Discuss in detail pericoronal abscess. [NTR]
12. Describe the aetiology, clinical features, differential diagnosis and treatment of myofacial dysfunction syndrome. [RGUHS]
13. Classify temporomandibular disorders and describe in detail about myofacial pain dysfunction syndrome. [RGUHS]

Short Essays

1. Drugs to relieve muscular spasm. [RGUHS]
2. Clinical features and management of degenerative arthritis of TMJ. [RGUHS]
3. Clinical features of TMJ subluxation. [MUHS]
4. Treatment plan for myofacial pain dysfunction syndrome. [MUHS]
5. Articular disc disorders of temporomandibular joint. [RGUHS]
6. Internal derangement of temporomandibular joint. [RGUHS]
7. Maxillary sinusitis. [NTR-OR]
8. Treatment of postirradiation mucositis. [BUHS]
9. Allergic manifestations of oral mucositis. [BUHS]
10. Subluxation of TMJ. [RGUHS]
11. Myofacial pain dysfunction syndrome. [RGUHS; NTRUHS]
12. Aetiology of myofacial pain dysfunction syndrome. [MUHS]

Short Notes

1. Internal derangement of temporomandibular joint. [RURS, TN]
2. Ankylosis of temporomandibular joint. [TN; RGUHS]
3. TMJ ankylosis. [NTRUHS]
4. Myofunctional pain dysfunction syndrome. [NTRUHS]
5. Enumerate the temporomandibular joint views. [RGUHS]
6. Four causes of trismus. [RGUHS]
7. Treatment of pericoronitis with trismus. [NTR-GR]
8. Subluxation of TMJ. [RGUHS]
9. Myositis ossificans. [RGUHS]
10. Trismus. [NTR-NR; NTRUHS]
11. Four causes of trismus. [RGUHS]
12. Temporomandibular joint ankylosis. [RGUHS]

IONIZING RADIATION AND REGRESSIVE ALTERATIONS OF THE ORAL CAVITY

Long Essays

1. Classify radiographic lesions of the jaws. Discuss the various radio-opacities in normal jaws. [NTRUHS]

Short Essays

1. Hypersensitive teeth. [MUHS]
2. Traumatic keratosis. [MUHS]
3. Ptyalism. [MUHS]
4. Radio-opaque landmarks in the mandible. [RGUHS]

Short Notes

1. Argyria. [TN]
2. Radiolucent landmarks of maxilla. [TN]
3. Stomatitis nicotina. [TN]
4. Dental fluorosis. [TN]
5. Dental hypersensitivity. [TN]
6. Pink tooth. [NTR-GR]
7. Resorption of roots. [NTR-GR]
8. Clinical features of internal and external resorptions of teeth. [BUHS]

9. Pink tooth. [RGUHS]
10. Pink tooth. [RGUHS]
11. Pink tooth of mummery. [RGUHS]
12. Osteoradionecrosis. [TN]
13. Dental management of hypertensive patient. [TN]
14. Denture sore mouth. [TN]
15. Name any four commonly used chemical agents responsible for oral mucosal bum. [MUHS]

ODONTOLOGIC DISEASES

Long Essays

1. Dens invaginatus. [MUHS]
2. Write briefly about the clinical features of:
   a. Erythema multiforme
   b. Dentinogenesis imperfecta. [BUHS; MUHS; TN]
3. Describe in detail developmental anomalies of teeth. [MUHS]
4. Anodontia. [MUHS]

Short Essay

1. Internal resorption. [NTRUHS]

Short Notes

1. Regional odontodysplasia. [RGUHS, NTR]
2. Dentinogenesis imperfecta. [RGUHS-BUHS; TN; RGUHS]
3. Enumerate briefly developmental anomalies of teeth. [RGUHS-BUHS]
4. Hutchinson's triad. [RGUHS; NTRUHS]
5. Fordyce's granules. [RGUHS; TN]
6. Anodontia. [NTR, RGUHS]
7. Talon's cusp. [RGUHS]
8. Dilaceration. [RGUHS]
9. Dens in dente. [RGUHS]
10. Turner's tooth. [RGUHS]
11. Dentinogenesis imperfecta. [NTR; TN]
12. Dens in dente. [BUHS; TN]
13. Turner's tooth. [RGUHS]
14. Enamel hypoplasia. [RGUHS]
15. Dilaceration. [BUHS; RGUHS]
16. Pulp polyp. [TN]
17. Benign migratory glossitis. [TN]
18. Halitosis. [TN]
19. Globulomaxillary cyst. [TN]
20. Mesiodens. [RGUHS]
21. Pathergy test. [NTRUHS]
22. Fordyce's spots. [RGUHS]
23. Pink tooth of mummery. [RGUHS]
24. Red teeth. [NTR-NR]
25. Concrescence. [RGUHS]
26. Regional odontodysplasia. [BUHS]
27. Causes of perforation of palate. [MUHS]
28. Macroglossia. [TN]
29. Dentine dysplasia. [TN]
30. Talon's cusp. [RGUHS]
31. Turner's hypoplasia. [NTRUHS]
32. Black hairy tongue. [NTRUHS]
33. Natal teeth. [NTRUHS]
34. Peutz-Jeghers syndrome. [NTRUHS]
35. Gingival cysts of infants. [RGUHS]
36. Fordyce's granules. [RGUHS]
37. Turner's tooth. [RGUHS]
38. Hereditary opalescent dentine. [RGUHS]
39. What is taurodontism and fusion? [MUHS]
40. Taurodontism. [RGUHS]
41. Oligodontia. [RGUHS]
42. Gardner's syndrome. [RGUHS]
43. Supernumerary teeth. [RGUHS]
44. Taurodontism. [RGUHS; NTRUHS]
45. Describe briefly the causes for early loss of teeth. [TN]
46. Acute pericoronal abscess. [TN]
47. Tori. [TN]
48. Median rhomboid glossitis. [TN; RGUHS]
49. Geographic tongue. [TN]

OROFACIAL PAIN

Long Essays

1. Photogenic pain. [MUHS]
2. Enumerate the various causes of trismus. How would you investigate a case of trismus? [TN]
3. Define pain. Describe the aetiology, clinical features and management of myofascial pain dysfunction syndrome. [TN]
4. Describe the clinical features differential diagnosis and treatment of trigeminal neuralgia. [BUHS]

5. Define trismus. Discuss the various causes and differential diagnosis of trismus. [NTRUHS]
6. Enumerate the causes of orofacial pain and write about the aetiology, diagnosis, clinical features and management of trigeminal neuralgia. [TN]
7. Define pain. Describe the aetiology, clinical features, differential diagnosis and treatment of trigeminal neuralgia. [TN]
8. Classify facial pain. Describe the aetiopathogenesis, clinical features and management of atypical facial pain. [TN]
9. Enumerate the clinical features, differential diagnosis and management of myofascial pain dysfunction syndrome. [BUHS]
10. Define pain. Give classification of orofacial pain. Describe aetiology, clinical features and management myofascial pain dysfunction syndrome. [MUHS]
11. Discuss the differential diagnosis of odontogenic pain. [MUHS]
12. Describe the clinical features differential diagnosis and treatment of trigeminal neuralgia. [RGUHS]
13. Classify facial pain. Describe in detail aetiology, clinical features, differential diagnosis and management of periodic migrainous neuralgia. [TN]
14. Classify orofacial pain. Discuss in detail the aetiology, clinical features, investigations and various treatment modalities for myofascial pain dysfunction syndrome. [TN]
15. Write differential diagnosis of orofacial pain. Write a note on aetiology, management of idiopathic trigeminal neuralgia. [RGUHS]
16. Describe aetiology, clinical features and management of trigeminal neuralgia. [RGUHS]
17. What is neuralgia? Describe different types of neuralgias of orofacial origin and add a note on management of orofacial neuralgia. [TN]
18. Define orofacial pain. Discuss in detail the aetiology, clinical features and management of trigeminal neuralgia. [TN]
19. Give the differential diagnosis of pain in and around the tooth. [NTR-OR]
20. Describe the 'pain in and around the tooth'. Mention the treatment. [NTR-NR]
21. Discuss neuralgias affecting maxillofacial region. How would you treat trigeminal neuralgias? [NTR-OR]
22. Classify facial pain. Describe aetiopathogenesis, clinical features and management of trigeminal neuralgia. [NTR-NR]
23. Define pain. Enumerate the causes of facial pain. Write clinical features and management of MPDS. [RGUHS]
24. Classify facial pain. Describe in detail the aetiology, clinical features and management of trigeminal neuralgia. [NTR-GR]
25. Define pain. Write briefly about trigeminal neuralgia. [BUHS]
26. Define trigeminal neuralgia. Mention aetiopathological causes and add a note on its management. [RGUHS]
27. Classify orofacial pain. Write in detail about the aetiology, clinical features, differential diagnosis and management of trigeminal neuralgia. [RGUHS; NTRUHS]

Short Essays

1. Treatment of myofascial pain dysfunction syndrome. [TN]
2. Trigeminal neuralgia. [TN; MUHS; NTRUHS]
3. Myositis ossificans. [NTRUHS]
4. Aetiology, signs and symptoms of Bell's palsy. [RGUHS]
5. Pain in migraine and periodic migrainous neuralgia. [RGUHS]
6. Aetiology, signs and symptoms of trigeminal neuralgia. [RGUHS]
7. Management of trigeminal neuralgia. [RGUHS]
8. Trans-electric nerve stimulation. [RGUHS]
9. Give the clinical picture and medical management of trigeminal neuralgia. [MUHS]
10. Give the differential diagnosis between pain characteristics of trigeminal neuralgia and acute pulpitis. [MUHS]

Short Notes

1. TENS therapy. [RGUHS]
2. Classification of headache. [RGUHS]
3. Postherpetic neuralgia. [RGUHS]
4. Treatment of myofascial pain dysfunction syndrome. [RGUHS]
5. Treatment of trigeminal neuralgia. [NTRUHS]
6. Subauricular pain. [NTR-NR]
7. Atypical facial pain. [NTR-OR; RGUHS]
8. Atypical facial neuralgia. [NTR-OR]
9. Trigeminal neuralgia. [NTR-OR; TN]
10. Management of the tic douloureux. [NTR-N; TN]
11. Management of myofascial pain dysfunction syndrome. [RGUHS; TN]
12. Alarm clock headache. [RGUHS]
13. Trigger zones. [BUHS]
14. Bell's sign. [RGUHS]
15. Burning mouth. [RGUHS]
16. Clinical features of Bell's palsy. [RGUHS]
17. Classify the neuralgias of orofacial origin. [NTR-OR]

18. Pain in migraine and periodic migrainous neuralgia. [RGUHS]
19. Discuss orofacial pain control measures. [BUHS]
20. Bell's palsy. [NTR-NR; TN]
21. Management of paroxysmal trigeminal neuralgia. [NTR-NR]
22. Glossodynia. [BUHS]
23. Clinical features of Bell's palsy. [RGUHS]
24. Drugs to relieve muscular spasm. [RGUHS]
25. Treatment of trigeminal neuralgia. [NTR-OR; TN; NTRUHS]
26. Management of trigeminal neuralgia. [NTR-QR; TN]
27. How do you manage a case of trigeminal neuralgia? [NTR-OR]
28. Describe briefly the classification and management trigeminal neuralgia. [NTR-OR]
29. MPDS. [NTR-OR]
30. Myolacial pain dysfunction syndrome. [NTR-OR; TN]
31. Burning mouth syndrome. [NTR-OR]
32. Enumerate the important differences between the paroxysmal neuralgias and atypical neuralgias. [NTR-OR]
33. Aetiology, signs and symptoms of Bell's palsy. [RGUHS]
34. Aetiology, signs and symptoms of trigeminal neuralgia. [RGUHS]
35. Give the treatment plan for trigeminal neuralgia. [RGUHS]
36. Postherpetic neuralgia. [RGUHS]
37. Glossopharyngeal neuralgia. [TN]
38. Tic douloureux. [TN]
39. Trismus. [TN; RGUHS]
40. Diagnosis and management of tic douloureux. [TN]

VIRAL AND INFECTIOUS DISEASES OF THE ORAL CAVITY INCLUDING AIDS

Long Esssays

1. Hutchinson's triad. [MUHS]
2. Oral changes in secondary syphilis. [MUHS]
3. Syphilis. [MUHS]
4. Investigations of syphilis. [MUHS]
5. Oral changes in syphilis. [MUHS]
6. Differential diagnosis between ANUG and primal herpes simplex lesions. [MUHS]
7. Acquired syphilis. [MUHS]
8. Oral manifestations of primary stage of syphilis. [MUHS]
9. Discuss the differential diagnosis of cervical lymph node enlargement. [TN]
10. What are the predisposing factors of acute necrotizing ulcerative gingivostomatitis? How will you diagnoses and treat a patient suffering from this disease? [TN]
11. Classify radiolucent lesions of the jaw. Write in detail about osteomyelitis—aetiology, clinical features, differential diagnosis and management. [TN]
12. What are the viral infections in the oral cavity? Write about the aetiology, clinical features, diagnosis and differential diagnosis of acute herpetic gingivostomatitis. [TN]
13. Classify osteomyelitis. Write in detail about the aetiology, clinical features, radiographic features and management of chronic suppurative osteomyelitis. [NTRUHS]
14. Enumerate the various causes of cervical lymphadenopathy. Write the differential diagnosis of cervical lymphadenopathy. [RGUHS]
15. Enumerate periapical radiolucencies and radiopacities. How would you diagnose systemic diseases with periapical changes in radiographs? [NTR-NR]
16. Discuss importance of lamina dura in dental radiographs and describe in detail periapical radiolucent areas. [RGUHS]
17. Radiographic changes of periapical region in systemic diseases—discuss in detail. [RGUHS]
18. Enumerate periapical lesions and describe in detail periapical cyst and abscess. [RGUHS]
19. Describe the aetiology, clinical features, radiographic feature and histological feature of periapical granuloma, and mention its sequel. [RGUHS]
20. What are the aetiological factors of osteomyelitis of mandible? [RGUHS]
21. Define osteomyelitis Describe various types, aetiology clinical features, diagnosis and management of osteomyelitis of mandible. [RGUHS]
22. What is meant by focal sepsis? Describe the systemic effects of oral sepsis. Evaluate the need for full mouth radiographic in oral sepsis. [RGUHS]
23. Enumerate viral lesions occurring in the oral cavity and discuss in detail about acute herpetic gingiva stomatitis. [TN]
24. Describe the aetiology, clinical features, radiographic features and histological features of periapical granuloma, and mention its sequel. [BUHS]
25. Define facial sepsis. Describe its local and systemic effects. [NTR-OR]

26. Describe the oral manifestations of secondary infected syphilis. [NTR-OR]
27. Describe oral manifestations of viral infections. [RGUHS]
28. List the common viral infections that may involve the oral cavity. Discuss in detail the differential diagnosis of herpes simplex. [RGUHS]
29. Enumerate the sexually transmitted diseases. Give oral manifestations for a full blow HIV-positive core. [MUHS]
30. AIDS. [MUHS]
31. Lab investigations for AIDS. [MUHS]
32. Describe the oral manifestations of viral infections. [RGUHS]
33. Clinical features and treatment of acute suppurative osteomyelitis. [RGUHS]
34. Describe the oral manifestations of HIV infection. What are the tests used to confirm the diagnosis. [TN]
35. Describe the clinical features and treatment of actinomycosis of jaw. [RGUHS]
36. Describe the clinical features and treatment of actinomycosis of the jaw. [BUHS]
37. What are the aetiological factors of osteomyelitis of mandible? Describe the clinical features and treatment of actinomycosis of the jaws. [BUHS]
38. What is meant by focal sepsis? Describe the systemic effects of oral sepsis. Evaluate the need for full mouth radiography in oral sepsis. [BUHS]
39. Enumerate sexually transmitted diseases. Describe in detail oral changes in AIDS. Add a note on cross-infection in dental clinic. [RGUHS]
40. Discuss differential diagnosis of chronic discharging sinus in mandibular angle region. [MUHS]
41. Ludwig's angina. [MUHS]
42. Differential diagnosis between periapical cysts and periapical abscess. [MUHS]
43. Describe differential diagnosis and mention the necessary investigations for periapical abscess and periodontal abscess. [MUHS]
44. Enumerate the sexually transmitted diseases. Discuss in detail the clinical pictures of acquired immunodeficiency syndrome and state the measures to control the spread of infection in a dental clinic. [MUHS]

Short Essays

1. Enumerate periapical lesions. [MUHS]
2. Pyogenic granuloma. [MUHS]
3. Differential diagnosis between periapical abscess and periodontal abscess. [MUHS]
4. Differential diagnosis between reversible and irreversible pulpitis. [MUHS]
5. Oral changes in secondary syphilis. [MUHS]
6. What is Hutchinson's triad. [MUHS]
7. Write distinguishing features between primary herpes and herpangina. [MUHS]
8. Cellulitis. [BUHS]
9. Focal sepsis. [RGUHS]
10. Lipschutz bodies. [RGUHS]
11. Chancre. [RGUHS]
12. Treponema pallidum. [BUHS]
13. Oral manifestations of syphilis. [BUHS; TN]
14. Clinical features of gumma in palate. [BUHS]
15. Behcet's syndrome. [NTRUHS]
16. Herpangina. [NTRUHS]
17. Juvenile periodontitis. [RGUHS]
18. Enumerate oral changes in AIDS. [MUHS]
19. Nonvital teeth. [RGUHS]
20. Herpetic gingivostomatitis. [RGUHS]
21. Periapical cyst. [RGUHS]
22. Hepatitis B. [RGUHS]
23. Herpes zoster infection. [BUHS]
24. Postherpetic neuralgia? [RGUHS]
25. Differences between herpes simplex and zoster? [BUHS]
26. Write the differential diagnosis of primal HSV and herpangina. [MUHS]
27. Treatment of candidiasis. [MUHS]
28. Predisposing factors of moniliasis. [MUHS]
29. How do you clinically distinguish primary herpes simplex infection from herpangina. [MUHS]
30. Treatment plan of herpes zoster. [MUHS]
31. Pyogenic granuloma. [RGUHS]
32. Oral manifestations of HIV infection. [RGUHS; RGUHS; NTRUHS]
33. Types of osteomyelitis and their features. [RGUHS]
34. Secondary stage of syphilis. [NTR-NR]
35. Clinical appearance of actinomycosis. [BUHS]
36. HIV. [RGUHS]
37. Tongue in AIDS. [RGUHS]
38. Oral hairy leukoplakia. [RGUHS]
39. Name oral changes in AIDS patients. [RGUHS]
40. Name two investigations to be carried out in a suspected HIV infection. [RGUHS]
41. Mention the oral changes in AIDS patients. [MUHS]
42. Diagnostic test for AIDS. [MUHS]
43. Oral changes in AIDS. [MUHS]
44. Differential diagnosis between periapical abscess and periodontal abscess. [MUHS]
45. Enumerate the various vesiculobullous lesion of oral cavity. Discuss in detail clinical features, differential diagnosis and treatment plan of primary herpes simplex infection. [MUHS]

46. Enumerate the various vesiculobullous lesion of oral cavity. Discuss in detail varicella zoster infection in detail. [MUHS]
47. Classify oral candidiasis. Describe the aetiology, clinical features, differential diagnosis and management of oral thrush. [MUHS]
48. Causes for cervical lymphadenopathy. [RGUHS]
49. Oral manifestations of acquired syndrome. [TN]
50. Necrotizing sialometaplasia. [TN]
51. ELISA tests for AIDS. [RGUHS]

Short Notes

1. Oral manifestations of syphilis. [RGUHS]
2. Clinical features of gumma in palate. [RGUHS]
3. Lamina dura. [NTR-OR]
4. Radiolucent lesions of periapical region. [NTR-NR]
5. How do you manage pulpitis and periodontitis. [NTR-NR]
6. Periapical abscess. [RGUHS]
7. Pyogenic granuloma. [RGUHS]
8. Radiographic features of periodontal diseases. [RGUHS]
9. Radiographic appearance of periapical granuloma and periapical cyst. [RGUHS]
10. Periapical cyst. [BUHS]
11. Hyperaemia of pulp. [BUHS]
12. Periapical cyst. [RGUHS]
13. Hyperaemia of pulp. [RGUHS]
14. Pink tooth of mummery. [RGUHS]
15. Clinical features of internal and external resorptions of teeth. [RGUHS]
16. Describe the differences of acute pulpitis and acute apical periodontitis. [RGUHS]
17. Enumerate any two differences between periapical abscess and periodontal abscess. [RGUHS]
18. HIV. [RGUHS]
19. Name two investigations to be carried out in a suspected HIV infection. [RGUHS]
20. Oral manifestations secondary of syphilis. [TN]
21. Chronic suppurative osteomyelitis. [TN]
22. Chronic retentive lymphoid hyperplasia. [TN]
23. Actinomycosis. [TN]
24. Acute and chronic pulpitis. [TN]
25. Oral manifestations of acquired immunodeficiency syndrome. [RGUHS]
26. Split papule. [RGUHS]
27. Window period. [RGUHS]
28. Structure of HIV. [RGUHS]
29. Koplik's spots. [RGUHS]
30. Herpangina. [RGUHS]
31. Garre's osteomyelitis. [RGUHS]
32. Koplik's spots. [RGUHS]
33. Name three specific infections of oral cavity. [RGUHS]
34. Four conditions associated with cervicofacial lymphadenopathy. [RGUHS]
35. Id reaction. [NTR]
36. Cellulitis. [RGUHS]
37. Focal sepsis. [RGUHS]
38. Hutchinson's triad. [RGUHS; TN; RGUHS]
39. Treponema palladium. [RGUHS]
40. Garre's osteomyelitis. [RGUHS]
41. Describe the differences of acute pulpitis and acute apical periodontitis. [BUHS]
42. Enumerate any two differences between periapical abscess and periodontal abscess. [RGUHS]
43. Mumps. [NTR; TN; RGUHS]
44. Hutchinson's triad. [NTR-OR; TN]
45. Serological test for syphilis. [NTR-OR]
46. Herpes zoster. [NTR-NB; TN].
47. Herpes labialis. [NTR-NR; RGUHS]
48. Herpes stomatitis. [NTR-OR]
49. How do you manage herpangina and herpetic stoma. [NTR-OR]
50. How do you manage a case of herpetic stomatitis. [NTR-OR]
51. Describe briefly the classification and management of acute infections of the oral cavity. [NTR-OR]
52. Herpangina. [RGUHS]
53. Differences between herpes simplex and herpes zoster infections. [BUHS]
54. Investigations and management of primary heretic gingivostomatitis. [RGUHS]
55. Hairy leukoplakia. [NTR-NR]
56. Oral manifestations of HIV. [RGUHS]
57. Oral manifestations of HIV infection. [RGUHS; NTR]
58. HIV. [NTR-NR]
59. Hairy leukoplakia. [NTR-NR]
60. Acyclovir. [RGUHS]
61. Acute dentoalveolar abscess. [TN]
62. Septicaemia. [TN]
63. Sialadenitis. [TN]
64. Shingles. [TN]
65. Oral manifestations of AIDS. [TN]
66. Secondary syphilis. [TN]
67. Acute necrotizing ulcerative gingivitis. [TN]
68. Sialadenosis. [TN]
69. Laboratory diagnosis of HIV infection. [TN]
70. Scrofula. [TN]
71. Juvenile periodontitis. [TN]

DISEASES OF THE ENDOCRINE AND RESPIRATORY SYSTEM, CVS, AND GIT

Long Essays

1. Discuss the role of oral diagnosis in diagnosing endocrinal disorders. [MUHS]
2. Hyperparathyroidism. [MUHS]
3. Dental management of rheumatic patient. [RGUHS]
4. Describe the oral manifestations of endocrine diseases. [NTR-NR]
5. Describe oral and dental manifestations of various endocrine disorders. [MUHS]
6. Acromegaly. [MUHS]
7. Oral manifestations of diabetes mellitus. [MUHS]
8. Grinspan's syndrome. [NTRUHS]
9. Grinspan's syndrome [NTRUHS]

Short Essays

1. Dental consideration for an ischaemic cardiac disease. [NTRUHS]
2. Management of cardiac patient in dental extraction. [NTRUHS; RGUHS]
3. Hyperparathyroidism. [NTRUHS]
4. Oral manifestations and dental considerations in diabetes mellitus. [RGUHS]
5. Koplik's spots. [RGUHS]
6. Endocarditis prophylaxis regimen for dental procedure. [RGUHS]
7. Oral manifestations of diabetes. [RGUHS]

Short Notes

1. Hyper parathyroidism—investigative. [NTR-NR]
2. Describe the oral manifestations of primary hyper parathyroidism. [NTR-OR]
3. Oral manifestations of diabetes mellitus. [NTR-NR]
4. Describe the oral manifestations of diabetes mellitus. [NTR-OR]
5. Oral manifestations and dental considerations in diabetic mellitus. [NTR-NR]
6. Addison's disease. [BUHS]
7. Hyper parathyroidism. [NTR-NR]
8. Oral manifestations of diabetes mellitus. [RGUHS]
9. Dental management of rheumatic patient. [BUHS]
10. Renal osteodystrophy. [RGUHS]
11. Hyper parathyroidism. [NTR]
12. Acromegaly. [BUHS]
13. Oral manifestations of diabetes mellitus. [BUHS]
14. Radiographic appearance of hyper parathyroidism. [RGUHS]
15. Dental considerations for a patient with a history of gastritis. [NTRUHS]
16. Koplik's spot. [RGUHS]

METABOLIC DISORDERS

Short Essays

1. What are the oral manifestations of hypovitaminosis? [RGUHS]
2. Describe the oral aspects of hypovitaminosis. [NTRUHS]
3. Discuss the oral manifestations of avitaminosis. [BUHS]
4. Describe in detail about rickets. [MUHS]
5. The medical management of acute infection of the oral cavity in a patient suffering from diabetes mellitus. [TN]

Short Notes

1. Hypervitaminosis A. [NTRUHS]
2. Uraemic stomatitis. [NTRUHS]
3. Renal rickets. [RGUHS]
4. Antibiotic sore mouth. [NTRUHS]
5. Anaphylactic shock. [NTRUHS]
6. Paget's disease. [NTRUHS]
7. Dental fluorosis. [NTRUHS]
8. Chemical bum. [NTRUHS]
9. NSAIDs which are safe to be used in pregnant women. [RGUHS]
10. Bence Jones protein. [NTR]
11. Hyperparathyroidism. [NTR]
12. Purpura. [RGUHS]
13. Precautions to be taken during dental treatment of cardiac patient. [NTR-NR]
14. Bronchial asthma. [RGUHS]
15. Renal osteodystrophy. [RGUHS]
16. Dental management of rheumatic patient. [BUHS]
17. Oral manifestations of pregnancy. [RGUHS]
18. Hyperparathyroidism. [RGUHS; TN]
19. Scurvy. [TN]

20. Dental considerations in pregnancy. [TN]
21. Laboratory diagnosis of diabetes mellitus. [TN]
22. Oral manifestations of vitamin A deficiency. [TN]
23. Scorbutic gingivitis. [TN]
24. Riboflavin deficiency. [TN]
25. Oral manifestations and dental considerations in diabetes mellitus. [TN]
26. Oral manifestations of diabetes mellitus. [TN; RGUHS; NTR]
27. Dental significance of diabetes mellitus. [NTRUHS]
28. Avitaminosis A. [NTRUHS]
29. Discuss oral manifestations of avitaminosis. [BUHS]
30. Oral manifestations of pregnancy. [BUHS]
31. Dental significance of hypertension. [RGUHS]
32. Dental considerations in asthmatic patients. [TN]
33. Management of cardiac patient in dental extraction. [NTR-NR]
34. Oral manifestations of vitamin C and D deficiencies. [BUHS]
35. Rheumatoid arthritis. [RGUHS]
36. Infective endocarditis. [RGUHS]
37. Bronchial asthma. [RGUHS]
38. Renal osteodysfunction. [RGUHS]
39. Discuss oral manifestations of avitaminosis. [RGUHS]
36. Oral manifestations of vitamin C and D deficiencies. [RGUHS]
37. Rheumatoid arthritis. [RGUHS]
38. Infective endocarditis. [RGUHS]

HAEMATOLOGIC DISEASES

Long Essays

1. Describe various types of anaemiae. Mention oral manifestations of anaemiae. [TN]
2. Discuss the importance of haematological investigations in the proper management of dental patients. [TN]
3. Under what conditions would you suggest blood studies for a dental patient and what are oral manifestations of purpura? [TN]
4. What are the aetiological factors for the spontaneous bleeding from gingiva? Describe the oral manifestation of myelogenous leukaemia? [TN]
5. Describe the oral manifestations of the different types of anaemiae. How would you manage angular cheilitis? [TN]
6. Describe oral manifestations of leukaemia. [TN]
7. Classify anaemiae. Describe clinical features and laboratory diagnosis of iron deficiency anaemia. [TN]
8. Discuss the oral manifestations of blood dyscrasias and add on their management. [TN]
9. Discuss tongue lesions in various anaemiae. [RGUHS]
10. Discuss the importance of haematological investigations in the proper management of dental patients. [RGUHS]
11. Under what conditions would you suggest blood studies for a dental patient and what are the oral manifestations of purpura? [RGUHS]
12. What are the aetiological factors for the spontaneous bleeding from gingiva? Describe the oral manifestations of myelogenous leukaemia. [RGUHS]
13. Describe the laboratory investigations for bleeding and clotting disorders. [TN]
14. Discuss differential diagnosis of bleeding gums along with laboratory investigations. [TN]
15. Define purpura. Discuss in detail the clinical features and investigations of purpura. [TN]
16. Classify anaemiae. Discuss in detail the oral manifestations, diagnosis and management of pernicious anaemia. [RGUHS]
17. Define and classify anaemiae. Discuss in detail about iron deficiency anaemia. [NTR UHS]
18. Enumerate the causes of cervical lymphadenopathy and give the clinical features of Hodgkin's diseases. [RGUHS].
19. Classify bleeding disorders of the mouse. How do you manage a case of myeloid race leukaemia patient visiting dental hospital? [TN]
20. Discuss tongue lesions in various anaemiae. [TN]
21. Enumerate the local and systemic causes of gingival enlargement. Describe the clinical features and oral changes seen in leukaemia and scurvy. [MUHS]
22. Bell's palsy. [MUHS]
23. Enumerate various causes of gingival bleeding. How would you manage a case of haemophilia. [MUHS]
24. What are the causes of bleeding from the gums? Discuss laboratory aids in the diagnosis of blood disorders. [MUHS]
25. Describe clinical manifestation and laboratory investigations for various types of anaemiae. [MUHS]

Short Essays

1. Purpura. [RGUHS]
2. Oral manifestations of leukaemia. [MUHS]
3. Cooley's anaemia. [MUHS; TN]

4. Thalassaemia major. [MUHS]
5. Bleeding and clotting time. [MUHS]
6. Thrombocytopaenic purpura. [MUHS]
7. Laboratory investigations of anaemiae. [RGUHS]
8. Clinical and laboratory diagnosis of anaemiae. [RGUHS]
9. Infectious mononucleosis. [RGUHS]
10. Diagnosis of pernicious anaemia. [RGUHS]
11. Oral manifestation of anaemia. [NTRUHS]
12. Pernicious anaemia. [NTRUHS]
13. Iron deficiency anaemia. [NTRUHS]
14. Pernicious anaemia. [MUHS]
15. Eosinophilia. [NTRUHS]
16. Leukaemia. [MUHS]
17. Oral manifestation of acute leukaemia. [MUHS]
18. Diagnostic tests for:
    a. Anaemia
    b. Thrombocytopenic purpura. [MUHS]
19. What is purpura? [MUHS]
20. Define purpura and petechiae. [MUHS]

Short Notes

1. Chronic lymphatic leukaemia. [RGUHS]
2. Haemophilia. [RGUHS]
3. Plummer-Vinson syndrome. [RGUHS]
4. Control of bleeding. [NTR]
5. Importance of asking DLC. [NTR]
6. Sideropenic dysphagia. [NTR]
7. Oral manifestations of haemophilia. [RGUHS]
8. Agranulocytosis. [RGUHS]
9. Laboratory investigations in bleeding disorders. [TN]
10. Schilling test. [TN]
11. Cyclic neutropaenia. [TN; RGUHS]
12. Humanisms. [TN]
13. Oral manifestations of neutropaenia. [TN]
14. Plummer-Vinson syndrome. [TN; RGUHS; NTRUHS]
15. Four oral manifestations of aplastic anaemia. [RGUHS]
16. Investigations to be carried out prior to extraction of a tooth in
    a. Leukaemia
    b. Purpura. [RGUHS]
17. Agranulocytosis. [NTRUHS]
18. Oral manifestations of leukaemia. [TN; NTRUHS]
19. Chronic lymphatic leukaemia. [NTR OS]
20. Oral manifestations of acute leukaemia. [RGUHS]
21. Iron deficiency anaemia. [TN]
22. Polycythaemia rubra vera. [NTRUHS]

DIAGNOSTIC LABORATORY PROCEDURES

Short Essays

1. Enumerate the importance of:
   a. Intravital staining
   b. Peripheral blood picture in oral medicine
   c. Role of immunoglobulin in oral medicine
   d. Bisecting techniques of intraoral radiographs. [NTR-OR]
2. What are the indications of following investigations in dentistry?
   a. Biopsy
   b. Sialography
   c. Exfoliative cytology [NTR-OR; RGUHS]
3. Describe the merits and demerits of using corticosteroids in oral lesions with suitable examples. [NTR-OR]
4. Biopsy. [MUHS]
5. Toluidine blue. [MUHS]
6. Glossodynia. [MUHS; TN]

Short Notes

1. Biopsy. [NTR-QR; TN; RGUHS]
2. Patch test. [NTR-NR]
3. Paget's test. [NTR-NR]
4. Schirmer's test. [NTR-NR]
5. Rose Waller test. [NTR-NR]
6. Paul-Bunnell test. [NTR-NR]
7. Exfoliative cytology. [NTR-OR; TN]
8. Oral exfoliative cytology. [NTR-OR; TN]
9. Role of intravital staining in oral medicine. [NTR-NR]
10. Describe the role of peripheral blood smear in oral medicine. [NTR-NR]
11. Brush biopsy. [RGUHS]
12. Schirmer's test. [RGUHS]
13. Paul-Bunnell test. [RGUHS; NTRUHS]
14. Exfoliative cytology. [RGUHS; TN]
15. Toluidine blue staining. [RGUHS]
16. Any two differences between direct and indirect immunofluorescence. [RGUHS]
17. Vitality tests. [NTR-NR]
18. Mid palatal swelling. [NTR-NR]
19. Clinical examination of ulcer. [NTR-NR]
20. Four conditions associated with cervicofacial lymphadenopathy. [RGUHS]
21. Age in examination. [RGUHS]
22. Causes for cervical lymphadenopathy. [RGUHS]

23. Brush biopsy. [RGUHS]
24. Toluidine blue staining. [RGUHS]
25. Any two differences between direct and indirect immunofluorescence. [RGUHS]
26. Patch test. [NTR-NR]
27. ESR. [BUHS]
28. Tzanck test. [RGUHS]
29. Erythrocyte sedimentation rate. [RGUHS]
30. Lip prints. [NTRUHS]
31. Bite marks. [NTRUHS]
32. Wound certificate. [NTRUHS; NTR-OR]
33. Bite-mark analysis. [NTRUHS]
34. Age determination methods. [NTRUHS]
35. Lip prints. [RGUHS]
36. Scope of forensic dentistry. [NTR-NR]
37. Wound certificate. [NTRUHS]
38. Tzanck smear. [RGUHS]
39. Nikolsky's sign. [BUHS; RGUHS]
40. Acid phosphatase. [RGUHS]
41. Alkaline phosphatase. [RGUHS]
42. 17-Ketosteroids in oral medicine. [NTR-OR]
43. Metronidazole. [BUHS]
44. Drugs to relieve muscular spasm. [RGUHS]
45. Oral penicillin. [BUHS]
46. Classification and uses of oral penicillins. [RGUHS]
47. Antinuclear antibody (ANA) test. [RGUHS]
48. Postprandial blood glucose technique. [RGUHS]
49. State purpose of toluidine blue staining. [RGUHS]
50. Antiviral drugs. [NTR-NR]
51. Antifungal drugs. [NTR-NR]
52. Anti-inflammatory drugs. [NTR-NR]
53. Corticosteroids in dentistry. [NTR-NR]
54. Antibiotics in oral diseases. [NTR-OR]
55. Paul-Bunnell test. [TN; RGUHS]
56. Intraoral exfoliative cytology. [TN]
57. Significance of haemogram. [RGUHS]
58. Bence Jones proteins. [RGUHS]
59. Aspiration biopsy. [RGUHS]
60. Schilling test. [RGUHS]
61. Uses and side-effects of oral penicillins. [RGUHS]
62. Indications and contraindications of corticosteroid therapy in dentistry. [RGUHS]
63. Drug allergic manifestations of oral mucosa. [BUHS]
64. Role of antibiotic therapy. [NTR-NR]
65. Fixed drug eruption. [BUHS]
66. Jarisch-Herxheimer reaction. [RGUHS]
67. Name the oral/systemic conditions in which corticosteroids are contraindicated. [RGUHS]
68. Write in brief about Toluidine blue test. [NTRUHS]
69. Diagnostic tests of bleeding disorders. [RGUHS]
70. Types and indications of biopsy in oral medicine. [RGUHS]
71. Western blot test. [RGUHS]
72. Biopsy versus exfoliative cytology. [TN]
73. Lab investigations for anaemiae. [TN]
74. Diagnostic test for HIV. [TN]
75. Pathergy test. [TN; NTR UHS]
76. Serum alkaline phosphatase. [TN]
77. Fine needle aspiration cytology. [TN]
78. Name any two conditions that show elevated serum alkaline phosphatase levels? [RGUHS]
79. Elevation of serum calcium. [RGUHS]
80. Bleeding time. [RGUHS]
81. Alkaline phosphatase. [RGUHS]
82. Write in brief about toluidine blue test. [MUHS]

MISCELLANEOUS

Long Essays

1. Corticosteroids in dentistry. [MUHS]
2. Allergic stomatitis. [MUHS]
3. What are the oral causes of halitosis? How are you going to treat a case of ANUG [BUHS]
4. Give the differential diagnosis of swelling in the midline of the palate? [NTR UHS]
5. Write the definitions of various basic lesions of oral mucosa. Write the names of three diseases for each of the basic lesion? [NTRUHS]
6. Define halitosis. What are the various causes leading to halitosis? Discuss any two of them in detail. [MHUS]

Short Essays

1. Anaphylaxis. [RGUHS]
2. Serum sickness. [RGUHS]
3. How will you manage a case of anaphylactic shock due to local anaesthesia. [BUHS]
4. Eagle's syndrome. [NTR-OR]
5. Trotter's syndrome. [NTR-NR]
6. Sjogren's syndrome. [NTR-NR]
7. Grinspan's syndrome. [NTR-OR]
8. Hereford's syndrome. [NTR-OR]
9. Pericoronitis. [NTRUHS]
10. Metronidazole. [RGUHS]

11. Oral penicillin. [RGUHS]
12. Drugs to relieve muscular spasm. [RGUHS]
13. Classification and uses of oral penicillins. [RGUHS]
14. Broad-spectrum antibiotics. [RGUHS]
15. Ramsay Hunt syndrome. [NTR-OR]
16. Burning mouth syndrome. [NTR-OR; TN; RGUHS]
17. Give one absolute and two relative contraindications for use of steroids. [MUHS]
18. Steroid in dentistry. [RGUHS]
19. Antifungal drugs in oral medicine. [RGUHS]
20. Melkersson-Rosenthal syndrome. [NTR-OR]
21. Ascher's syndrome. [RGUHS]
22. Albright's syndrome. [RGUHS]
23. Sturge-Weber syndrome. [RGUHS]
24. Uses and side-effects of oral penicillins. [RGUHS]
25. Indications and contraindications of corticosteroid therapy in dentistry. [RGUHS]
26. Syncope. [NTR; RGUHS]
27. Anaphylactic shock. [NTR-NR]
28. Bite marks. [NTR]
29. Steroids in dentistry. [RGUHS]
30. Papillon-Lefevre syndrome. [BUHS; RGUHS]
31. Eagle's syndrome. [NTR-NR]
32. Battered baby syndrome. [NTR-NR]
33. Definition of erythema dose. [MUHS]
34. Allergic stomatitis. [NTRUHS]
35. Patch test. [MUHS]

Short Notes

1. Papillon-Lefevre syndrome. [RGUHS]
2. Ethics in dental profession. [NTRUHS]
3. Adverse effects of ibuprofen. [RGUHS]
4. Target lesions. [RGUHS]
5. Alkaline phosphatase. [RGUHS]
6. Fixed drug eruption. [RGUHS]
7. Moth-eaten appearance. [RGUHS]
8. Name two conditions that show elevated serum alkaline phosphate levels. [RGUHS]
9. How will you manage a case of anaphylactic shock due to local anaesthesia. [RGUHS]
10. Trotter's syndrome. [RGUHS]
11. Eagle's syndrome. [RGUHS]
12. Ascher's syndrome. [RGUHS]
13. Albright's syndrome. [RGUHS]
14. Grinspan's syndrome. [RGUHS]
15. Sturge-Weber syndrome. [RGUHS]
16. Ramsay Hunt syndrome. [RGUHS]
17. Halitosis. [RGUHS]
18. Dysgeusia. [NTR]
19. Auspitz's sign. [NTR; RGUHS]
20. Nikolsky's sign. [NTR]
21. Mucous patches. [NTR]
22. Metallic stomatitis. [NTR]
23. Stomatitis venenata. [NTR]
24. Midpalatal swelling. [NTR]
25. Periapical osteofibrosis. [NTR]
26. Various types of periosteal reactions in sarcoma. [NTR]
27. T lymphocytes. [NTR-NR]
28. Epithelial dysplasia. [NTR-NR]
29. Soap-bubble appearance. [RGUHS]
30. Onion-skin appearance. [RGUHS]
31. Name four conditions that show onion-peel appearance. [RGUHS]
32. Paul-Bunnell test. [RGUHS]
33. Van den Berg test. [TN]
34. Corticosteroids in dentistry. [MUHS; TN]
35. Mouth washes in oral mucosal lesions. [TN]
36. Natural protective mechanism of the body against infection. [TN]
37. Pathergy test. [RGUHS]
38. Patch test. [RGUHS]
39. Frictional keratosis. [RGUHS]
22. Stony hard lymph node. [NTR-NR]
23. Cleidocranial dysostosis. [NTR-NR]
24. Lipschutz bodies. [RGUHS]
25. Koplik's spots. [RGUHS]
26. Cafe-au-lait spots. [RGUHS]
27. Moth-eaten appearance. [RGUHS]
28. What is Gorlin's sign? [NTRUHS]
29. Antibiotic sore mouth. [NTRUHS]
30. Line of Ennis. [RGUHS]
31. Diclofenac sodium. [RGUHS]
32. Diazepam. [RGUHS]
33. Vasovagal syncope. [RGUHS]

RADIATION PHYSICS

Long Essays

1. Describe with a neat and labelled diagram, production of X-rays. [MUHS]
2. Describe the construction and working of the X-ray tube. Add a note on collimation. [TN]
3. Define ideal radiograph and discuss the factors affecting the X-ray beam. [MUHS]

4. What are the parts of an X-ray tube? Describe the working of the X-ray tube and add a note on Bremsstrahlung radiation. [RGUHS]
5. Describe the factors controlling X-ray beam. [TN]
6. With a neatly labelled diagram explain the principle, construction and working of an X-ray tube, with the significance of each component. [MUHS]
7. Write an essay on the production of X-rays, their properties, intraoral radiographs and their techniques. [TN]
8. Describe the parts of an X-ray tube and add a note on properties of X-rays. [RGUHS]

Short Essays

1. Filtration. [RGUHS; NTRUHS]
2. Define ideal radiograph and discuss the factors affecting the X-ray beam. [MUHS]
3. Definition of roentgen. [MUHS]
4. Limitations of radiology. [MUHS]
5. Ideal requirements of target material. [MUHS]
6. Requirements of a darkroom. [MUHS]
7. Name the principles of shadow casting. [MUHS]
8. Name any four properties of X-rays. [MUHS]
9. Principles of projection geometry. [RGUHS; MUHS]
10. Production of X-rays. [RGUHS; TN]
11. Bremsstrahlung radiation. [RGUHS]
12. Electromagnetic spectrum. [RGUHS; MUHS; TN]
13. The role of fibre, gird and collimation in diagnostic radiography. [TN]
14. Diagnostic property of X-rays. [TN]
15. Rare earth substances. [NTR-UHS]
16. Electromagnetic spectrum. [NTR]
17. X-ray tube. [RGUHS]
18. Diagnostic properties of X-rays. [MUHS]
19. Properties of X-rays. [RGUHS; MUHS; NTR; TN]
20. Radiolysis of water. [RGUHS]
21. Collimation and filtration. [RGUHS; NTR; TN]
22. Types and uses of filtration. [RGUHS]
23. What are the properties of X-rays? Discuss the use£of OPG in dentistry. [RGUHS; BUHS]
24. Filters and collimation in radiography. [NTR-OR]
25. Bremsstrahlung radiation. [TN]

Short Notes

1. Draw a neat labelled diagram of an X-ray tube. [RGUHS]
2. Inverse square law. [RGUHS]
3. Filtration. [RGUHS]
4. Electromagnetic spectrum. [RGUHS; MUHS]
5. Collimation. [RGUHS; NTR; TN]
6. Anode in X-ray machine. [NTRUHS]
7. Focal trough. [NTRUHS; MUHS]
8. Name any four properties of X-rays. [MUHS]
9. Why is tungsten used as a target material in an X-ray tube? [MUHS]
10. Ionization. [RGUHS]
11. Inverse square law. [RGUHS]
12. Write Short Notes on:
    a. Properties of X-rays
    b. KVP [NTR-OR; NTR-UHS; RGUHS]
13. Collimation of X-ray beam. [RGUHS]
14. Radiology and roentgenology. [NTR-OR]
15. Generation of X-rays. [NTR-NR]
16. Characteristics of radiation. [NTR-OR]
17. Filters and collimators. [NTR-OR]
18. Collimators. [NTR-OR; TN]
19. Factors controlling X-ray beam. [TN]
20. Tungsten application in X-ray machine. [NTR-UHS]
21. Filtration and collimation in dental radiography. [MUHS]
22. Filters and collimators. [TN]
23. Filtration of X-ray beam. [MUHS]
24. Filters. [TN]
25. Define frequency. [MUHS]
26. What represents the particulate radiations? [MUHS]
27. Compton effect. [NTR]
28. Filtration of X-ray beam. [MUHS; TN]
29. What is the line focus principle? [MUHS]
30. Write two uses of collimation. [MUHS]
31. Gray. [RGUHS]
32. X-ray tube. [NTR-GR; NTR-NR; TN]
33. Coolidge tube. [NTR-GR]
34. Resolution. [NTR-NR]
35. X-ray timer. [TN]
36. Filtration in X-ray tube. [TN]
37. Uses and properties of X-rays. [TN]
38. Collimation and filtration. [NTR]

RADIATION BIOLOGY, HAZARDS OF RADIATION AND RADIATION PROTECTION

Long Essays

1. Discuss adverse effects of therapeutic radiation on oral tissues. [RGUHS]
2. Enumerate hazards of radiation. Discuss the effects of radiation on oral tissues. [NTR-OR; RGUHS]
3. What are the effects of radiation in the oral cavity? Write about osteoradionecrosis. [RGUHS]

4. Describe the radiation hazards in orofacial region and mention its preventive measures. [NTR-OR]
5. Discuss radiation hazards. Describe the various methods to protect the patient and operator from the haz-ards. [NTR-OR]
6. What are the hazards of radiation seen on oral cavity and measures to protect operative from radiation hazards. [MUHS]
7. Discuss radiation protection. [NTR-NR]
8. Enumerate various techniques of taking intraoral radiography. Discuss the various procedures taken to protect the operator and the patient during radiography. [NTR-NR]
9. Mention radiation hazards affecting body. How would you protect from them while taking intraoral radiographs. [TN]
10. Enumerate the effects of radiation on oral tissues. Discuss the measures of radiation protection in dental radiology. [RGUHS]
11. Describe radiation protection measures. [RGUHS]
12. What are the biologic effects of radiation in the oral cavity [RGUHS]
13. Discuss radiation protection. [MUHS]
14. Discuss the biological properties of X-rays. [MUHS]
15. What are the hazards of radiation seen on skin and bones? Discuss protection from radiation. [MUHS]
16. Discuss the effects of radiation on orofacial tissues. Write on the radiation protection measures in dental radiology. [TN]
17. Write about the effects of radiation on the living tissues. Add a note on prevention and management of osteoradionecrosis. [TN]
18. Discuss the methods of radiation safety and protection of the operator, patient and public. [TN; RGUHS]
19. Write an essay on the effects of ionizing radiation on the living tissues. Add a note on radiation safety. [TN]
20. Write on radiation hazards and the protective measures to be taken by the operator and the patient. [TN]
21. Discuss the different methods of radiation protection of the patient and personnel (operator) in oral radiography. [TN]
22. Write about harmful effects of radiation on body. [NTR]

Short Essays

1. Radiation protection from X-rays. [MUHS]
2. Radiation protection for the operator. [MUHS; NTR; TN]
3. Radiation protection of patient. [MUHS; NTR]
4. TLD. [MUHS]
5. ALARA. [MUHS]
6. Enumerate the various means to reduce the exposure to the patient while taking diagnosis radiograph. [MUHS]
7. Radiation dosimetry. [RGUHS; TN]
8. Osteoradionecrosis. [RGUHS; NTRUHS; TN]
9. Effects of radiation in the oral cavity. [RGUHS]
10. Biological effects of radiation in oral cavity. [RGUHS]
11. Thermoluminescent dosimeter. [NTR-NR]
12. X-ray monitoring devices. [MUHS]
13. Dosimetry. [RGUHS]
14. Write about osteoradionecrosis. [MUHS]
15. Clinical features and management of osteoradionecrosis. [RGUHS]
16. Postirradiation mucositis. [BUHS]
17. Radiation dosimetry. [RGUHS; TN]
18. Osteoradionecrosis. [RGUHS; NTRUHS; TN]
19. Effects of radiation in the oral cavity. [RGUHS]
20. Biological effects of radiation in oral cavity. [RGUHS]
21. Thermoluminescent dosimeter. [NTR-NR]
22. X-ray monitoring devices. [MUHS 1986]
23. Dosimetry. [RGUHS]

Treatment of postirradiation mucositis. [BUHS]

24. Types of the radiation caries. [RGUHS]
25. Write on radiation caries. [BUHS]
26. Write on radiation hazards in dentistry. [BUHS]
27. Describe radiation hazards and its prevention. [BUHS]
28. Protection from radiation hazards in dental radiography. [TN]
29. Radiation caries. [NTR]
30. Scattered radiation. [NTR]

Short Notes

1. Radiation mucositis. [RGUHS]
2. Thermoluminescent dosimeter. [RGUHS; MUHS; TN]
3. Effects of radiation on developing tooth. [RGUHS]
4. Dosimetry. [NTR-UHS; NTR-OR; TN; RGUHS]
5. Enumerate the various means to reduce the exposure to the patient while taking diagnostic radiograph. [MUHS]
6. Discuss radiation protection. [MUHS]
7. Measure to protect the patient from radiation hazard. [MUHS]
8. Discuss radiation protection. [MUHS]
9. Definition of erythema dose. [MTHS]
10. Film badge. [RGUHS; BUHS]
11. Postirradiation mucositis. [RGUHS]
12. Types of the radiation caries. [RGUHS]
13. Write on radiation caries. [RGUHS]
14. Treatment of postirradiation mucositis. [RGUHS]
15. Describe radiation hazards and its prevention. [RGUHS]
16. Write radiation hazards in dentistry. [RGUHS]

17. Osteoradionecrosis. [NTR-OR; TN]
18. Radiation caries. [NTR-OR; TN]
19. Radiation hazards of jaws. [NTR-NR]
20. Hazards of radiation. [NTR-NR]
21. Radiation hazards of teeth, oral mucosa and the jaws. [NTR-NR]
22. Radiolysis of water. [RGUHS]
23. Effects of radiation in the oral cavity. [RGUHS]
24. Clinical features and management of osteoradionecrosis. [RGUHS]
25. Radiation protection. [NTR-OR]
26. Radiosensitive and radioprotective. [TN]
27. Definition of roentgen and erythema dose. [TN]
28. Limitations of radiography. [NTR]
29. Radioresistant cells. [RGUHS]
30. ALRA principle. [RGUHS]

X-RAY FILMS AND ACCESSORIES

Long Essays

1. What is the composition of the radiographic film? Describe the mechanism of image formation. Add a note on the constituents of developing and fixing solution. [RGUHS]

Short Essays

1. Intensifying screens. [RGUHS; MUHS; NTR; TN; RGUHS]
2. Grid. [MUHS; NTR; TN; RGUHS]
3. Radiographic film. [MUHS; NTR]
4. State the functions of lead foil in the X-ray film packet. [MUHS]
5. What is the function of grid? [MUHS]
6. Uses and types of grids. [RGUHS]
7. Composition and uses of intensifying screens. [RGUHS; TN]
8. Composition and functions of intensifying screens. [RGUHS]
9. Types and uses of intraoral radiographs. [RGUHS]
10. Dental X-ray film. [TN]
11. Radiographic accessories. [RGUHS]
12. Moving grid. [TN]
13. Intraoral periapical film. [RGUSH]

Short Notes

1. Storage of X-ray films. [RGUHS]
2. Composition of intensifying screen. [RGUHS]
3. Composition of X-ray film. [RGUHS]
4. Describe the composition of X-ray film. [MUHS]
5. Give two advantages of paralleling technique. [MUHS]
6. Speed of intraoral film. [MUHS]
7. Enumerate types of grids. [MUHS]
8. What is grid? Where is it used? [MUHS]
9. Enumerate various types of intraoral films. [MUHS]
10. State the functions of lead foil in the X-ray film packet. [MUHS]
11. Advantages of bitewing radiographs. [MUHS]
12. X-ray film. [RGUHS; NTR]
13. Occlusal film. [RGUHS; NTR]
14. Intensifying screen. [RGUHS; NTR]
15. Write notes on radiographic films. [RGUHS]
16. X-ray film packet. [NTR-NR]
17. Potter-Bucky diaphragm. [NTR-OR]
18. Composition of intraoral periapical film. [NTR-GR]
19. Occlusal radiograph. [NTR-GR]
20. Indications of occlusal films. [NTR-NR]
21. Features of an ideal intraoral periapical radiograph. [TN]

PROCESSING OF X-RAY FILMS

Long Essays

1. What is the composition of radiographic film? Describe the mechanism of image formation. Add a note on the composition of developing and fixing solution and their functions. [NTR-NR; TN]
2. Write the composition and actions of developer and fixer used in dental radiography. [TN]
3. Describe processing of X-ray films. [MUHS]
4. Describe the formation of 'lateral image' and darkroom chemistry. [MUHS]

Short Essays

1. Composition of developer solution. [NTR]
2. Types of X-ray film processing. [RGUHS]
3. Automatic processing. [RGUHS; TN]
4. Developing solution. [NTRUHS; TN]

5. Composition and actions of developing solution. [TN]
6. Fixing solution. [MUHS; NTR; RGUHS]
7. Processing errors of radiographs. [MUHS]
8. Composition and functions of developing solution. [RGUHS; TN]
9. Composition of fixer. [NTR]
10. X-ray fixing solution. [NTR-OR]
11. Automatic film processing. [NTR-NR]
12. Processing of X-ray films. [NTR-NR]
13. Processing of an intraoral film. [NTR-OR]
14. Requirements of darkroom. [NTR-NR]
15. Composition and action of fixer solution. [NTR-OR; TN]
16. Coin test. [NTR]
17. Requirements of a darkroom. [MUHS]

Short Notes

1. Composition of developer solution. [RGUHS; TN]
2. Resolution. [RGUHS]
3. Replenisher. [RGUHS]
4. Fixing solution. [RGUHS]
5. Composition and action of developing and fixing solutions. [RGUHS; NTR; MUHS]
6. Replenisher. [RGUHS]
7. What is the composition of developer solution? [MUHS]
8. Radiographic dyes. [RGUHS-BUHS]
9. Fixer and developer. [RGUHS-BUHS]
10. Image dislocation in X-ray. [RGUHS]
11. X-ray developer and fixer. [RGUHS-BUHS]
12. Four causes for dark radiographs. [RGUHS]
13. Write about developing solution. [RGUHS-BUHS]
14. Describe the faulty radiographs. [RGUHS]
15. Contents of fixing solution. [TN]
16. Automatic film processing. [TN]
17. Processing. [NTR]
18. Storage of X-rays films. [RGUHS]
19. Requirements of darkroom. [RGUHS]
20. Composition of intraoral radiographic films. [NTR]
21. Speed of intraoral film. [MUHS]

IMAGE PRINCIPLES: X-RAY QUALITY CONTROL

Long Essays

1. Describe artifacts, blemishes and fault in dental radiography. [RGUHS]
2. Discuss the causes of faulty radiograph. How would you avoid it? [NTRUHS; TN]
3. Discuss the faults in dental radiograph and prevention of these faults. [MUHS]
4. Discuss factors responsible for obtaining an ideal radiograph. [RGUHS]
5. Discuss basic principles involved in taking intraoral X-rays. [RGUHS]
6. What is an ideal radiograph? Describe all the factors influencing the diagnostic quality of a dental radiograph. [MUHS]
7. Discuss the causes of faulty radiographs. [NTR-QR]
8. Discuss the procedure of intraoral radiographic technique. [TN]
9. Write about the different causes of faulty radiograph. [TN]
10. Discuss the causes of distortion of images in the radiographs. [TN]
11. What is an ideal radiograph? Enumerate the various factors influencing the quality of radiograph. Describe the role of processing procedures on the quality of radiograph. [TN]
12. Discuss faulty IO radiographs? [NTR-NR]
13. Define an ideal radiograph. Describe basic principles to obtain an ideal radiograph. [TN]
14. Discuss various causes for faculty radiographs and measures to rectify them. [RGUHS]

Short Essays

1. Artifacts on a radiograph. [RGUHS]
2. Light radiograph. [RGUHS]
3. Localization technique. [RGUHS]
4. What is latent image? [RGUHS]
5. Latent image on radiograph. [MUHS]
6. Define an ideal radiograph. Discuss the factors required to obtain an ideal radiograph. [RGUHS]
7. Faulty X-rays. [BUHS]
8. Dark radiograph. [RGUHS]
9. Image dislocation in X-rays. [BUHS]
10. Four causes for dark radiographs. [RGUHS]
11. Film fog. [NTR]
12. Write note on image receptors. [RGUHS]

Short Notes

1. Cone-cut. [RGUHS]
2. What is latent image? [MUHS]
3. What are the causes of fog on radiograph? [MUHS]

4. Latent image. [MUHS]
5. Describe the faulty radiographs. [BUHS]
6. Artefacts. [TN]
7. Density and contrast in radiology. [NTR]
8. SLOB technique. [RGUHS]
9. Radiographic density. [RGUHS]
10. Dark and light radiographs. [RGUHS]
11. Faulty X-rays. [RGUHS]

INTRAORAL RADIOGRAPHIC TECHNIQUES

Long Essays

1. Write the principles of imaging and discuss the bisecting angle technique. [RGUHS]
2. Describe the bisecting angle technique of intraoral periapical radiography. [RGUHS]
3. Enumerate the types of intraoral radiographs. Describe the technique of obtaining intraoral periapical radiograph of maxillary central incisors. [RGUHS]
4. Intraoral radiographic techniques. [RGUHS]
5. Define ideal radiograph. Describe the technique for intraoral periapical radiographs with merits and demerits. [MUHS]
6. Define ideal radiograph. State the rules of projection geometry and describe the relative merits and demerits of bisecting angle technique and paralleling technique (short cone and long cone techniques). [MUHS]
7. Describe the principle of short cone technique. What are the merits and demerits of the same? [MUHS]
8. Differentiate bisecting angle technique and paralleling technique. [MUHS]
9. What is an ideal radiograph? State the rules of projection geometry. Describe the principles, advantages and disadvantages of bisecting angle technique and paralleling technique. [MUHS]
10. Describe the advantages, disadvantages, limitations and technique of bitewing radiographs. [MUHS]
11. Give differential diagnosis of perforation of palate, mention radiographic technique for the same. [MUHS]
12. What are the uses of occlusal X-ray? Describe the techniques of occlusal X-ray of maxillary palate. [RGUHS-BUHS]
13. What are indications for occlusal radiographs? Describe the radiographic techniques in taking maxillary and mandibular cross-sectional occlusal radiographs. [RGUHS]
14. Composition of intraoral periapical films. [NTR-OR]
15. Enumerate intraoral radiographic technique. Describe the procedure of localizing an impacted left maxillary canine. [NTR-OR]
16. Describe the angulations for full-mouth periapical radiographs. [RGUHS]
17. How will you take intraoral radiograph of upper permanent molar. [NTR-OR]
18. Describe the procedure of periapical radiograph of the mandibular central incisor using short cone technique. [NTR-OR]
19. Compare bisecting angle or short cone technique and long cones technique of radiography. Describe technique of lower third molar. [NTR-OR]
20. What are the various factors affecting the dental radiographs. Describe the placement of film in periapical intraoral radiography. [NTR-OR]
21. Describe the five principles of image production in relation to periapical radiography. [NTR-NR]
22. Describe the advantages, disadvantages and shortcomings of short cone and long cone techniques in periapical radiography. [TN]
23. Describe a technique for taking bitewing radiograph for the posterior teeth. [TN]
24. Define an ideal radiograph. Describe the technique to take periapical radiograph of upper central incisors.[TN]
25. Discuss the merits and demerits of the technique. [TN]
26. Describe advantages and limitations of bisecting angle technique of periapical radiography. [TN]
27. Discuss techniques of intraoral periapical radiographs and their advantages and disadvantages. [NTR]
28. Discuss basic principles involved in taking intraoral X-rays. [RGUHS]

Short Essays

1. Localization technique. [RGUHS]
2. Occlusal radiograph. [RGUHS; MUHS; TN]
3. Indications and inteipretation of Clark's technique. [RGUHS]
4. Clark's rule. [RGUHS]
5. Bitewing radiography. [MUHS; RGUHS-BUHS]
6. Radiographic technique to study the following:
   a. Globulomaxillary cyst [MUHS]
   b. Midline cyst of palate [MUHS]
   c. Keratocyst [MUHS]
   d. Nasopalatine cyst [MUHS]

7. Give the indications of true occlusal radiograph. [MUHS]
8. Give two advantages of paralleling technique. [MUHS]
9. Enumerate various types of intraoral films. [MUHS]
10. Indication and angulation of bitewing radiograph for posterior region. [MUHS]
11. Give the indications of bitewing X-ray. [MUHS]
12. Advantages of bitewing radiographs. [MUHS]
13. Principle and indications for Clark's technique or shift cone technique. [RGUHS]
14. Types and uses of intraoral radiographs. [RGUHS]
15. Indications and radiographic technique for maxillary standard occlusal view. [RGUHS]
16. What are the uses of the following radiographs:
    a. Periapical film
    b. Bitewing film [BUHS]
17. Target film distance. [NTR-NR]
18. Long cone technique. [NTR-NR]
19. Occlusal view radiography. [NTR-NR]
20. Angulation of upper molar. [NTR-OR]
21. Indications of transorbital view. [NTR-NR]
22. Enumerate the importance of bisecting techniques of intraoral radiographs. [NTR-OR]
23. Bisecting angle technique. [TN; RGUHS]
24. Write indications for occlusal radiographs and technique for topographical occlusal view. [RGUHS]

Short Notes

1. Indications of bitewing radiographs. [RGUHS; NTR]
2. Name four indications for bitewing radiographs. [RGUHS]
3. Enumerate the advantages of paralleling technique. [MUHS]
4. Indications of true occlusal view. [MUHS]
5. Buccal object rule method of localization. [MUHS]
6. Indications for a mandibular occlusal radiographs. [RGUHS]
7. Advantages of paralleling technique. [MUHS]
8. Disadvantages of the bisecting angle technique. [MUHS; RGUHS]
9. Give indications of bitewing radiographs. [MUHS; RGUHS]
10. How will you manage the problem of gagging in a patient during the periapical technique. [MUHS]
11. Enumerate the anatomical landmarks seen on maxillary anterior periapical film. [MUHS]
12. Give indications of true occlusal radiograph. [MUHS]
13. Bisecting angle technique. [NTR]
14. Write Short Notes on occlusal X-ray. [RGUHS; BUHS]
15. What are the uses of following radiographs:
    a. Orthopantomograph
    b. PNS view. [RGUHS]
16. Bisecting technique. [RGUHS-BUHS]
17. Write notes on bisecting techniques for intraoral roentgenograms. [RGUHS-BUHS]
18. Timer. [NTR-NR]
19. Angulation. [NTR-DR]
20. Compton effect. [NTR-DR]
21. SLOB. [NTR-NR]
22. SLOB formula or principle. [NTR-OR; NTR-NR]
23. Indications of topographic and cross-sectional occlusal radiography. [TN]
24. ALARA. [NTR-NR]
25. Occlusal film. [TN]
26. Short cone technique. [TN]
27. Intraoral film. [TN]
28. Miller's technique. [TN]

EXTRAORAL RADIOGRAPHIC TECHNIQUES

Long Essays

1. Describe the transcranial and transpharyngeal radiographic techniques of TMJ. [MUHS]
2. Describe anatomy of TMJ. Discuss various disorders of the TMJ. [MUHS]
3. Enumerate the radiographic techniques to study temporomandibular joint and describe any two. [MUHS]
4. Describe the radiology procedure used for localization of foreign body in maxillary sinus. [MUHS]
5. Describe the principle, indications and limitations of panoramic radiography. [RGUHS]
6. Write the radiographic technique used for viewing the maxillary sinus. Give the radiographic diagnosis of important pathological entities involving the antrum. [MUHS]
7. Enumerate radiographic techniques to study temporomandibular joint. Give advantages and disadvantages of orthopantomography. [MUHS]
8. Describe the procedure about talking lateral oblique view radiograph. [RGUHS-BUHS]
9. How will you take a lateral oblique radiograph of the mandible? Mention normal radiographic landmarks in the same radiograph. Draw necessary diagrams. [TN]

10. Write indications of panoramic radiography. Discuss theory of tomography. [TN]
11. How will you take lateral oblique view of mandible and ive interpretations to that? [NTR-OR]
12. Enumerate various skull radiographs and discuss posteroanterior, paranasal sinus and submentovertex view of skull. [TN]
13. Discuss the principle, technique, advantages and disadvantages of panoramic imaging. [TN]
14. What are the indications of panoramic radiography? Discuss the theory of tomography. [NTR]

Short Essays

1. Technique for better visualization of paranasal air sinus. [RGUHS]
2. Oblique lateral radiograph of mandible. [RGUHS]
3. Waters projection. [RGUHS]
4. Temporomandibular joint radiography. [RGUHS]
5. Posteroanterior and Water's view. [RGUHS]
6. Bregma-Mentum view. [NTRUHS]
7. Panoramic radiography. [MUHS; RGUHS-BUHS]
8. Advantages of OPG. [MUHS]
9. Radiographs to study the following:
   a. Fractures of the angle of mandible [MUHS]
   b. Fracture in symphysis region [MUHS]
   c. Zygomatic arch fracture [MUHS]
10. Mention the disadvantages of orthopantomography. [MUHS]
11. Define focal trough and write any two principal advantages of panoramic radiograph. [MUHS]
12. Principle and indications of panoramic radiograph. [RGUHS]
13. Indications for paranasal sinus view. [RGUHS]
14. Indications and radiographic technique for paranasal sinus view. [RGUHS; TN]
15. Disadvantages of orthopantomograph. [NTR]
16. Mention the uses of lateral oblique view. [BUHS]
17. Indications of PA view skull. [NTR-NR; RGUHS]
18. PNS view. [NTR]
19. What are the uses of following radiographs:
   a. Orthopantomograph [NTR; RGUHS]
   b. Panoral radiography [NTR]
20. Technique of transcranial view of temporomandibular joint. [NTR]

Short Notes

1. Principle. of panoramic radiography. [RGUHS]
2. Advantage of panoramic radiography. [MUHS]
3. Transorbital view. [MUHS]
4. Give uses of lateral skull projection. [MUHS]
5. Name two radiographic techniques to study temporomandibular joint. [MUHS]
6. Name any two techniques for temporomandibular joint radiography. [MUHS]
   a. Periapical film
   b. Bitewing film [RGUHS]
7. Mention the uses of lateral oblique view. [RGUHS]
8. Mention the uses of Water's view. [RGUHS-BUHS]
9. Describe one radiographic technique to study-maxillary sinusitis. [RGUHS-BUHS]
10. PA view radiograph. [NTR-GR]
11. Submentovertex view. [NTR-NR]
12. Radiographic appearance of hyperparathyroidism joint. [RGUHS]
13. Water's view. [TN]
14. Submentovertex radiographic projection. [TN]
15. Paranasal sinus radiographic projections. [TN]
16. Indications for panoramic radiograph. [TN]
17. Lateral oblique view of mandible. [TN]
18. Miller's technique (radiographic). [TN]
19. Extraoral radiographs. [RGUHS]
20. OPG. [MUHS]

SPECIALIZED IMAGING TECHNIQUES

Long Essays

1. Describe sialography and write on its significance in various salivary gland disorders. [RGUHS; NTR]
2. Sialography: Describe the indications, contraindications of sialography and the technique. [RGUHS]
3. Enumerate various diseases of the salivary gland. Discuss how you will locate a calculus in the Wharton's duct. [MUHS]
4. Define sialography. What are the indications and contraindications of sialography? Give the ideal requirements of the contrast media used in sialography. [MUHS]
5. Describe sialography and its significance in various diseases of salivary glands. [RGUHS-BUHS]
6. Clinical features differential diagnosis and management of functional disturbance of salivary glands. [RGUHS]

7. Describe the procedure for sialography of parotid gland. [NTR-OR]
8. Discuss the indications and contraindications of sialography. Describe the contrast media and the stepwise procedure for submandibular salivary gland sialography. [TN]
9. What is contract radiography? Discuss the technique of sialography and add a note on its interpretation in various diseases of salivary glands. [RGUHS]

Short Essays

1. Digital radiography. [RGUHS; TN]
2. Applications of ultrasound in dentistry. [RGUHS]
3. CT in dentistry. [RGUHS]
4. Scintigraphy. [RGUHS]
5. Radiograph to study:
   a. Salivary calculus. [MUHS]
6. Sialography. [MUHS; NTR; TN]
7. Write two indications and contraindications of sialography. [MUHS]
8. Contrast radiography. [NTR-OR]
9. Magnetic resonance imaging. [NTR-OR]
10. Radionuclide imaging. [NTR]
11. SLOB formula. [NTR]
12. Temporomandibular joint radiography. [RGUHS]

Short Notes

1. Two indications and contraindications of sialography. [RGUHS]
2. Contraindications of sialography. [RGUHS]
3. Digital radiography (radiovisiography). [NTR-UHS]
4. Indications and contraindications of sialography. [MUHS; RGUHS]
5. What are the requirements of ideal contrast medium used for sialography. [MUHS]
6. Sialolithiasis. [MUHS]
7. Stereoradiography. [RGUHS-BUHS]
8. Write notes on xeroradiography. [RGUHS-BUHS]
9. Indications of sialography. [RGUHS-BUHS]
10. Contrast media. [TN]
11. Xenoradiography. [TN]
12. Sialography. [NTR]
13. Indications of CT in oral and maxillofacial region. [NTR]
14. Object localization. [RGUHS]

RADIOGRAPHIC INTERPRETATIONS

Long Essays

1. Radiographic features of fibro-osseous lesions of the jaws. [RGUHS]
2. Discuss the differential diagnosis of periapical radiolucencies. [RGUHS; TN]
3. Describe the normal anatomical landmarks in intraoral radiographs. [RGUHS]
4. Describe the radiolucent and radiopaque anatomic landmarks of the mandible. [MUHS]
5. Define ideal radiograph. Discuss the factors to obtain an ideal radiograph. [MUHS]
6. Describe in short various radiographic landmarks of the maxilla. Why is it important to know radiographic landmarks of maxilla? [MUHS]
7. Name the malignant tumours of the jaws. Describe the radiographic appearance of the same. [MUHS]
8. Describe various radiopaque lesions at the root of mandibular premolar. [MUHS]
9. Give clinical and radiographic features of osteomyelitis of jaws. [MUHS]
10. Describe various radiopaque lesions at the root of mandibular premolar. [MUHS]
11. Name the malignant tumours of the jaws. Describe the radiographic appearance of carcinoma and sarcoma of the jaws. [MUHS]
12. What is an ideal radiograph? Describe all the factors influencing the diagnostic quality of a dental radiograph. [MUHS]
13. Enumerate periapical radiolucencies and radiopacities. How would you diagnose systemic diseases with periapical changes in radiographs? [RGUHS]
14. Define an ideal radiograph. Discuss the factors required to obtain an ideal radiograph? [BUHS]
15. Enumerate the periapical radiolucencies and radiopacities. How would you diagnose systemic diseases with periapical changes in radiographs? [NTR-NR]
16. Discuss importance of lamina dura in dental radiographs and describe periapical radiolucent areas. [RGUHS]
17. Discuss radiographic changes of periapical region in systemic diseases. [RGUHS]
18. Enumerate periapical lesions and describe periapical cyst and abscess. [RGUHS]
19. Describe the radiographic appearance of different cysts of maxilla and mandible. [NTR-NR]

20. Describe the radiographic appearance of different stages of osteomyelitis of jaws. [NTR-NR]
21. Write the differential diagnosis of radiopacities of maxillary antrum. [NTR-OR]
22. Enumerate the various radiographic techniques for the diagnosis of fracture of mandible. [NTR-NR]
23. Discuss the differential diagnosis of radiolucencies on coronal part of the teeth. [NTR-OR]
24. Describe the differential diagnosis of radiolucent lesions in posterior part of the body of the mandible. [NTR-OR]
25. Describe the radiographic appearance of various odontomes and give the differential diagnosis. [TN]
26. Enumerate the radiopaque lesions of the jaws. Discuss the radiological features of cementoma. [TN]
27. Discuss radiolucent lesions of jaw. [TN]
28. Discuss the role of radiography in the diagnosis and management of periodontal disease. [TN]
29. Give a suitable classification of cysts of the jaws. Describe the clinical features, radiographic appearance and differential diagnosis of dentigerous cyst. [TN]
30. Give the differential diagnosis of periapical lesions laying stress on the radiographic interpretation. [TN]
31. Discuss the multilocular lesions of the mandible. [TN]

Short Essays

1. Periapical radiolucencies. [RGUHS]
2. Multilocular radiolucencies. [RGUHS; NTR]
3. Radiotherapy. [RGUHS]
4. Radiographic appearance of ameloblastoma. [RGUHS; NTR; TN]
5. Radiographic features of fractures of the jaw. [RGUHS]
6. Radiographic features of periodontal disease. [RGUHS]
7. Radiographic features of fractures of the teeth. [RGUHS]
8. Types of X-ray film processing. [RGUHS]
9. Importance of lamina dura in radiographs. [RGUHS]
10. Complications of radiotherapy in orofacial region. [RGUHS]
11. Broken needle in the pterygomandibular space. [MUHS]
12. Radiographic appearance of incisive foramen. [MUHS]
13. Landmarks seen on periapical maxillary X-rays. [MUHS]
14. Radiographic technique to study:
    a. The initial proximal caries. [MUHS]
15. Radiographic technique to study proximal caries. [MUHS]
16. Radiographic technique to study incipient interproximal callus radiology. [MUHS]
17. Radiography in periodontal disease. [MUHS]
18. Moth-eaten appearance. [RGUHS; NTR]
19. Potter-Bucky diaphragm. [RGUHS]
20. Describe the radiographic appearance of following:
    a. Invaginated odontome [MUHS]
    b. Periapical osteofluorosis (cementoma) [MUHS]
    c. Odontomes [MUHS]
21. Radiographic appearance of the following:
    a. Adenomatoid odontogenic tumour [MUHS]
    b. Periapical osteofibrosis [MUHS]
    c. Multiple myeloma [MUHS]
    d. Adenoameloblastoma [MUHS]
    e. Ameloblastoma [MUHS; RGUHS]
22. Radiographic appearance of:
    a. Osteogenic sarcoma [MUHS]
    b. Adenocystic carcinoma [MUHS]
    c. Squamous cell carcinoma [MUHS]
23. Describe radiographic appearance of:
    a. Periapical osteofibrosis [MUHS]
    b. Cherubism [MUHS]
    c. Periapical cemental dysplasia [MUHS; RGUHS]
24. Describe the radiographic appearance of:
    a. Maxillary sinus [MUHS]
    b. Localization of a root in the maxillary sinus [MUHS]
    c. Paranasal sinuses [MUHS]
    d. Maxillary sinusitis [MUHS]
    e. Pansinusitis [MUHS]
25. Differential diagnosis of unilateral radiopacity of maxillary sinus. [MUHS]
26. Enumerate the landmarks seen on the intraoral periapical view of upper 3rd molar region. [MUHS]
27. Describe the radiographic appearance of chronic osteomyelitis. [MUHS; RGUHS]
28. Radiographic features of chronic osteomyelitis. [MUHS]
29. Radiography appearance of dental caries. [NTR]
30. Discuss the radiological appearance of periodontitis and periodontosis. [BUHS]
31. Discuss the importance of radiographs in the detection of periodontal disease. [BUHS]
32. Radiographic appearance of odontogenic keratocyst. [NTR-NR]
33. Describe the radiographic appearance of myxoma. [NTR-OR]
34. Radiographic appearance of periapical cyst. [RUHS]
35. Radiographic appearance of osteosarcoma. [RGUHS]
36. Describe the radiological appearance of jaws in osteogenic sarcoma. [BUHS]
37. Radiographic appearance of Paget's disease. [NTR-NR]
38. Describe the radiological appearance of fibrous dysplasia. [NTR-OR; TN]
39. Discuss the radiological appearance of acute and chronic osteomyelitis. [BUHS]

40. Clinical features and radiographic appearance of osteosarcoma. [RGUHS]
41. Multilocular radiolucencies of jaw bone. [NTR-NR; TN]
42. Radiographic appearance of dental caries. [RGUHS]
43. Differential diagnosis of unilocular radiolucencies. [RGUHS]
44. Radiographs to evaluate mandibular third molars. [RGUHS]
45. Faulty radiographs. [RGUHS]
46. Periapical radio opacities. [RGUHS]
47. Differential diagnosis of periapical radiopacities. [RGUHS]

Short Notes

1. Cotton-wool appearance on radiograph. [RGUHS]
2. PDL space. [RGUHS]
3. Radiation caries. [RGUHS; NTR]
4. Onion-peel appearances on a radiograph. [RGUHS; TN]
5. Radiographic appearance of ameloblastoma. [RGUHS]
6. Name four conditions showing soap-bubble appearance on skull radiograph. [RGUHS]
7. Radiographic appearance of osteogenic sarcomas. [RGUHS]
8. Brach therapy. [RGUHS]
9. Dark radiograph. [RGUHS]
10. Cotton-wool appearance. [RGUHS]
11. Radiographic appearance of periapical abscess.[RGUHS]
12. Radiographic appearance of compound composite odontomes. [RGUHS]
13. Radiographic classification of proximal caries. [RGUHS]
14. Onion-skin appearance. [RGUHS]
15. Enumerate the landmarks seen on the intraoral periapical view of upper 3rd molar region. [MUHS]
16. Mention any four radiolucent normal anatomical landmarks of maxilla. [MUHS]
17. Radiographic appearance of dentigerous cyst. [MUHS]
18. What is radiographic appearance of globulomaxillary cyst. [MUHS]
19. Radiographic appearance of chronic osteomyelitis. [MUHS]
20. Write about radiographic appearance of adenomatoid odontogenic tumour. [MUHS]
21. Radiograph appearance of adenomatoid odontogenic tumour. [MUHS]
22. Radiographic features of squamous cell carcinoma. [MUHS]
23. Enumerate periapical lesions. [MUHS]
24. Enumerate the anatomical landmarks seen on maxillary anterior periapical film. [MUHS]
25. Radiopaque lesions of jaws. [RGUHS-BUHS]
26. Normal radiolucent landmark in maxilla and mandible. [RGUHS-BUHS]
27. Discuss radiopaque lesions of mandible in the premolar region. [RGUHS-BUHS]
28. Write notes on localization of radiopaque lesions in the mandibular body. [RGUHS-BUHS]
29. Discuss the importance of radiographs in the detection of dental caries. [RGUHS]
30. Discuss the importance of radiographs in the detection of periodontal disease. [RGUHS-BUHS]
31. Discuss the radiological appearance of periodontitis and periodontosis. [RGUHS]
32. Radiographic appearance of periapical granuloma. [RGUHS]
33. Describe the radiographic appearance of teeth and jaws in periapical granuloma and cyst. [RGUHS-BUHS]
34. Describe the radiological appearance of:
a. Ameloblastoma [NTR]
b. Cementoma [RGUHS-BUHS]
c. Dentigerous cyst [RGUHS]
35. Get the radiographic appearance of the following:
a. Ameloblastoma
b. Garre's osteomyelitis
c. Cementoma [RGUHS-BUHS]
36. Discuss the radiological appearance of hypercementosis and cementoma. [RGUHS-BUHS]
37. Radiographic appearance of mandibular fracture. [RGUHS]
38. Radiographic view to detect fractured zygomatic arch. [RGUHS]
39. Describe one radiographic technique to study the following:
a. Impacted maxillary canine [BUHS]
b. Fracture at the right angle of mandible [RGUHS-BUHS]
40. Name four conditions showing onion-peel appearance on skull radiographs. [RGUHS]
41. Radiographic appearance of hyperparathyroidism. [RGUHS]
42. Describe the radiological appearance of jaws in hyperparathyroidism. [RGUHS]
43. Describe the radiographic appearance of teeth and jaws in hyperparathyroidism. [RGUHS]
44. Radiographic appearance of:
a. Fibrous dysplasia [RGUHS; NTR]
b. Aneurysmal bone cyst [MUHS]
c. Odontogenic keratocyst [MUHS; RGUHS]
d. Radicular cysts [MUHS]
e. Dentigerous cyst [MUHS]

45. Radiographic techniques to study TMJ ankylosis. [MUHS]
46. Describe the radiological appearance of jaws in fibrous dysplasia. [RGUHS]
47. Describe the radiographic appearance of teeth and jaws in fibrous dysplasia. [RGUHS]
48. Lamina dura. [NTR-OR; TN]
49. Radiopaque lesions of the jawbones. [NTR-OR]
50. Describe the radiopaque lesions of the jawbones. [NTR-OR]
51. Radiographic appearance of periapical cemental dysplasia. [NTR-NR]
52. Radiolucent lesions of periapical region. [NTR-NR]
53. Describe the radiological appearance of jaws in fibrous dysplasia. [BUHS]
54. Radiographic features of fibrous dysplasia. [RGUHS]
55. Radiographic appearance of hyperparathyroidism. [RGUHS]
56. Sunray appearance. [NTR-NR]
57. Soap-bubble appearance. [RGUHS]
58. Onion-skin appearance. [RGUHS]
59. Name four conditions that showing onion-peel appearance. [RGUHS]
60. Radiographic diagnosis of osteomyelitis. [TN]
61. X-ray appearance of metastatic carcinomas. [TN]
62. Significance of lamina dura in oral and systemic disorders. [TN]
63. Role of radiograph in periodontal disease. [TN]
64. Radiographic features of osteomyelitis. [TN; RGUHS]
65. Herring bone pattern. [TN]
66. Radiopaque landmarks of maxilla. [TN; RGUHS]
67. Periapical osteofibroma. [TN]
68. Radiographic interpretation of dental caries. [NTR]
69. Radiographic appearance of jaws in fibrous dysplasia. [NTR]
70. Radiographic appearance of osteosarcoma. [NTR]
71. Radiological features of odontoma. [RGUHS]
72. Periapical radiopacities. [RGUHS]